introduction to
clinical medicine

The National Medical Series for Independent Study

introduction to clinical medicine

Janice L. Willms, M.D., Ph.D.

Associate Professor
Department of Medicine
University of Connecticut
*   School of Medicine*
Farmington, Connecticut

Judy Lewis, M.Phil.

Assistant Professor
Departments of Community Medicine
*   and Pediatrics*
University of Connecticut
*   School of Medicine*
Farmington, Connecticut

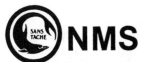**NMS**

National Medical Series from Williams & Wilkins
Baltimore, Hong Kong, London, Sydney

Harwal Publishing Company, Media, Pennsylvania

Williams & Wilkins

Editor: Jane Edwards
Production coordinator: Keith LaSala
Illustrators: Wieslawa Langenfeld and Jack Crane
Compositor: TeleComposition, Inc.

Library of Congress Cataloging-in-Publication Data

Introduction to clinical medicine / [edited by] Janice L.
    Willms. Judy Lewis.
        p.   cm.—(The National medical series for
            independent study)
    Includes index.
    ISBN 0-683-06212-3 (pbk. : alk. paper)
    1. Clinical medicine—Examinations, questions,
etc.   I. Willms, Janice L. II. Lewis, Judy,
1946-   . III. Series.
        [DNLM: 1. Clinical Medicine—examination
            questions.   WB 18 I635]
    RC58.I59   1991
    616.0076—dc20
    DNLM/DLC
    for Library of Congress   91-7054
                                                   CIP

10 9 8 7 6 5 4

Contents

Contributors

Paula S. Algranati, M.D.
Assistant Professor
Department of Pediatrics
University of Connecticut
    School of Medicine
Attending Physician
John Dempsey Hospital
Farmington, Connecticut

Anthony J. Ardolino, M.D.
Assistant Professor
Department of Medicine
University of Connecticut
    School of Medicine
Farmington, Connecticut

Linda R. Benedetto, M.D.
Pediatric Resident
Department of Pediatrics
University of Massachusetts
    Medical Center
Worcester, Massachusetts

Judy Lewis, M.Phil.
Assistant Professor
Departments of Community Medicine
    and Pediatrics
University of Connecticut
    School of Medicine
Farmington, Connecticut

Polly J. Macpherson, M.S.
Instructor in Residence
Department of Community Medicine
University of Connecticut
    Health Center
Farmington, Connecticut

Carrie S. Mukaida, M.S.
Nutritionist
Nutrition Counseling Service
University of Connecticut
    Health Center
Farmington, Connecticut

Linnie Newman, M.S.
Assistant Professor
Department of Family Medicine
University of Connecticut
    School of Medicine
Farmington, Connecticut

Carol A. Pfeiffer, Ph.D.
Assistant Professor
Department of Medicine
Director, Clinical Skills
    Assessment Program
University of Connecticut
    School of Medicine
Farmington, Connecticut

Anne E. Schick, M.A.
Director of Clinical Education
University of Connecticut
    School of Medicine
Farmington, Connecticut

Henry Schneiderman, M.D.

Associate Professor
Departments of Medicine and
   Pathology
University of Connecticut
   School of Medicine
Attending Physician
Associate Director, Internal Medicine
   Residency Training Program
University of Connecticut
   Health Center
Farmington, Connecticut

Nancy A. Stilwell, Ph.D.

Assistant Professor
Department of Behavioral Sciences
Director, Program in Personal and
   Professional Development
University of Connecticut
   School of Dental Medicine
Farmington, Connecticut

Eileen Storey, M.D.

Assistant Professor
Departments of Medicine
   and Community Medicine
University of Connecticut
   School of Medicine
Director, Occupational Medicine
   Program
University of Connecticut
   Health Center
Farmington, Connecticut

Janice L. Willms, M.D., Ph.D.

Associate Professor
Department of Medicine
University of Connecticut
   School of Medicine
Farmington, Connecticut

Preface

Beginning students of medicine must acquire a set of skills that prepare them to become clinicians. This includes establishing rapport and a therapeutic relationship with the patient, basic interviewing, the specific conduct and content of medical data collection (the history and the physical examination), formulation of a problem list and diagnostic hypotheses, documentation and record-keeping, and communication with others involved in the patient's care. An introduction to these skills during the first 2 years of medical school focuses on the basics of data collection and information synthesis rather than the specifics of disease, diagnosis, and treatment—that is, the emphasis is on process rather than specialized content.

There are many fine texts that provide detailed discussions of the medical history and physical examination. This book is not intended to replace these comprehensive approaches but rather to summarize methods and outline the basic principles essential to data collection.

The authors of this book have all been involved in teaching the Introduction to Clinical Medicine course at the University of Connecticut. Their experience has informed the problem-based approach used in this book. This book is structured to allow students to review a set of skills that will enable them to approach undifferentiated medical problems systematically and with confidence in preparation for clinical clerkships.

Janice L. Willms
Judy Lewis

Acknowledgments

The editors and contributing authors would like to acknowledge Dr. Eugene Sigman, Dean of the University of Connecticut School of Medicine, for his continuing commitment to improving clinical education. We would also like to thank Pat Giomblanco, Anna Fazio, and Cindy Pearson for their support in the preparation of the manuscript.

We are grateful to Harwal Publishing Company/Williams & Wilkins, particularly Matt Harris, who initiated this project, Jane Edwards for her editorial contributions, and Keith LaSala for production.

To the Reader

Since 1984, the *National Medical Series for Independent Study* has been helping medical students meet the challenge of education and clinical training. In today's climate of burgeoning information and complex clinical issues, a medical career is more demanding than ever. Increasingly, medical training must prepare physicians to seek and synthesize necessary information and to apply that information successfully.

The *National Medical Series* is designed to provide a logical framework for organizing, learning, reviewing, and applying the conceptual and factual information covered in basic and clinical sciences. Each book includes a comprehensive outline of the essential content of a discipline, with up to 500 study questions. The combination of an outlined text and tools for self-evaluation allows easy retrieval of salient information.

All study questions are accompanied by the correct answer, a paragraph-length explanation, and specific reference to the text where the topic is discussed. Study questions that follow each chapter use the current National Board format to reinforce the chapter content. Study questions appearing at the end of the text in the Comprehensive Exam vary in format depending on the book. Wherever possible, Comprehensive Exam questions are presented as clinical cases or scenarios intended to simulate real-life application of medical knowledge. The goal of this exam is to challenge the student to draw from information presented throughout the book.

All of the books in the *National Medical Series* are constantly being updated and revised. The authors and editors devote considerable time and effort to ensure that the information required by all medical school curricula is included. Strict editorial attention is given to accuracy, organization, and consistency. Further shaping of the series occurs in response to biannual discussions held with a panel of medical student advisors drawn from schools throughout the United States. At these meetings, the editorial staff considers the needs of medical students to learn how the *National Medical Series* can serve them better. In this regard, the Harwal staff welcomes all comments and suggestions.

1
Physician–Patient Relationship and Professional Socialization

Judy Lewis
Linda R. Benedetto
Janice L. Willms

I. ROLE SHIFTS. Adopting a set of values and a professional identity is an important part of a professional education.

A. Types of transition

1. **Layperson to medical professional.** There are many rites of passage that comprise the transformation of a layperson into a medical professional. These involve an increase in knowledge, a change in identity, as well as a familiarity with the events that define the profession (e.g., anatomy and dissection of the human body, access to intimate information about patients, and performance of invasive procedures).

2. **Student to worker**
   a. **The preclinical curriculum** is a traditional learning environment. It is highly structured and largely dependent on lectures and conferences, providing little individual attention. The passive nature of the student's role within this structured environment fosters a feeling of anonymity, involves relatively little risk-taking, and lacks a sense of consequence for individual actions.
   b. **The clinical curriculum** is based on the student as a worker in the health care setting. All the learning is directed toward collecting data as well as acquiring diagnostic and management skills. During the clinical rotations, students begin to develop a clear sense of individual responsibility for patient care and to their contribution to the team.
   c. As students progress through training, they become increasingly responsible for their educational experience. They are no longer told what to study but must identify informational needs and know how to attain them.

B. Lack of knowledge. In the process of becoming medical professionals, students must acquire a large body of knowledge. Overwhelming feelings of incompetence often plague students when confronting new situations, particularly during the transition from the preclinical to the clinical years.

1. **Unfamiliar language.** Both the technical terms and the jargon used among medical professionals can be intimidating to students. Learning to use the appropriate anatomic terminology and standard abbreviations in describing a patient's symptoms, laboratory assessments, and diagnoses can be major difficulties for most students.

2. **New settings**
   a. The hectic pace and variety of physical settings may be stressful to most students.
   b. Adjusting to the different organizational, professional, and hierarchical relationships in the health care environments can be difficult.
   c. Flexibility concerning accepted procedures in one hospital, which may not be accepted in another, may be difficult to maintain.

3. **Conflicting values.** Students often enter medicine with very high ideals and struggle to accommodate to the reality they see in the practice of clinical medicine. The ideal of medicine in which the clinician is the compassionate and caring healer is at times contradicted by the cynical attitudes of some clinicians and clinicians-in-training encountered by students. Patients who have engaged in behaviors which have contributed to their medical problems (e.g., alcohol- or drug-related) are often not treated with the respect that student-clinicians have been taught is essential to a therapeutic relationship.

4. First experiences. Medical education is a continuum of first events, such as the first patient interview, the first time wearing a white coat or using a stethoscope, the first "code," or the first lumbar puncture. Although exciting, each first experience may be accompanied by performance anxiety as well as concern about how to answer questions from patients, such as, "Is this your first time?" Considerable debate surrounds the issue of how directly a student should inform patients when they are performing procedures for the first time.

5. Style of clinical teaching. The clinical setting can be threatening to students because it provides the potential for group exposure or humiliation in contrast to the individual feedback previously received on examinations or papers.

6. Hospital and clinical hierarchy. Students are at the bottom of the power structure in the clinical setting, which can result in a sense of alienation and inadequacy.

C. Dealing with emotions. As students increase their interactions with patients, they more frequently encounter situations in which they must confront patients' feelings and their own responses.

1. Intimate information. Patients often share intimate information with clinicians about family difficulties, sexual relationships, and fears about disability and death. It is important that student-clinicians develop strategies for responding appropriately to the patient's needs as well as their own. This should include identifying peers, faculty, or significant others with whom to discuss feelings. Many medical schools have peer support groups or special sessions in ICM to deal with issues of intimacy that may arise.

2. Lack of legitimacy. Students often feel that they are somehow just "playing" at being clinicians and that the patients with whom they work might just as well share intimate information with the person in the next bed. This is often compounded by "looking young" and having patients question their role as student-clinicians. This is one of the most difficult rites of passage in becoming a clinician. Students can manage these situations by:
   a. Explaining their stage of training and level of responsibility—for example, "I am a first-year medical student, and I am here to interview you as part of our medical history course"
   b. Developing confidence about data collection skills and an awareness that new and important information may be discovered

3. Conflict between education and patient care. Some students feel a tension between attaining educational objectives and providing patient care. They are often concerned that they are "using patients" when they repeat examinations that are clinically unnecessary. However, students should not overlook the fact that:
   a. They may discover something new and important.
   b. Most patients are pleased that they have something worthwhile to teach students.
   c. Many patients appreciate the extra attention and benefit from the additional time that students spend listening to their histories.

4. Patients with self-inflicted problems. Frequently, clinicians encounter patients who have acquired diseases or disabilities from high-risk behaviors, such as alcohol abuse, resulting in liver failure; heavy cigarette consumption, resulting in emphysema or lung cancer; and intravenous drug use, resulting in endocarditis, osteomyelitis, or acquired immune deficiency syndrome (AIDS). While these patients may engender feelings of anger or frustration in health care professionals, they still require sensitive and medically appropriate care.

5. Patients with terminal illness. Student-clinicians must explore their feelings about death and dying so that they can better attend to terminally ill patients and their families. Many schools have courses that deal with these issues. The commonest reactions to death and dying are:
   a. Withdrawal from the patient to avoid emotional involvement or sadness about the impending loss
   b. Anger over "treatment failure"
   c. Feelings of inadequacy in caring for the patient
   d. Denial (see Chapter 4 IX D)

6. Regimentation and loss of sense of self
   a. Because medical school is a highly structured educational environment, it may feel like a regression to high school; students are in class 8 hours a day, 5 days a week, with everyone taking the same courses.
   b. Other medical students are the main source of social interaction as non–medical student friends may not understand the time constraints of medical school. Leisure pursuits, such as exercise, recreational reading, or playing a musical instrument, may be lost.

    c. While many students chose medicine because of a desire to work with people, they often feel more isolated in the first 2 years than at any other point in their lives.

D. Attitudes and values. Student clinicians are constantly exposed to professional attitudes and values, which they must incorporate into their practice of medicine (see Chapter 5).

    1. Tolerance for uncertainty. After the emphasis on facts and memorization of the basic science curriculum, it is often difficult for students in clinical rotations to accept their inability to "know everything."

    2. Clinical experience. Because the extent of a clinician's clinical experience is an important element in both the status hierarchy and knowledge base of clinical medicine, students are constantly reminded of their status as a novice.

    3. Responsibility versus fear of making mistakes. Many students find that while it is easier to retain information about patients and their illnesses when they are responsible for patient care, they are often afraid that they will make a mistake that will result in injury or even death. However, the early clinical experience of medical students is closely supervised by the nursing staff, interns, residents, and attending clinicians so that students are not in a position to cause harm. Student-clinicians are only gradually given responsibility for patient care.

    4. Detached concern/affective neutrality. Genuinely caring for patients without becoming overly involved or losing objectivity is a goal that is often difficult to attain. It is for this reason that clinicians do not usually treat family members or close friends. Students may be devastated by the death of patients with whom they have become close and, thus, need to develop coping strategies for these stressful events.

    5. Idealism versus cynicism. While the ideal values of medicine are laudable, they are often difficult to sustain on an everyday basis. As the new and exciting world of clinical medicine becomes more routine and exhausting, cynicism may provide a break from the continuous exposure of caring. However, a balance between cynicism and idealism is necessary for the health of the clinician and the patient.

    6. Assumption of professional self-image. The point at which student-clinicians see themselves as clinicians-in-training is a gradual process. As Engle (1973) has stated, "The desire to help others and to alleviate suffering, which underlies the career choice of most medical students, also helps them to assume the role of a physician as they begin their clinical work. When a student feels concern for the patient, he or she is already beginning to act like a physician." This transition in identification and self-confidence is necessary to becoming a partner in the therapeutic relationship.

E. Coping strategies. Professional socialization is often a process that requires successful coping strategies.

    1. Anticipatory problem-solving involves identifying areas of potential difficulty and developing an approach to manage the problem. It might involve advice from faculty and peers.

    2. Distancing. Stepping aside and trying to view a given situation objectively can provide perspective. Distancing is an important coping strategy, which medical students must acquire early, so that they can analyze their interactions with patients, peers, and preceptors.

    3. Self-control. Learning to control immediate emotional reactions is important for functioning well in clinical encounters. Although the immediate emotional response to a situation may not be appropriate to communicate to the patient, it should always be analyzed and discussed (see I E 1, 4).

    4. Seeking social support. Developing support systems is important so that the student-clinician does not feel completely isolated and can engage help during the stressful periods of medical education.

    5. Positive reappraisal. Reframing a stressful situation to determine the areas of learning is another positive strategy.

    6. Confrontation. Examining the causes of discomfort or seeking clarification from faculty about areas of conflict can help students to deal positively with stress. Students often need to learn how to approach confrontation in an assertive rather than aggressive way.

7. Escape or avoidance. Sometimes escape through fantasy or exercise allows individuals to re-group and reexamine the stressful situation at a later, less intense, time. Continuous avoidance or denial of stress is not a constructive coping mechanism, however.

II. PATIENT PERSPECTIVE. To provide appropriate care, clinicians must have an understanding of the perspective patients bring to the health care encounter.

A. Social context. Patients and clinicians are influenced by and act on the expectations of the society of which they are a part.

1. Sick role. In 1951, Parsons, a sociologist, developed a theoretical perspective on the func-tional meaning of being sick in Western societies. From his perspective, illness is a socially undesirable state, which prevents a person from performing ordinary tasks and roles and which must be remediated as soon as possible. There are four major components to the sick role, two "rights" and two "duties."

   a. Rights of the sick role

     (1) Recognition that the sick person is not responsible for his or her state and, therefore, cannot be blamed

     (2) Exemption from work obligations and normal social responsibilities

   b. Duties of the sick role

     (1) Obligation to "want to get well" and, therefore, cooperation in any therapeutic effort

     (2) Obligation to seek competent and appropriate treatment

2. Illness response factors. The decision to seek medical care usually involves the patient's at-tempts to act on symptoms and health concerns in accordance with the obligations discussed in the sick role.

   a. Patients must first make sense of the problem and define it within the constraints of their cognitive ability and social and cultural milieu.

   b. The patient's definition of illness and treatment may not be compatible with that of the clinician, and this discrepancy may result in considerable miscommunication between the clinician and the patient.

   c. Mechanic (1968) defined several dimensions within which the patient determines the im-portance of acting upon an illness.

     (1) Visibility, recognizability, or perceived immediacy of signs and symptoms

     (2) Perceived seriousness of symptoms; that is, the patient's estimate of the present and future likelihood of danger

     (3) Extent of disruption of normal activities, involving family, work, and other social ac-tivities

     (4) Frequency of symptoms or episodes of illness

     (5) Tolerance to symptoms of patients, their families, and the social environment

     (6) Knowledge, understanding, and cultural assumptions about the signs and symptoms

     (7) Basic needs competing with illness responses or affecting perception of symptoms

     (8) Competing explanations for symptoms

     (9) Availability of treatment resources, distance to treatment, and psychological and mon-etary costs of taking action

B. Disease factors. Once a disease has been diagnosed, there are aspects of the condition that in-fluence how a patient responds to clinicians in the health care encounter, including the duration and severity of the condition as well as the effectiveness of available treatment.

1. Acute disease. Diseases that are self-limited or that can be easily diagnosed and treated are usually easier for the clinician and patient to manage.

   a. Data collection involves events with a short chronology, making it easier for students to organize questions and responses.

   b. While patients may be anxious about the presenting symptoms, the short duration aids in presenting the chronology and usually enhances the validity of information.

   c. There will be little or no history of contact with other clinicians regarding the present con-dition.

2. Chronic disease. Chronic diseases may present problems for both clinicians and patients in terms of remembering the chronology of the illness, effective management, or compliance with treatment.

    a. Students may have difficulty keeping track of a long history, which may irritate some patients.

    b. Patients with chronic disease often have a history of previous encounters with clinicians, some of which may have been negative, thus influencing the present interaction.

    c. Clinicians should try to get some sense of the patient's previous experience with the health care system.

  3. Serious or terminal illness may cause considerable discomfort for clinicians, and patients are extremely sensitive as to how issues are explored and handled. Patients are also concerned with how clinicians deal with emotional and family matters.

C. Context. The physical environment and terms of the interaction are very important to the physician–patient relationship. Most interactions take place on the clinician's turf—hospitals, clinics, and office settings. Clinicians usually establish the tone of the encounter and the flow of information. To maintain a trusting relationship, it is critical that clinicians let patients know who is involved in their care and the level of training of these individuals.

  1. Educational setting. In academic environments, most patients are aware of being in a "teaching hospital" but still must be informed when the interaction is primarily educational rather than related to their ongoing care. Most patients are willing to participate in the educational activities if they are well-informed and given a choice.

  2. Family issues. The family should be informed of the level of training and the responsibility of those involved in the care of the patient.

  3. Home setting. Home visits by clinicians, although rare, can provide invaluable information for patient care. They present a good opportunity to see how the individual functions outside the medical environment.

D. Patient as teacher. A basic tenet of the physician–patient relationship is that the patient is always a teacher—that is, it is the patient who experiences the illness and, therefore, has the most information about the symptoms and their impact on daily life.

III. CONFIDENTIALITY

A. Definition. All communication between patient and clinician is privileged and legally protected. Without the written consent of the patient, this information may be shared only with individuals who are involved in the patient's care.

B. Maintenance of confidentiality. Confidentiality is one of the key elements of the profession of medicine and the delivery of health care.

  1. Use of initials or anonymity. To preserve confidentiality, it is standard practice to use either initials or general descriptors (e.g., L. K. is a 55-year-old female Caucasian postal worker with a 10-year history of hypertension) in the presentation of case information.

  2. Professional exchange of information. It is standard and appropriate practice that information obtained from the patient may be shared with other health professionals under specific circumstances.

    a. Patient care. Other professionals involved in the ongoing care of patients may need to know information collected from the patient by another professional. In this instance, the name of the patient is necessarily used.

    b. Educational purposes. When patients agree to participate in an educational activity, confidentiality should be maintained in any verbal or written presentation, using initials or general descriptors as described above.

  3. Patient's family and friends. Information collected from patients should not be shared with their family or friends unless the patient indicates that this is acceptable. A demand from a family member to know about drug use or sexual behavior of an adolescent child or a spouse is a typical example of the type of conflict that may occur.

  4. Clinician's family and friends. Difficult situations encountered by clinicians in the course of patient interactions may affect their emotional health if they are not shared with family or friends who can offer support. Thus, it is unrealistic to expect that clinicians will never share their patient experiences. However, confidentiality should be protected. Such "debriefing" may not be appropriate in small communities.

C. Limitations. Two exceptions to the rule of confidentiality concern the professional responsibility of clinicians and student-clinicians to guard the safety and well-being of the patient and others.

   1. When patients threaten suicide or other immediately self-destructive behavior, clinicians have a responsibility to intervene.

   2. When patients threaten to harm others, clinicians have a responsibility to take action.

IV. TOUCHING

A. Touching—a professional issue. Touching of strangers is an act laden with cultural interpretation, one that must be carefully considered by individuals embarking on a career in which it is demanded. Parish reminds us that "Medicine is a delicate blend of science and art. The clinician's approach may, on occasion, be the patient's only source of hope. To touch or lay on the hands may convey human warmth, perhaps even an act of compassion. Touching can be a valuable therapeutic measure, especially when utilized in diseases of less than certain origin." Consideration of the ways in which touching becomes a part of the professional role is part of a medical student's education.

   1. Concept of personal space. Each individual has personal views of the concept of "personal space," which is established very early in life. It is essential to understand and to respect the differences among individuals in connection with this concept.

   2. Fear of touching. Concerns about touching can be overcome by developing an understanding of the value of touching, as well as its boundaries. Fear of touching may be the result of:
   a. The clinician's background or sense of personal space
   b. Fear of sexual arousal
   c. Concern that the patient might not want to be touched

   3. Fear of being touched. Some patients fear being touched, perhaps as a result of being hurt by a clinician's touch or perhaps because they are stridently protective of personal space. A patient's feelings about being touched should be anticipated, using a "sixth sense" that is developed with time and experience.

B. Types of touching

   1. Diagnostic touch. It is impossible to conduct a physical examination without direct physical contact.
   a. After the initial introduction and handshaking, the least intrusive parts of the examination, such as taking a pulse or blood pressure, are a good introduction to crossing the personal space barrier. Warm hands and a gentle approach, maintaining conversation and explaining each step, help to relax the patient about being touched.
   b. Patients should be warned before being touched deeply, as in an abdominal examination. They should be encouraged to indicate discomfort. The patient's face should be watched carefully for signs of distress.
   c. The examination should be a mutual affair, a partnership in assessing the patient's problems. Before clinicians perform some unusual act, such as stroking the sole of the foot for a plantar reflex, they should warn patients and explain what they can expect to feel.
   d. Certain parts of the physical examination require gloves. In most instances, patients will appreciate gloves, such as for examination of body cavities or external genitalia or obtaining body fluid samples; however, clinicians should explain that they are wearing gloves for the protection of all patients, particularly when Universal Precautions are enforced.

   2. Hurtful touch. Clinicians must occasionally hurt patients with their touch, such as when they draw blood, do lumbar punctures, or palpate inflamed body parts. Pain cannot always be avoided, but apprehension and anger can be minimized by communication with the patient in two ways:
   a. Warning. The patient should be warned if touching is expected to cause discomfort or pain. The pain should not be minimized as surprises are not appreciated.

   b. **Getting permission.** Permission should be obtained before doing something that will be unpleasant or painful. This "contract," or agreement, gives the patient a sense of control and is essential for the successful accomplishment of the mutual goal of the patient and clinician.

3. **Healing touch.** From the initial handshake of greeting to the final resolution of the medical problem, the method of touching is a part of the relationship. If the patient is in distress, a touch on the hand conveys understanding and empathy. Sometimes patients need a hug or need to have their hand held in sympathy. Learning how much of the clinician's touch is healing, and when it becomes harmful to the professional relationship, requires constant reassessment.

V. LANGUAGE. Clinical language is full of abbreviations, jargon, and anatomic terms used to describe data collection and diagnosis, which can intimidate the student.

A. Basic definitions

1. **Symptoms** are any problems experienced by the patient that may be related to a health condition. Symptoms usually are used to identify the underlying pathology.

2. **Signs** are physical indications of the disease or syndrome. They may be visible to anyone or specifically to the clinician in the course of the examination.

3. **Diagnosis** is a determination of the underlying cause of a symptom or sign or set of symptoms or signs.

4. **Prognosis** is the predicted course of a disease—that is, its duration, progression, and outcome.

5. **Genogram** is a diagram of a family tree with specific reference to health conditions.

6. **Activities of daily living (ADLs)** are a measure of a patient's level of functioning. They can be used to assess the function levels of all patients, but they are most often used to evaluate chronically ill and geriatric patients.

B. Abbreviations. There are multiple abbreviations used in clinical situations; the most commonly used abbreviations are defined in the Appendix. The accepted definitions for the components of the medical history and the physical examination are discussed in Chapters 3 and 6.

C. Sensitivity of words and labels

1. The phrase, "patient denies alcohol use" or "denies any history of . . ." implies that the patient is not telling the complete truth. While many clinicians use this phraseology, there are other nonjudgmental ways of describing the patient's behavior, such as "the patient reports, states, or indicates."

2. Negative or implied responsibility is also inherent in certain medical diagnoses, such as "incompetent" cervix, which can easily be misunderstood by the patient, although it is standard medical usage. Such terms should be discussed with the patient to ensure that there is no implication of judging the patient or the condition.

3. Precise information and avoidance of labeling is also important in describing patient behaviors. Thus, it is more precise to say "The patient reports consuming 6 beers each day" rather than "The patient is an alcoholic."

STUDY QUESTIONS

Directions: Each of the numbered items or incomplete statements in this section is followed by answers or by completions of the statement. Select the **one** lettered answer or completion that is **best** in each case.

1. Changes occurring as the student progresses through training include all of the following EXCEPT

(A) increased responsibility for patient care
(B) more active role in determining personal educational needs
(C) more guidance of all management decisions by superiors
(D) tendency to take for granted the performance of actions that were previously considered novel
(E) trend toward tempering idealism with realism

2. Constructive approaches to the care of patients with self-inflicted problems include all of the following EXCEPT

(A) the clinician's recognition of any personal hostility
(B) distinction between patient as a person and patient's behavior
(C) realization that all people have a right to medical care
(D) withholding care from the patient until the patient displays health-promoting behavior
(E) presentation of options to help the patient discontinue the self-destructive habit or behavior

3. The sick role includes all of the following rights and responsibilities EXCEPT

(A) seeking help
(B) not being responsible for getting sick
(C) knowing the cause of the symptoms
(D) release from work
(E) cooperating in treatment

4. Patients are likely to seek medical care for a condition if it has all of the following characteristics EXCEPT

(A) it is caused by a virus
(B) it keeps them from working
(C) it has a spiritual basis
(D) it attracts attention
(E) it will get worse if not treated

5. Confidentiality can be breached in all of the following circumstances EXCEPT

(A) talking to another professional
(B) the patient's life is in danger
(C) the patient threatens someone else's life
(D) talking to the mother about her 2-year-old child
(E) talking to a nurse who provides care to the patient

6. Gloves for a physical examination are absolutely indicated in all of the following situations EXCEPT palpation of

(A) tongue and floor of mouth
(B) dry skin lesions
(C) prostate gland
(D) uterine cervix
(E) moist skin lesions

7. All of the following are symptoms EXCEPT

(A) pain
(B) fear
(C) shortness of breath
(D) hypertension
(E) agitation

Directions: Each item below contains four suggested answers of which **one or more** is correct. Choose the answer

    A if **1, 2, and 3** are correct
    B if **1 and 3** are correct
    C if **2 and 4** are correct
    D if **4** is correct
    E if **1, 2, 3, and 4** are correct

8. Factors that reinforce students' feelings of incompetence include

(1) frequently changing work settings and practice procedures
(2) patients' questions about looking young and lack of experience
(3) isolation from students who may be having similar difficulties
(4) increasing responsibility for decision-making

9. Students who doubt the legitimacy of their role in patient care might be reassured by which of the following?

(1) The contribution that the student makes to the patient's well-being simply by listening to the patient's story
(2) The importance to the patient of being valued as a teacher
(3) The patient's belief that anyone in a white coat is a member of the health care team
(4) The possibility that the student will uncover a previously unknown aspect of the history

10. A resident is observing while a third-year medical student prepares to do an arterial blood gas on a patient. The patient asks, "Is this the first time you have done this?" Reasons the student may feel uncomfortable in this situation include

(1) heightened awareness of lack of experience
(2) fear of causing unnecessary pain due to lack of dexterity
(3) public nature of the success or failure of the procedure
(4) passivity of the student's role with little opportunity for feedback

ANSWERS AND EXPLANATIONS

1. The answer is C. [*I A 1, 2, B 3*] Like any initiation, the transition from student to clinician is one in which activities that were previously considered novel become commonplace. Students moving from the pre-clinical to the clinical curriculum assume greater responsibility for patient care and for their own education. Their increased experience enables them to make management decisions more independently. In addition, with continual exposure to the stresses of patient care and to the cynicism of senior colleagues, students begin to find a balance between their earlier idealism and a more realistic perspective.

2. The answer is D. [*I B 3, C 4*] Many clinicians find it difficult to care for patients who have acquired illnesses as a result of self-destructive habits or practices. In dealing with these patients, it may be helpful for the clinician to distinguish the behavior that is objectionable from the patient who is worthwhile and for the clinician to identify any personal negative feelings to avoid acting on unrecognized hostility. It is essential to remember that everyone has a right to health care. Clinicians cannot decide which patients deserve health care based on their behaviors. Most health care professionals advocate maintaining the physician–patient relationship with patients who engage in self-destructive behaviors and providing excellent health care by urging the patient to discontinue the self-destructive habits and offering a plan to make this possible.

3. The answer is C. [*II A 1 a, b*] The sick role provides a framework for examining the rights and duties of the patient. These include the duties of seeking appropriate help and cooperating in treatment and the release from normal responsibilities, such as work, as well as not being blamed for the illness condition. It does *not* include knowing the reason for the illness or the cause of the symptoms.

4. The answer is C. [*II A 2 a–c*] If patients define an illness as having a cause outside the realm of scientific medicine, they will probably seek help within their cultural belief system (e.g., spiritualist, church, traditional healer). Patients, however, are likely to seek medical care for all of the other reasons listed in the question—that is, if the condition is a virus, if they miss work, if other people take notice of the condition, or if the condition worsens without treatment.

5. The answer is A. [*III B 2 a, C*] Talking to another professional is not a justified breach of confidentiality unless the professional is directly involved in the patient's care. Exceptions to the rule of confidentiality include situations in which patients present a danger to themselves or others.

6. The answer is B. [*IV B 1 d*] Obviously dry and nonexudative skin lesions may be palpated with ungloved hands since there is no hazard to the patient or examiner of transmission of infection. On the other hand, moist or weeping lesions should be examined with gloves because of the potential for secondary infection or spread of existing infection to the examiner or via the examiner to another patient. Mucosal surfaces should always be palpated with the gloved hand only.

7. The answer is D. [*V A 1*] Symptoms are any problems experienced by the patient that may be used to identify the underlying pathology. Hypertension is not something the patient directly experiences; it is a sign measured through a blood pressure cuff.

8. The answer is A (1, 2, 3). [*I B 2, 4, C 2, 6*] Many stressors encountered during medical education contribute to the student's feelings of incompetence. Students participating in new activities may lack dexterity or skill, which may arouse the patients' concerns about "being used as guinea pigs." Also, students who look young may be viewed with distrust since some patients equate looking young with a lack of experience. Students may have to adapt to new locations and new coworkers as frequently as every month as they change rotations; thus, whatever level of comfort students have attained is quickly removed. One way of coping with these stresses is to seek support from students who may be having similar experiences; isolation may compound stress. Although increased responsibility for decision-making may provide anxiety, it is actually recognition of the student's increased competence.

9. The answer is E (all). [*I C 2, 3*] Students often feel that they are just "playing" at being clinicians, a feeling that is often compounded by patients who question their roles as student-clinicians. Students are also concerned that they are "using patients" when they repeat clinically unnecessary examinations. However, students should be reminded that in redoing examinations they may, indeed, discover something new. Patients may not be familiar with the medical hierarchy and assume that all people in white coats have equal responsibility for their medical care. In addition, most patients like their role of teaching the student, and almost all patients appreciate the extra attention.

10. The answer is A (1, 2, 3). [*I C 2, 3*] Learning to perform medical procedures, some of which are invasive and painful, is part of becoming a health care professional. Patients' questions about whether or not this is a first experience highlight the fact that the student appears young or inexperienced. In the example in the question, if blood is not obtained immediately after the needle is introduced, it will be quite obvious to the resident, the student, and the patient that the procedure has been unsuccessful; the public nature of this failure can increase the student's anxiety. Also, unsuccessful attempts may be unpleasant for the patient, so the student often worries about causing the patient pain because of inexperience.

2
Interviewing Skills

Anne E. Schick
Judy Lewis

I. ESTABLISHING A THERAPEUTIC RELATIONSHIP. A therapeutic relationship promotes healing and is the basis of all physician-patient interactions. The **basic components** of a therapeutic relationship are **rapport, mutual respect,** and **genuineness**. Even the early stages of student interviewing can be therapeutic as the very act of expressing a problem can be beneficial to patients (therapeutic listening).

A. Purpose and benefits. A therapeutic relationship is an end in itself. It is also essential for collecting valuable information from patients. If rapport is established and patients are treated with respect, it is more likely that they will provide a complete and accurate description of their problems.

1. **Effective data collection.** A therapeutic relationship helps to put patients at ease and, thus, facilitates the collection of data, particularly information that is sensitive or painful.

2. **Patient compliance and satisfaction** are improved when there is a good physician-patient relationship.

B. Techniques to develop therapeutic relationships

1. **Establishing respect and acknowledging the patient's beliefs.** Clinicians should accept the beliefs of their patients even if they conflict with their own. Clinicians should respect the integrity of their patients even when the patients may contribute to their own health problems through neglect or self-abuse. The clinician's role does not include making moral judgments about patient behavior.
   a. **Introduction and purpose.** The clinician should introduce him- or herself and provide a clear statement of the purpose of the interview, how long it will take, the types of physical examinations to be performed, and the expected outcomes.
   b. **Form of address.** The clinician should ask each patient the name by which he or she wishes to be called.
   c. **Understanding the patient's perspective.** The clinician should encourage each patient to express his or her beliefs about the cause of the illness and how the illness or problem has affected daily life.
   d. **Reinforcing and acknowledging the patient's experience.** The clinician should support the experience of the patient and validate what has happened or what has been felt.
   e. **Providing feedback.** The clinician should provide feedback to let the patient know what he or she thinks about the presenting problem. This also enables the patient to correct any misperceptions on the part of the clinician.

2. **Establishing rapport with patients**
   a. **Expressing concern for the patient.** The clinician can demonstrate interest in the patient as an individual by indicating interest in the presenting problem and the patient's general life situation. This will assure the patient that the clinician identifies him or her as more than just an illness. Additionally, the clinician may learn valuable information about the effect of the illness on the patient's life and may see how the environment affects the patient's functioning.
   b. **Allowing the patient to speak.** Open-ended questions should be used to encourage the patient to use his or her own words to describe feelings and problems. Open-ended questions let the patient tell his or her own story without assumptions being made by the clinician. For example, the statement "Please tell me about your shortness of breath" allows

the patient to qualify the extent of the shortness of breath. If the clinician uses his or her own words to describe what the patient is saying, the patient may feel that it is acceptable to use only the clinician's description.

c. **Offering empathy.** The clinician can provide a supportive setting in which the patient can talk about anger, frustration, or loss, empathizing with the patient's feelings and reactions. Examples include: "That must have been a difficult time for you." "You must be concerned." "That sounds like a frustrating situation." Empathetic remarks are useful in helping patients continue with their story.

d. **Sharing common experiences.** Often personal interests and opinions are revealed in the course of the interview to which the clinician can respond to enhance rapport. However, this technique should not be used extensively because it can detract from the data collection activity.

e. **Conveying genuine concern for the patient's well-being.** Clinicians must express a real caring for patients. This does not mean that clinicians must like each patient, but it does mean that they must care about helping each patient. It is essential for the clinician to keep in mind the best possible outcome for each individual patient, according to the patient's defined goals.

f. **Drawing the patient out.** The clinician can put a patient at ease and encourage him or her to elaborate on specific points by using nonverbal cues (e.g., leaning forward, giving a questioning look) or by direct verbal communication (e.g., asking the patient to continue talking). The clinician must try a variety of methods to obtain a complete history.

g. **Validating the patient's experience.** The clinician should try to understand what is happening from the patient's perspective. If the clinician does not understand the patient's perspective, the issues that are most important to the patient may not be addressed even if the "illness" is treated. If the patient's experience is acknowledged and accepted, the patient is more likely to cooperate and be satisfied with the treatment.

C. Problems in establishing a therapeutic relationship

1. **Time constraints.** Often the time allotted for an interview and physical examination is limited and does not allow for the exploration of all issues covered in the course of the interview. If the patient is concerned about a certain topic, the clinician should give this priority and organize the rest of the interview to ensure the collection of essential information. Detail about less relevant parts of the interview can be scheduled for another time. Most importantly, the clinician should not appear rushed and should always remain attentive to the patient's needs.

2. **Environment.** Busy clinics and hospital wards often do not provide an appropriate atmosphere in which to collect personal data from patients. Interruptions disrupt the flow of information and interaction, and privacy is difficult to maintain when there may be only a curtain separating the patient from others in the room. Extraneous elements should be controlled or eliminated, whenever possible, by closing doors, turning off televisions and radios, sitting close to the patient, and concentrating on the interview.

3. **Cultural differences.** Clinicians must be aware of different norms of behavior among cultures, including body space, manner of expression, and degree of emotionality and dependence about illness. A general respect and effort to obtain the patient's perspective will help in the initial interaction with patients from different cultural backgrounds. Seeking information about cultural norms from a community member or staff member familiar with the population is also useful.

4. **Language barriers.** It is very difficult to establish rapport with patients whose first language is not the same as that of the clinician. These patients are not able to describe problems easily. The clinician should become familiar with the primary foreign languages spoken in the local patient population. While it may not be possible to become fluent in all of these languages, a few brief words of introduction and polite conversation can help to break down barriers.

II. COMMUNICATION.
Good communication refers to the exchange of information—both giving and receiving. The clinician must understand a patient's frame of reference and communication style to understand what he or she intends to say as well as to be able to relate information and phrase questions in a manner that is understandable to the patient. Techniques in both verbal and nonverbal communication are discussed below.

A. Body language. Body language is the transmission of meaning, feeling, or intent by physical act or manner.

  1. Interpretation. The clinician may gain additional clues about a patient's problems, including particular physical problems and fears a patient may have about health and other areas of his or her life by observing body language. The mood of the patient may be indicated by body language, which may also aid in deciphering contributing problems.

  2. Presentation. The patient interprets the clinician's body language to assess the clinician's level of comfort, confidence, and genuineness.

B. Techniques of presenting and interpreting body language

  1. Posture is the way in which an individual sits, stands, and holds his or her arms and head.
    a. Interpretation. The clinician should assess the body posture of the patient to determine whether the patient is feeling protective (shoulders over and arms crossed) or angry (shoulders back, arms crossed, or hands clenched) and use this information to explore further concerns. The patient should not be confronted with this interpretation, but the clinician should try to validate feelings and discuss origins. Positive feelings are evidenced by shoulders down and arms at sides or crossed casually in the lap with hands held loosely.
    b. Presentation. The clinician should attend to his or her own posture, demonstrating attention and interest. The most encouraging words will lose their effect if the clinician appears fidgety or bored.

  2. Position. The way in which individuals place themselves in a room relative to others may indicate their level of comfort and the nature of the relationships. A therapeutic relationship does not benefit from a situation in which the clinician has power over the patient. The relationship should certainly include acknowledgment of the clinician's medical skill and knowledge but should not diminish the equal humanness of the clinician and patient.
    a. Interpretation. The patient may sit far away from the clinician, near the door, or in a corner, indicating discomfort with the situation or the clinician.
    b. Presentation. The clinician often controls the positioning in the interview and examination.
      (1) Standing over a patient in a hospital bed, a wheelchair, or an examination table imposes the clinician's authority and diminishes the patient's humanness and comfort level.
      (2) Clinicians who sit behind big desks may create distance between themselves and the patient.
      (3) Standing near the door may communicate disinterest or lack of time for listening.

  3. Eye contact. This is an area in which cultural norms play a very strong role; for example, in Native American and Latino cultures, a lack of eye contact is a sign of respect for elders and professionals. The examples below are limited to the culturally accepted behavior of Anglo-European Americans.
    a. Interpretation. Patients who avert their eyes for most of the interview may be concealing information or expressing discomfort. Staring too steadily may be an expression of aggression or hostility.
    b. Presentation. The clinician should establish and maintain eye contact with the patient at a level that is comfortable for both. Good eye contact helps to form a connection that enhances communication. Patients who feel positively about their health care providers are more likely to be cooperative and compliant with their care.

  4. Mirroring is a subtle copying of body posture in social interactions. [It may also apply to verbal communications (see II D 7).]
    a. Interpretation. The patient who mirrors the body posture of the clinician generally indicates a high level of comfort with the interaction.
    b. Presentation. Clinicians can help make the patient more comfortable by mirroring the patient's body posture (e.g., leaning forward, crossing legs) with slight variations until the patient's comfort seems greatest. This can and should be done very subtly since obvious copying would be rude.
      (1) Mirroring is most important when patients are ill at ease.
      (2) Mirroring is often natural when there is already rapport.

5. **Gestures** are the specifics of body language, such as pointing, nodding, and arm waving.
   a. **Interpretation.** Gestures can indicate a patient's mood, expressiveness, and style of interacting. Patients who tap their fingers may be showing nervousness or fear. Patients who keep pointing away from themselves may be trying to disown their physical problems.
   b. **Presentation.** Clinicians can help to make the patient feel at ease and indicate interest and attentiveness by such gestures as nodding affirmatively while the patient speaks. It may also be appropriate to use a reassuring gesture, such as a light touch on the hand or arm when the patient is clearly upset; however, the patient's ability to accept this type of contact must be carefully assessed.

6. **Double-bind messages** occur when there is incongruent behavior between verbal communication and body language.
   a. **Interpretation.** Body language often takes precedence over spoken language when interpreting a patient's behavior. The spoken language may reflect what patients think clinicians want to hear, while the body language or gestures may indicate what they actually feel. For example, the patient may say that he or she is comfortable with what the clinician is saying, while holding his or her arms tightly across the chest.
   b. **Presentation.** Clinicians must learn to assess the congruency of their own body language with spoken language. Verbal expressions of interest and concern can easily be undermined by a lack of eye contact or constantly checking the time.

C. **Problems in interpreting and presenting body language**

1. **Nervousness** on the part of either the clinician or the patient may mask other feelings.
   a. **Nervous patient.** The nervousness of patients who are fearful about their well-being may inhibit a good therapeutic relationship. It is the clinician's responsibility to put the patient at ease by the techniques discussed in this chapter.
   b. **Nervous clinician.** Nervousness in a clinician usually occurs when the clinician is inexperienced and concerned about performance. Concentrating on the needs of the patient will help the clinician to overcome this self-consciousness.

2. **Cultural norms.** Accepted behaviors among cultures vary considerably, particularly body language because it is not as consciously used as spoken language. When clinicians work with patients from other cultures, they should make every effort to learn how to interpret behavior as well as how to make appropriate changes in presenting themselves in the interaction.

3. **Clinician awareness of self-presentation.** Videotaping can provide an excellent way for clinicians to observe how they appear to patients. If videotaping is not a reasonable option, watching tapes of others may sensitize clinicians to some of the major interactional areas on which to focus.

D. **Verbal communication.** Spoken language is the primary means of communicating in almost all physician-patient interactions. How questions are asked often determines the response. Specific interviewing techniques for the facilitation of data collection and furthering the therapeutic relationship are discussed below.

1. **Open-ended questions.** The clinician should begin each interview with open-ended questions, allowing the patient to state the problem in his or her own words. Questions such as "Tell me about your problem," "What kind of pain was it?" and "What else did you notice that was different?" are nonjudgmental and do not lead the patient in any particular direction.

2. **Closed-ended questions.** This type of question should be restricted to clarify information after a sufficient data base has been collected; for example, "Was it a stabbing pain or a throbbing pain?" and "Did you fall when you felt dizzy?" These questions may also be used when the patient has been unable (or unwilling) to describe something adequately or when the clinician is searching for a new direction in which to go.

3. **Feedback.** Clinicians should let patients know that they hear and understand what is being said by providing comforting words about difficult situations (e.g., the death of a parent, child, or spouse) and summarizing what patients have said to make sure that the information is accurate. Clinicians should not parrot everything patients say but should summarize essential information at the end of each major portion of the interview.

4. **Pacing.** The interview should allow adequate time and pacing of topics to cover all the necessary data in a manner that flows smoothly and is comfortable for the patient. Silence is not always a disruption of the interview. A patient may need a moment or two to gather thoughts,

and this must be respected. The clinician should make sure that the patient is not uncomfortable but merely thinking. The clinician may need to collect his or her thoughts or consider other lines of inquiry but should avoid prolonged silences.

5. **Vocabulary.** The level of language and terminology used must be set by the educational and cultural background of the patient. This is essential for accurate data collection and problem assessment.
   a. **Avoidance of jargon.** Technical terminology and medical jargon should be avoided with all but patients who are clinicians. In those rare instances where the terminology is essential, it should be explained as fully and simply as possible. For example, a patient who needs a series of tests may be told the technical and appropriate names of the tests, provided a simple, nontechnical explanation of their purpose is given. Patients should not be spoken to in a condescending fashion, and they should not be expected to have the same level of knowledge as clinicians.
   b. **Neutrality.** Terms should also be selected for their neutrality lest clinicians unintentionally appear judgmental; for example:
      (1) Sexual preference and family planning are sensitive issues that must be handled accordingly. Clinicians should not assume that everyone is heterosexual or that all pregnancies are unwanted if unplanned.
      (2) Assuming that all people over a certain age are no longer sexually active and that all people under a certain age have never been sexually active is naive. Judgmental words such as "yet" or "still" must not be used when inquiring about sexual activity.

6. **Flexibility.** If the clinician does not understand what the patient is saying, a *different* way of eliciting the information must be found. For example, "Have you been dizzy?" can be expanded to "Did the room spin?" "Did you lose your balance?" "Did your vision change?" or "Did you become nauseated?"
   a. **Repetition** alone is unlikely to be helpful. "How did you get here?" may seem like a simple question, but if the patient says "by ambulance" instead of responding with the reason why he or she came to the hospital, simply repeating the question exactly the same way will not help.
   b. **Facilitation of interaction.** Finding a new way to express something should help the clinician avoid being labeled as "incompetent" or labeling the patient as "resistant."

7. **Representational systems** are identifiable styles of describing how people feel or think about things. The clinician may find it helpful to "mirror" the system used by the patient to improve rapport; for example, a patient who says, "There is a dark cloud hanging over me," is apt to feel more rapport with a clinician who responds, "I understand that everything seems bleak, but we will work on brightening things up for you," rather than "Yes, you have every right to feel like you are carrying more than your share of the load."
   a. **Visual.** People who use a visual representational system use words that express their feelings in terms of visual imagery. For example, "It is clear to me now," "All is darkness ahead of me," "She has a sunny disposition," and "My heart seems to flash on and off."
   b. **Kinesthetic.** People who use kinesthetic language use words that have a physical nature. For example, "I feel weighed down by everything," "I feel buoyant," and "My heart was fluttering."
   c. **Auditory.** An auditory representational system is used less frequently. The words used to describe what the person feels are words used for sounds. For example, "It rings true," or "My heart was rumbling."

8. **Paralinguistics.** The tone of the interaction can affect the interpretation of what is being communicated. A kind word delivered in a harsh or abrupt style can be interpreted as uncaring because the tone overshadowed the meaning of the words.

9. **Word choice.** Clinicians must choose their words carefully. Qualifiers such as "just" and "only" tend to diminish the patients' statements. For example, "So your pain only lasted 2 hours," or "It was just a dry cough." Patients can be put off by thoughtless terminology that contradicts the perceived severity of their problem.

III. STRUCTURED INTERVIEW. The structured interview is one for which the clinician has a plan. There should be a sense of what needs to be accomplished and how to proceed in attaining the goal in the most useful way. The basic format should be adapted to the needs of the patients as well as with time constraints. The basic structure of comprehensive and focused clinical interviews is provided in Chapter 3. Specific content and problems in interviews are discussed in Chapters 4 and 5.

A. Purpose. Clinicians need to learn how to conduct a structured interview to ensure that all pertinent information is gathered.

B. Components of a structured interview

    1. Clinicians need to monitor their own conversational habits.

    2. The interview must be patient-centered.

    3. The content of the interview must be focused yet maintain flexibility and rapport in the collection of information.

    4. Note-taking should be minimized. Clinicians are able to listen to patients and follow nonverbal cues better if there is little or no note-taking.

    5. Clinicians must have an outline and goals in mind for each interview so that the process is natural, the responses of the patient can be followed up, and the interview can be adjusted to fit the needs of the individual patient.

    6. Clinicians should have a sense of the amount of time available for the interview so that the pace and content can be adjusted as needed.

    7. Clinicians should inform patients of the various components or stages of the interview and give a brief statement to inform them that the topic of the interview is changing. For example, statements such as, ''I am now going to ask some questions about your family's health,'' or ''Now I would like to ask you a few questions about your past health'' allow the history to be evenly paced.

C. Problems in keeping to a structured interview

    1. Confused patients can disrupt the time allotted for questions.

    2. Interruptions by others in the clinical setting can throw the clinician off the structure of the interview.

    3. Time constraints can make it difficult to cover information logically and thoroughly. Anticipating the time constraints, however, necessitates the prioritizing of data to be collected (e.g., limiting the amount of information, not the interactive quality, rapport, and specific data relevant to the patient's condition).

STUDY QUESTIONS

Directions: Each of the numbered items or incomplete statements in this section is followed by answers or by completions of the statement. Select the **one** lettered answer or completion that is **best** in each case.

1. Reinforcement and acknowledgment help to establish rapport by

(A) convincing the patient that the clinician is correct
(B) making the patient feel at ease and, therefore, more cooperative
(C) acknowledging the clinician's lack of knowledge
(D) showing the patient that the clinician has had similar experiences

2. The clinician should provide feedback to the patient for all of the following reasons EXCEPT to

(A) give the patient the opportunity to correct any misperceptions
(B) establish control of the interaction
(C) make sure the patient understands what information is most important
(D) check on the patient's understanding of the disease process
(E) show the patient that the clinician is hearing what the patient says

3. Clinicians must be aware of double-bind messages in their communications with patients because the

(A) patient might be overwhelmed by receiving too much information
(B) clinician will reveal his or her lack of interest in the patient
(C) patient will be confused by the conflicting meanings
(D) clinician will need to pursue more information

4. Closed-ended questions are appropriate for all of the following situations EXCEPT when

(A) the patient refuses to answer other types of questions
(B) the patient is rambling, and the clinician needs to control the situation
(C) the clinician needs to learn details of issues raised by the patient
(D) time is a problem and the interview must be limited in length

Directions: The item below contains four suggested answers of which **one or more** is correct. Choose the answer

A if **1, 2, and 3** are correct
B if **1 and 3** are correct
C if **2 and 4** are correct
D if **4** is correct
E if **1, 2, 3, and 4** are correct

5. Mirroring body language or vocabulary is best used to

(1) figure out the physical problems of the patient by copying them
(2) establish rapport by subtly using similar language or gestures
(3) get the patient to see similarities between the clinician and patient
(4) help the patient stay calm when he or she is stressed

Directions: The group of items in this section consists of lettered options followed by a set of numbered items. For each item, select the **one** lettered option that is most closely associated with it. Each lettered option may be selected once, more than once, or not at all.

Questions 6–10

For each of the case scenarios listed below, select the aspect of the therapeutic relationship that it best illustrates.

(A) Lack of observation of a patient's body language
(B) Sharing common experiences appropriately
(C) Offering empathetic remarks
(D) Personal story telling by the clinician
(E) Use of jargon

6. A 42-year-old man comes into the clinic with a CC of "severe headaches that keep me from work and feel like a vise around my head." The clinician says, "That sounds terrible. Headaches can be the worst pain for some people. I will do what I can to help right away."

7. A 56-year-old woman presents after 3 days of lower back pain. The clinician says, "My cousin had terrible lower back pain from lifting on the job. Actually, he worked in an office, but whenever supplies were delivered, he always offered to carry the package or box to the right place. . . ."

8. A 50-year-old man is waiting in an examining room. When the clinician enters, the man is standing in the far corner of the room, close to the wall with his arms folded across his chest. The clinician says, "Hi, how are you today? It is really a beautiful day. I am sure you are looking forward to going back outside."

9. A 35-year-old woman comes to the office complaining of a sore throat that started 3 days ago. The clinician says, "That must feel awful; it is very red. The last time I had something like that, I was miserable. Can you swallow?"

10. A 65-year-old man complains of chest pain. His clinician asks, "Do you have angina?"

ANSWERS AND EXPLANATIONS

1. The answer is B. [*I B 1 d*] A therapeutic relationship is the basis of all physician-patient interactions. Techniques to develop therapeutic relationships include establishing respect, acknowledging the beliefs of patients, and establishing rapport. If clinicians try to understand the patient's perspective and acknowledge his or her experience, the patient is more likely to cooperate and be satisfied with the treatment.

2. The answer is B. [*I B 1 e; II D 3*] Feedback does not help the clinician to establish control of the interaction but provides an opportunity for both the clinician and the patient to monitor the progress of the interview. It allows the clinician to let the patient know what he or she thinks about the presenting problems, and it allows the patient to correct any misperceptions on the part of the clinician.

3. The answer is C. [*II B 6*] Double-bind communications occur when body language and verbal communication are incongruent with each other. For example, verbal expressions of concern can be easily negated by a lack of eye contact or by looking at one's watch.

4. The answer is D. [*II D 2; III C 3*] Closed-ended questions should be restricted to situations where clarification is needed, the patient is unable or unwilling to answer open-ended questions, or the clinician is searching for a new direction for further questioning. Time should not be the determining factor as the quality of the interaction should be maintained in brief as well as long interviews.

5. The answer is C (2, 4). [*II B 4*] Presentation of similar body posture or language by the clinician can help reduce the patient's nervousness or discomfort in the clinical situation as well as help to establish rapport. Mirroring is most important when patients are ill at ease and is often natural when there is already rapport.

6–10. The answers are: 6-C, 7-D, 8-A, 9-B, 10-E. [*I B 2 c, d; II A 1, D 5 a*] Empathetic remarks can help to provide a supportive atmosphere in which the patient can discuss anger, frustration, or loss. Empathetic remarks may also help a patient continue with his or her story.

Often personal interests or experiences are revealed in the course of an interview to which clinicians may respond to enhance rapport. However, excessive personal stories from the clinician can detract from the purpose of the encounter.

Clinicians can gain information about a patient's problems or mood by observing the patient's body language. The clinician should assess the body posture to determine the comfort level of the patient with the encounter.

Any kind of technical language should be avoided unless the patient is a clinician. If terminology cannot be avoided, it should be explained as fully and as simply as possible.

Basic Components of the Medical History

Linnie Newman

I. COMPONENTS OF THE (ADULT) COMPREHENSIVE MEDICAL HISTORY. The medical history is the foundation upon which diagnosis and treatment are made. It is the basis upon which hypotheses are built and tests ordered. Without a medical history, the clinician works in a vacuum. The medical history provides a place for the establishment of the physician–patient relationship; at the time of the history, rapport is created and trust begins.

A. Chief complaint (CC)

1. **Definition and elicitation.** The medical history usually begins with a determination of the patient's CC, which is the patient's perception of the problem or symptom for which he or she has sought a health care provider.
   a. The CC is usually elicited immediately after introductions by asking one of the following questions; for example, "What brought you here today?" "What problem brought you to the hospital?" "What symptoms cause your distress?"
   b. Patients often give short, succinct responses, such as, "I had chest pain," or "My diabetes was out of control."

2. **Hidden agendas.** Patients with hidden agendas may offer vague or misleading symptoms when asked about their CC instead of their true concern, such as, "I have been feeling tired lately," or "My body hurts."
   a. Embarrassment, denial, fear, or loneliness may contribute to a nonspecific response.
   b. Patients often feel that there must be a medical reason for entry into the system when in fact some common hidden agenda, such as depression or other psychological problem, sexual problem, or a desire to acquire something from the clinician, such as a specific medication or a disability letter, is responsible for the visit.

3. **Recording.** The CC is described in both the written history and the oral presentation by using the patient's exact words: "I fell over the curb and broke my leg." The clinician *must not* paraphrase the CC and write "broken leg."

4. **Relationship to other problems.** In most cases, the CC gives the clinician a clear understanding of the patient's major concern. However, the clinician may discover from the history or the physical examination that the patient has another or more serious medical problem. For example, the patient's CC may be "My knee has been hurting," but on examination, the clinician may find that the patient has asymptomatic hypertension. This does not alter the CC. The clinician must deal with the hypertension as well as the painful knee.

B. Identifying data

1. **Definition and recording**
   a. Identifying data give the reader or listener a mental picture of the patient, including the name, age, sex, and occupation, eventually leading to the CC. Some clinicians also include the number of admissions to the hospital. Examples follow:
      (1) Mr. Young is a 59-year-old steelworker with the CC: "I need another operation on my hand."
      (2) This is the seventh hospital admission for Mr. Young, a 59-year-old steelworker with the CC: "I need another operation on my hand."
   b. **Ethnicity** is not included in the identifying data unless this information is essential to the diagnosis; for example, certain diseases are more prevalent in certain racial or ethnic

groups, such as sickle cell disease in blacks. In this instance, the clinician might write, James Foster is a 5-year-old black child with the CC: "My fingers hurt."

2. Supplementary content

    a. Identifying data can also include medical facts that influence the remainder of the medical history (especially the history of the present illness); for example:

        (1) Knowing that a patient has diabetes may alter the treatment; for example, Mrs. O'Connor is a 59-year-old accountant with a 40-year history of insulin-dependent diabetes mellitus (IDDM) who comes into the hospital with the CC: "I have a sore on my foot."

        (2) A fever may be much more significant in a patient on chemotherapy than in a healthy individual; for example, Mr. Bradley is a 67-year-old, retired salesperson who is currently receiving chemotherapy at home and now comes to the hospital with the CC: "I have a fever."

    b. Reliability of the patient is assessed throughout the history. This judgment is based upon the patient's recall and reproducibility of facts rather than the interviewer's inexperience or lack of ability in obtaining data.

    c. Third-party informant. If someone besides the patient contributed to the history, it should be noted as: Informant—patient's wife who had minimal recall of events before 1987.

C. History of present illness (HPI)

  1. Overview

    a. Patient's description of symptoms. The HPI should include only symptoms—that is, information that the patient reports about changes in function, appearance, or sensation. A **symptom** is a **subjective** description. The HPI should **not include signs,** which are any abnormalities discovered by the clinician on direct observation or examination—that is, an **objective** indicator. The student may ask the patient about symptoms concerning something that he has observed (a sign): "I notice that your fingers do not move. Could you tell me about that?" In the HPI, the clinician reports **only the symptoms that the patient describes**. Objective descriptions are part of the physical examination.

    b. Acquiring primary data

        (1) Primary information. The student should investigate the patient's primary symptoms rather than accept third-hand information as fact. For example, if the patient reports, "The doctors said I have a gallbladder problem," the student must obtain a complete history (see I C 2). Only primary information belongs in the history.

        (2) Secondary information is data obtained from sources other than the patient, such as laboratory values or old records.

        (3) Tertiary information is information related verbally by the patient as if it had come from another source, such as, "My doctor told me I have gallbladder disease."

    c. Nonjudgmental attitude. The history should not reflect a bias. It should be obtained in a manner that does not impose the interviewer's values, beliefs, or prejudices about the patient or his problem. The phraseology of the questions can have a marked influence on the patient's response; for example, "You have never had venereal disease, have you?" A patient questioned this way is unlikely to say "Yes." In sensitive areas, such as the alcohol, drug, or sexual history, the clinician frequently will inadvertently slant the questions, make assumptions, and fail to ask pertinent questions. Examples include:

        (1) The clinician assumes that a married woman has only one sexual partner and fails to ask about sexually transmitted diseases.

        (2) The clinician assumes that a patient over 80 years of age cannot give an accurate history.

    d. Presence of third party. Occasionally, a patient's spouse, child, or friend is present during the interview. This individual can add information or remind the patient of dates or the chronology of a problem.

        (1) The clinician must be careful not to direct all questions to a third party, since the history should be the patient's view of the problem.

        (2) It may be difficult to ask sensitive questions in the presence of another individual. These questions can be deferred or posed during the physical examination, when the clinician is alone with the patient.

        (3) If the third party is not a close family member or intimate friend, it is appropriate to ask the visitor to leave while the history and physical examination are conducted.

        (4) The patient's preference should guide the interviewer in the decision to allow a third party to be present during the acquisition of the history.

e. **Unreliable patients.** The patient's inability to remember facts or to give a consistent story should be documented. Old records and interviews of the patient's family or friends may be necessary to acquire complete and reliable information.

2. **Seven parameters of each symptom** are needed to complete the HPI (see a–g below). Often asking the patient an open-ended question, such as, "Take me from the time you noticed the back pain until today and describe what happened," will provide the clinician with most of the parameters. Details can then be obtained by asking additional questions.
   a. **Chronology** of the symptom from the time it first started to the present time must be determined.
      (1) The chronology of an **acute symptom,** such as dysuria, may only encompass a few days.
         (a) Within that time, the pattern, severity, and any changes in the symptom should be described. Asking an open-ended question, such as, "Take me from the first time you felt the pain, and tell me what has happened since," will often provide the needed information.
         (b) The clinician must ascertain if an acute symptom has ever occurred before.
      (2) The chronology of a **chronic symptom** can span decades, such as diabetes or intermittent back pain for 10 years. The emphasis should not be on a day-to-day description of the problem but a gestalt of the disease over the years; for example, "The patient was asymptomatic until approximately 12 years ago when increased blood sugar was discovered on routine screening. The patient did well on diet and exercise without medication until approximately 5 years ago when symptoms of polyuria, polydipsia, and polyphagia occurred. The patient is regulated on 20 units NPH insulin and has been stable without complications or hospitalization until now."
      (3) An **acute exacerbation** of a problem should be described first (using the parameters listed below). The clinician then goes back to the onset of the problem and describes the entire chronology up to the acute event.
   b. **Quality.** The quality of a symptom is a detailed description of what exactly the symptom is.
      (1) Vague terms, or terms that have different meanings for different people, such as dizziness or diarrhea, should be clarified.
      (2) As many adjectives as possible should be used to describe the symptom; for example, "Sudden, sharp, knife-like chest pain," or "Hacking cough with about a teaspoon of greenish phlegm, which prevents sleep at night" are clearly descriptive.
      (3) Analogies to describe the symptom can be helpful, such as, "Heavy pain like an elephant sitting on my chest."
   c. **Quantity** of a symptom is the magnitude or intensity.
      (1) A common mistake is to take the patient's "a lot" or "not much" as sufficient. These terms are too vague and often misleading.
      (2) It helps to quantify a symptom by relating it to the person's activities of daily living (ADLs); for example, "Shortness of breath has increased so that the patient can now climb only five steps without stopping," or "Pain keeps the patient from sleeping."
      (3) Some interviewers ask patients to rate the symptom of pain on a scale from 1 to 10, which works if the scale is defined. If the patient says the pain was an "8 out of 10," and "10" was natural childbirth, that tells the clinician a great deal. On the other hand, if the patient has no context for a "10," then saying the pain was an "8" is not a helpful quantification.
      (4) It is necessary to quantify any symptom throughout its chronology; for example, "The loose stools occurred only once a day for 3 days, then increased to four to five times a day for a week, and now are occurring about every 4 hours."
      (5) The chronology of a chronic disease should be carefully documented; for example, "The knee pain began 5 years ago. Initially the pain only occurred when the patient had to torque the right knee when playing sports. Gradually, about 3 years ago, the patient began to get pain when climbing up and down stairs and doing minimal activity, such as mowing the lawn, but the pain ceased when the patient stopped the activity. The frequency of the pain has increased in the past 3 months so that the patient experiences it when walking about one-quarter mile, and it no longer goes away with the cessation of activity."
   d. **Location.** It is important that the patient identify where the symptom is located.

(1) The patient may point to a particular place but use incorrect anatomic terms; for example, he or she may point to the left lower quadrant of the abdomen and say, "I had stomach pains." It is the clinician's job to interpret this correctly.

(2) It is important to learn:

(a) If the symptom radiated anywhere

(b) If the symptom is generalized or can be pinpointed to one particular spot

(c) If touching or other maneuver of the area produces the symptom

e. Setting is the context in which the symptom occurs.

(1) It is important to know that the abdominal pain occurred 2 hours after eating spicy foods, that a patient who is allergic to cats had difficulty breathing within 5 minutes of entering a house with two cats, or that a patient has chest pain after physical activity.

(2) The setting also includes information, such as:

(a) Contact with other people who have the same symptoms (i.e., all the people in the house have the same rash)

(b) Travel to areas where such symptoms are known to be endemic (i.e., patient just returned from Mexico where symptoms began)

(c) Occupational risks (i.e., symptoms occur only on work days)

(3) Any factor that may affect how or when the symptom occurs must be sought.

f. Alleviating and aggravating factors include any activity, event, or attempted remedy that makes the symptom better or worse; for example, "The swelling went away in about 2 hours after elevating the leg," or "Walking on a cold winter day made my shortness of breath worse."

(1) If any medication has been tried, its effectiveness should be determined; for example, "I tried two extra strength aspirin (ASA) for the headache without relief." "The chest pain stopped 2 minutes after using nitroglycerine."

(2) Open-ended questions may expedite a full answer; for example, "Did anything you tried make the itching better?" Patients may, however, not be conscious of what specifically helped or did not help.

(3) As students learn more medicine, they will be able to ask **specific questions** if open-ended questions are not helpful. Specific questions may help the patient recall some event and provide positive or pertinent negative responses.

g. Associated symptoms are other symptoms that occur with or during the course of the problem being described. For example, the patient may have had a cough for 2 days and developed a fever of 102° F on day 3. The fever may be construed as a symptom associated (in time) with the cough.

(1) It is often difficult to ascertain whether or not associated symptoms are pathophysiologically related; for example, in a patient with burning on urination who subsequently develops a vaginal discharge and lower back pain, the clinician must determine whether the latter two symptoms are related to the dysuria or whether they need to be developed individually.

(2) Novice interviewers should separate the problems unless they feel confident in putting them together. As students learn more about the constellation of symptoms that comprise certain illnesses, decisions will become easier; for example, once students understand diabetes mellitus, they will consider weight loss, polyuria, and polydipsia as symptoms related to a single disease process.

h. Complications. Predictable complications of any extant chronic disease should be sought, although they are not considered one of the seven parameters. Some complications are serious and may need to be presented separately; for example, a patient may have renal failure as a complication of diabetes mellitus.

i. Summary. After all seven parameters have been covered by the clinician, it is helpful to summarize the information that has been obtained.

(1) This provides an opportunity for both clinician and patient to check the information for completeness and accuracy.

(2) Additional questions may be asked once the summary has been completed.

j. If the patient is loquacious, the clinician may instruct him or her to wait until the summary is completed to clarify or correct any information.

3. Patient's perception of causality

a. Asking patients if they have any preconceived ideas about what is causing the problem can be enlightening. A patient complaining of headaches may fear a brain tumor.

    b. Patients may have concerns or phobias that need to be addressed; for example, a 50-year-old patient may believe that a heart attack is imminent if one or both parents died from heart attacks when they were 50 years of age.

    c. Asking patients if there is anything they wish to add that has not already been covered may provide additional information about which the patient may not have felt comfortable discussing earlier.

4. Multiproblem HPIs. Patients can have multiple concurrent symptoms or problems.

    a. Any problem or symptom for which patients are currently being treated should be included in the HPI. The HPI of the patient with a presenting complaint of "shortness of breath" who also has arthritis and diabetes should list each of the three problems separately in the HPI with the seven parameters determined for each.

    b. Problems that occurred in the past, have been resolved, and have no impact on the patient today belong in the past medical history.

5. Controlling the interview. The greatest difficulty for most interviewers is directing the interview so that the patient talks about each problem separately. One tactic that can be used when a patient deviates from his shortness of breath to his abdominal pain is to say, "I am very interested in the abdominal pain, but let us finish discussing shortness of breath first and then you can tell me all about your abdominal pain." The clinician should then return to the abdominal pain: "You mentioned abdominal pain earlier; could you tell me about it now?"

D. Personal profile (PP)

1. Definition and significance. The PP should give the interviewer some insight into the **patient as a person**. It defines who (if anyone) provides the patient with support. It describes the patient's life-style and how the current hospitalization or health problem affects him or her. With this information, caregivers should be able to distinguish between the two 55-year-old men in the coronary care unit with the diagnoses of "heart attack."

2. Overview

    a. Note-taking should cease while taking a PP since eye contact is critical to rapport.

    b. Open-ended questions usually elicit the maximum information. Since most people like to talk about themselves, "Tell me a little about yourself," is often sufficient to get the ball rolling. Occasionally, the patient needs a few guidelines, such as, "Tell me a little about yourself, about the people who are closest to you, about your work, and what you do with your free time." This allows patients to talk about issues that they consider significant.

    c. Some clinicians begin the PP by asking the patient to describe a typical day.

3. Content. A PP will not necessarily include all of the possibilities listed (see a–e below). Variations will depend upon the patient and the interviewer. If the clinician already has a relationship with the patient, much of the PP may already be known. Additional information may be acquired as the clinician gets to know the patient over time.

    a. Significant others. It is important to determine with whom the patient lives and who provides emotional and physical support.

        (1) This may be the appropriate time to take a sexual history if it has not already been done as part of the HPI (for details of the sexual history, see Chapter 4 II).

        (2) With children, this is the point at which to determine how they get along with parents, siblings, and peers.

    b. Occupation. Assess the type of work, current and past employment, stress levels, and effect of illness on job status. Ask about health insurance and the potential financial impact of this illness.

    c. Effect of illness on the patient may be insignificant in the case of a 23-year-old man who is recovering from an appendectomy and will be back at a desk job in 10 days. On the other hand, the effect of illness may be a major problem for a 57-year-old man with chronic obstructive pulmonary disease (COPD) who is unable to work, too young for Medicare, and whose wife must now seek employment for the first time since their marriage.

    d. ADLs. Clinicians should attempt to learn what, besides work, patients do—that is, to which hobbies or organizations are they attracted. Clinicians may also ask about habits, such as exercise, diet, alcohol, cigarettes, and recreational drugs.

    e. Patient concerns. Any concerns, fears, anxieties (whether or not related to the illness) should also be elicited, such as fear of divorce, concern about a diagnosis, or grief surrounding a recent loss.

E. Past medical history (PMH)

1. **Definition and significance.** The PMH is obtained to ascertain any medical information from the patient's past that may have an impact on the present or future. The patient should be told that the interviewer plans to focus on major health problems. Clinicians should provide guidelines to direct the patient toward their agenda, which must be met in the PMH.

2. **Content**
   a. **Childhood illnesses**
      (1) The questions vary depending upon the age of the patient. For example, knowing that a 5-year-old child has had chicken pox is relevant. Learning if a woman in her childbearing years has been vaccinated against rubella is important, but this same information is less crucial in a 78-year-old woman.
      (2) Major childhood problems should be reviewed. To trigger a patient's memory, the interviewer may ask if the patient stayed home from school for long periods of time or was hospitalized during childhood.
      (3) With elderly patients, illnesses that have continued from childhood into adulthood (e.g., asthma) are important. Spending time determining whether or not a 70-year-old person had measles or mumps is not useful.
   b. **Adult illnesses.** This includes problems that have been resolved and are not currently causing any symptoms nor being treated in any way (i.e., by medication or diet).
      (1) A potential pitfall for students is their tendency to lump all of the patient's problems, other than those related to the CC, into the PMH.
      (2) There are two major hazards in following this format:
         (a) The clinician is responsible for being aware of all the patient's problems. For example, although the patient may be in the hospital for a total hip replacement, the clinician cannot ignore COPD and diabetes, which need constant monitoring and medication.
         (b) Problems may be interrelated; for example, in the patient with diabetes who is admitted for total hip replacement, the glucose level, amount of insulin needed, and type of intravenous fluids are affected by the stress of surgery and the recovery period.
      (3) Problems that do belong in the PMH include:
         (a) Tuberculosis treated in 1964 with isoniazid (INH), streptomycin, and para-aminosalicylic acid (PAS) for 2 years with no sequelae. The last chest x-ray in 1984 was reported as "unchanged since 1979."
         (b) Asthma attacks two to three times a year until age 25 with no symptoms since
   c. **Surgical procedures.** The following information should be obtained about all surgical procedures:
      (1) **Date of surgery** or, if not known, approximate age of patient at time of surgery
      (2) **Place of surgery,** especially for recent surgeries and those related to any current problems
      (3) **Reason for surgery,** which is obvious in some cases (e.g., appendectomy) but less so with others (e.g., hysterectomy). The symptoms that led to the operation should be determined.
      (4) **Sequelae.** Any complications during or after surgery should be determined.
   d. **Accidents and injuries**
      (1) Accidents, their causes, and all medical problems relevant to the accident should be listed with any sequelae; for example, a fall from a tree while playing that resulted in a fractured tibia or a car accident that resulted in headaches for 3 weeks.
      (2) Occasionally, there is a repetitive nature to these accidents. Clinicians should be attuned to the possibility of physical abuse or substance use and ask appropriate questions (see Chapter 4 III, VII).
   e. **Occupational history** (see Chapter 4 IV)
   f. **Immunizations**
      (1) The type of information to be acquired is age-dependent. Immunization for many of the childhood communicable diseases is relatively recent; therefore, it is not relevant to the history of an elderly patient.
      (2) Until the student is conversant with all the vaccines and ages at which they should be given, it is probably safe to ask mothers of young patients if their "shots" are up-to-date and whether they had any problems with immunizations.

(3) The clinician should ask adults about the date of the latest tetanus shot.

(4) Elderly patients and any adult or child with chronic medical problems should be asked about pneumonia and influenza immunization.

g. Obstetric history. Although most interviewers would not expect the obstetric history to be a sensitive or emotional part of the overall history, sometimes sad memories are relived. Acknowledgment or other personal response can be helpful. Regardless of the marital status of the patient, the clinician should inquire about the following:

(1) Number of pregnancies (gravida)

(2) Number of live births (para)

(3) Number of abortions, either spontaneous or induced

(4) Types of delivery, either vaginal delivery or cesarean section

(5) Problems with pregnancies, such as high blood pressure, placenta previa, or premature birth

(6) Sequelae, such as postdelivery hemorrhage

h. Psychiatric history. There is still a stigma associated with seeing a psychiatrist.

(1) Nonjudgmental ways of asking about a psychiatric history are: "Have you ever seen, or felt the need to see, a counselor or psychiatrist?" "Have you ever been hospitalized for an emotional problem?"

(2) If the patient has a serious, debilitating, or fatal disease, the clinician may also open up the potential need for counseling by saying, "It must be very difficult to be so young with a disease like lupus; do you think it would help to talk with someone?"

(3) These same questions, if indicated, could be asked during the HPI or the PP.

i. Medications. Many people take medications without knowing their names or why they were prescribed; therefore, it is important to ask for the following information:

(1) **Current prescribed medications**

(a) Names

(b) Doses

(c) Reasons for use

(2) **Nonprescription medications.** Any over-the-counter medication (i.e., analgesics, antacids, or antihistamines) may cause problems for individual patients. For example, certain antihistamines interact with blood pressure medication; ASA may alter the effect of warfarin; some sodium-containing antacids may complicate congestive heart failure (CHF).

(3) **Recreational (illicit) drug use** must be explored with all patients in a nonjudgmental manner. No assumptions should be made on the basis of the patient's age or economic and social position.

j. Health habits

(1) **Exercise.** Any formal or regular exercise or sports should be noted.

(2) **Diet.** Information is most easily obtained by asking the patient to describe what was eaten on a particular day. (For more in-depth dietary history, see Chapter 4 V.)

(3) **Alcohol** is such a prevalent and accepted part of our society that the clinician may ask, "During an average week, how much beer, wine, or hard liquor do you drink?" Patients often give vague answers, such as "I only drink socially," or "I drink no more than usual." These answers are inadequate. It is the clinician's responsibility to elicit a more detailed history. At times, it may help to overestimate the amount consumed and let the patient make corrections. The clinician should learn what type of alcohol and how much is consumed each day or week (see Chapter 4 III).

(4) **Tobacco**

(a) All patients should be asked if they smoke cigarettes, cigars, or a pipe. Clinicians must also determine how much tobacco is smoked and for what duration. Cigarette consumption is usually recorded as the number of packs smoked each year (pack/years).

(b) Often people who have smoked two to three packs a day for 20 or more years and stopped recently deny smoking unless asked about past smoking history. Thus, the past smoking history should be obtained, including the date of cessation.

k. Allergies

(1) **Medication.** Patients should be asked if they are allergic to any medication.

(a) Patients must be asked specifically what happens when the medication is taken. This will help the clinician to differentiate a true allergic response from an adverse reaction, such as an upset stomach with some antibiotics. This information may become crucial if the patient should need a particular medication. The clinician may choose to deal with the patient's "upset stomach" and give the needed antibiotic but would not opt for that antibiotic if the patient had a history of difficulty breathing, which required epinephrine.

    (b) **Penicillin allergies** are common; therefore, patients should be asked about this particular medication.

  (2) **Foods.** The patient must be asked about any food allergies.

    (a) This will avert problems in ordering a hospitalized patient's diet.

    (b) It will avert prescribing certain medications, which may be made from the allergenic product, such as porcine insulin in the pork-allergic patient.

  (3) **Other.** Seasonal allergies, bee-sting reactions, and animal dander allergies should all be elicited and information obtained about the symptoms of the reaction.

F. Family history (FH)

1. Definition and elicitation. The FH gives clues to familial or genetic diseases that may have an impact on the patient now or in the future.

  a. Having this information could alter a clinician's treatment or decision to screen for certain diseases; for example, if women have a strong FH of breast cancer, clinicians are likely to prescribe mammography earlier and more often than they do for patients with no FH of breast disease.

  b. The FH may be introduced by saying, "I would like to spend a few minutes finding out about the health of your blood relatives to see if any illnesses run in the family." Without this transition, the patient may still be thinking about earlier questions or may ramble on about the health of nonfamily members.

  c. If a patient is adopted and has no knowledge of biologic parents or siblings, then there is no relevant FH; in this instance, record a simple explanation under FH in the patient's medical record.

  d. **Content.** The extent of the FH is age-dependent.

    (1) Clinicians are concerned with parents, grandparents, and potentially great-grandparents of a child.

    (2) The medical history of parents and siblings is sufficient for a 78-year-old patient.

  e. **Unexpected emotional issues.** Although typically a relatively short part of the interview, the FH may become involved if any new or past sad memories are revived.

    (1) Recent deaths, or even memories of a relative who died years ago, can upset the patient, even to the point of tears.

    (2) A patient may also want to talk about a spouse who is presently ill or who has died. Even though the spouse's health is not part of the FH, the clinician should heed the patient's needs.

2. Specific components

  a. **Blood relatives**—grandparents, parents, siblings, and children

    (1) Ages now, if alive, or age at death

    (2) Any major medical problems for each and reason for death

  b. **Additional components.** In addition to the above information, the FH should include common genetic and familial diseases, as well as problems that the patient has identified as his or her own, such as "migraine headache" or "anemia." Diseases specifically sought by most clinicians are **hypertension, diabetes mellitus, cancer** (with primary site, if known), **stroke, heart disease,** and **sickle cell disease** or **trait** in blacks.

G. Review of systems (ROS)

1. Definition and elicitation. The ROS is the final part of the history. Its purpose is to determine that no major problems have been missed.

  a. To avoid hearing about every cold or case of hemorrhoids during a pregnancy 15 years ago, specific guidelines are given to the patient as part of the introduction, such as, "I am interested in knowing about any unusual problems in the last year." There are, however, patients who, despite instructions, relate minor past problems in great detail and must be redirected.

  b. It is important to let the patient know that, unlike the prior parts of the history, the ROS will be acquired by means of multiple closed-ended ("yes" or "no") questions.

  c. Occasionally, the ROS will identify another problem for which the seven parameters must be pursued.

2. **Specific components.** The following list is a sample of a typical ROS. The clinician asks these questions in a language that the patient will understand—that is, "difficulty breathing" rather than "dyspnea." If the interviewer does not know the medical significance of a positive response, he may need to acquire the full seven parameters.
   a. **General.** Usual weight, recent weight change, weakness, fatigue, and fever
   b. **Skin.** Rashes, lumps, itching, dryness, color change, and changes in hair or nails
   c. **Head.** Headache and head injury
   d. **Eyes.** Vision, glasses or contact lenses, last eye examination, pain, redness, excessive tearing, double vision, glaucoma, and cataracts
   e. **Ears.** Hearing, tinnitus, vertigo, earaches, infection, and discharge
   f. **Nose and sinuses.** Frequent colds, nasal stuffiness, hay fever, nosebleeds, and sinus trouble
   g. **Mouth and throat.** Condition of teeth and gums, bleeding gums, last dental examination, sore tongue, frequent sore throats, and hoarseness
   h. **Neck.** Lumps in neck, "swollen glands," goiter, and pain in the neck
   i. **Breasts.** Lumps, pain, nipple discharge, self-examination, and data from last mammogram
   j. **Respiratory.** Cough, sputum (color and quantity), hemoptysis, wheezing, asthma, bronchitis, emphysema, pneumonia, tuberculosis, pleurisy, tuberculin test, and last chest x-ray
   k. **Cardiac.** Heart trouble, high blood pressure, rheumatic fever, heart murmurs; dyspnea, orthopnea, paroxysmal nocturnal dyspnea, edema; chest pain, palpitations; and past electrocardiogram (EKG) or other heart tests
   l. **Gastrointestinal.** Trouble swallowing, heartburn, appetite, nausea, vomiting, vomiting blood, indigestion, frequency of bowel movements, change in bowel habits, rectal bleeding or black tarry stools, constipation, diarrhea, abdominal pain, food intolerance, excessive belching or passing of gas, hemorrhoids; jaundice, liver or gallbladder trouble, and hepatitis
   m. **Urinary.** Frequency of urination, polyuria, nocturia, dysuria, hematuria, urgency, hesitancy, incontinence, urinary infections, and stones
   n. **Genitoreproductive**
      (1) **Male.** Discharge from or sores on penis, history of venereal disease and its treatment, hernias, testicular pain or masses; and frequency of intercourse,* libido, and sexual difficulties
      (2) **Female**
          (a) Age of menarche; regularity, frequency, and duration of periods; amount of bleeding, bleeding between periods or after intercourse, or last menstrual period; dysmenorrhea; and age of menopause, menopausal symptoms, or postmenopausal bleeding
          (b) Discharge, itching, venereal disease and its treatment; and last Pap smear.
          (c) Number of pregnancies, deliveries, and abortions (spontaneous and induced); complications of pregnancy; birth control methods; and frequency of intercourse,* libido, and sexual difficulties
   o. **Musculoskeletal.** Joint pains or stiffness, arthritis, gout, and backache (if present, describe location and symptoms, such as swelling, redness, pain, stiffness, weakness, and limitation of motion or activity); and muscle pains or cramps
   p. **Peripheral vascular.** Intermittent claudication, cramps, varicose veins, and thrombophlebitis
   q. **Neurologic.** Fainting, blackouts, seizures, paralysis, local weakness, numbness, tingling, tremors, and memory
   r. **Psychiatric.** Nervousness, tension, mood, and depression
   s. **Endocrine.** Thyroid trouble, heat or cold intolerance, excessive sweating, diabetes, and excessive thirst, hunger, or urination
   t. **Hematologic.** Anemia, easy bruising or bleeding, past transfusions, and possible reactions

H. **Closure to the medical history.** Before proceeding with the physical examination, the clinician and the patient need some closure to the history. The clinician can ask if there is anything else the patient would like to discuss. The patient should be given another opportunity to add or correct historical information prior to the next step in the acquisition of data—the physical examination.

---

*Note that a sexual history is usually most effectively acquired while discussing life-style or, if pertinent, in the HPI; it may, however, be asked by default during the ROS.

II. PROBLEM-ORIENTED (OR FOCUSED) MEDICAL HISTORY

A. Components. There are situations in which the comprehensive history is not appropriate because of the timing, setting, or acuteness of the problem. Under these circumstances, the clinician must focus on the immediate complaint and the parameters that help to define it for specific action.

   1. Clinical setting. The need for the focused medical history and physical examination (see Chapter 6 V) arises in a variety of physical settings.

   a. Emergency rooms. The patient who comes into the emergency room often has an acute, circumscribed problem, which requires immediate attention. In this circumstance, clinicians must attend to the presenting complaint to achieve an efficient and timely diagnosis and treatment.

   b. Outpatient department, office, or ambulatory clinic. Frequently, the patient who comes into any of the above health care settings has a specific problem for which he or she seeks attention. The clinician should determine the immediacy of the need and be attentive to the **patient's agenda** before going beyond the presenting complaint.

   c. Other settings. The walk-in, or immediate-care center, is one solution to the busy lives of most patients. Individuals usually present to this setting with a clear agenda: Hear my problem and attend to it now. The clinician has a responsibility to respond to this agenda so long as it does not compromise the patient's health.

   2. The focused history should be directed toward the organ system suggested by the presenting complaint. If the patient presents with a CC of earache, the history should cover the seven parameters of this complaint and any attendant past history of the same complaint without spending time on an effort to be comprehensive.

   3. The HPI is the core of the focused history. The clinician must attend to the organ system suggested, the PMH that is specific to this organ system, and the PP, FH, or ROS only if they relate to the CC.

B. Associated organ systems

   1. Questions about organ systems other than those suggested by the CC need be asked only if this is necessary to rule out other possible systems.

   2. Questions about life-style, family diseases, and allergies should only be pursued if the interviewer perceives that they are relevant to the CC. Some clinicians include current medications, allergies, and use of tobacco and alcohol in even the most focused history.

C. Clinical examples

   1. "Shortness of breath." The focused history for this situation involves at least two systems, cardiovascular and pulmonary.

   a. Seven parameters should be obtained, followed by the ROS, covering the two organ systems involved.

   b. Tobacco use history, allergies, and occupational and environmental histories may be pertinent under some circumstances.

   2. "Headache." This complaint suggests the nervous system as the organ system involved.

   a. Seven parameters of the CC, possible stressors from the PP, and all the questions from the ROS that relate to the central nervous system should be elicited.

   b. If the novice cannot make a diagnosis, he or she can go to the clinical preceptor with the key information, which will direct the physical examination to the correct focus—the neurologic examination.

D. Limitations of the problem-oriented history

   1. Potential for error. Focus upon, or limited direction toward, a single symptom and its implied organ system must be approached with caution. This focus implies a level of **premature closure,** which is potentially hazardous. The clinician must be aware of the possibility of error in confining the history to a limited pursuit. If the **physical examination,** which flows from the focused history, fails to confirm or clearly deny the initial impressions growing out of the focused history, it may be necessary to expand the history further. It is important to remain flexible.

2. **Lack of comprehensive understanding of the patient.** The absence of a full history obviously limits the clinician's full appreciation of the patient as an individual, or of the other elements of his or her life. This is a trade-off that must be accepted under the circumstances that require the **problem-oriented history**.

STUDY QUESTIONS

Directions: Each of the numbered items or incomplete statements in this section is followed by answers or by completions of the statement. Select the **one** lettered answer or completion that is **best** in each case.

1. A 49-year-old, previously healthy but overweight, black, male, bank executive comes in with the CC: "I have a cough." He admits to smoking two packs of cigarettes a day. The man claims to be happily married and lives in Simsbury with his wife and two children. He is not taking any medication. Which of the following best illustrates the identifying data?

(A) A 49-year-old bank executive who smokes two packs of cigarettes a day presents with the CC: "I have a cough"
(B) A 49-year-old black bank executive presents with the CC: "I have a cough"
(C) A 49-year-old previously healthy bank executive presents with the CC: "I have a cough"
(D) A 49-year-old smoker from Simsbury presents with the CC: "I have a cough"
(E) A 49-year-old happily married man with two children presents with the CC: "I have a cough"

2. A 70-year-old retired baker has a broken leg, hypertension, heartburn, IDDM, myopia, decreased hearing, and COPD. The HPI should include how many of these problems?

(A) 3
(B) 4
(C) 5
(D) 6
(E) 7

3. A 54-year-old electrician comes in with the CC: "I have carpal tunnel syndrome." The best response is to find out

(A) when the carpal tunnel syndrome began
(B) the chronology of the carpal tunnel syndrome
(C) what symptoms the patient has
(D) how the carpal tunnel syndrome has affected the ADLs
(E) if this is the first episode

4. All of the following are components of the HPI EXCEPT

(A) recurrences
(B) change over time
(C) effects on the ADLs
(D) etiology of symptom
(E) location

5. Vague words that should be clarified by the clinician while taking the medical history include all of the following EXCEPT

(A) tired
(B) dizzy
(C) hiccups
(D) sick
(E) socially

6. While taking a PMH, the clinician learns that a patient is taking digoxin, a cardiac medication. The clinician should

(A) list the digoxin in the PMH
(B) find out about the cardiac symptom and put it in the PMH
(C) find out how long the patient has been taking the digoxin
(D) find out about the cardiac symptom and put it in the ROS
(E) find out about the cardiac symptom and put it in the HPI

7. In a PP, the category that best differentiates patients with cancer is

(A) primary site of cancer
(B) place of employment
(C) number of children
(D) response to disease
(E) type of treatment

8. For an 85-year-old woman, all of the following components of the PMH are crucial EXCEPT

(A) allergies
(B) childhood history
(C) medication
(D) surgical history
(E) alcohol use history

9. All of the positive findings listed below belong in the ROS of a 65-year-old man EXCEPT

(A) occasional chest pains
(B) occasional headaches
(C) occasional knee stiffness
(D) hay fever
(E) decreased hearing

10. Based on the FH illustrated below, the clinician should ask about all of the following conditions EXCEPT

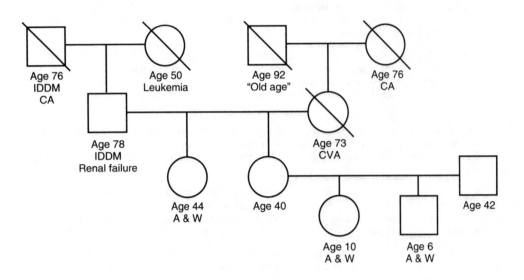

IDDM = insulin-dependent diabetes mellitus; CA = cancer; CVA = cerebrovascular accident; and A & W = alive and well.

(A) primary site of cancer
(B) any other diabetes mellitus
(C) any hypertension
(D) any traumatic deaths
(E) cause of renal failure

Directions: Each group of items in this section consists of lettered options followed by a set of numbered items. For each item, select the **one** lettered option that is most closely associated with it. Each lettered option may be selected once, more than once, or not at all.

Questions 11–15

For each description of pain that follows, select the part of the HPI in which it belongs.

(A) Chronology
(B) Quantity
(C) Aggravating factors
(D) Setting
(E) Quality

11. The pain starts when doing aerobics

12. The pain lasts for 10 minutes

13. The pain is like a dull, achy pressure

14. The pain occurs nightly, two or three times a week for the past 3 weeks

15. The pain increases if the patient does not stop aerobics

ANSWERS AND EXPLANATIONS

1. The answer is A. [*I B 1, 2 a*] Identifying data should be short, succinct sentences with a name, age, sex, occupation, and occasionally any pertinent medical information that will help in hearing or reading the HPI. In the case presented in the question, the smoking history is related to the CC of cough. Ethnicity is not an issue with this CC and should not be included. Although marital and living status are appropriate to the PP, they are not essential to the identifying data.

2. The answer is B. [*I C 1 a, G 1 a*] Fractured leg, hypertension, IDDM, and COPD are all active problems. Although it is safe to assume that the fractured leg is the acute problem, the three chronic problems need monitoring and treatment. The myopia, decreased hearing, and heartburn are important to note in the ROS, but unless there is some acute pain or exacerbation, they do not need the seven parameters to be explored.

3. The answer is C. [*I C 1 b*] The clinician should not accept tertiary information. Before obtaining the seven parameters of a symptom, the clinician must clarify and verify that the syndrome or disease stated in the CC is true. Without this knowledge, the clinician may miss a diagnosis and prescribe incorrect treatment.

4. The answer is D. [*I C 1 a, 2 a–h*] The etiology of a symptom is not information that is sought from patients for inclusion in the HPI. The etiology is hypothesis-verified by the history, physical examination, and laboratory results. The seven parameters of each symptom reported by the patient, including recurrences, changes over time, effects of the ADLs, and location, are necessary to complete the HPI.

5. The answer is C. [*I C 2 b (1), c (1)*] Vague words often have different meanings for different people. These words must be clarified so that the clinician and patient know exactly what is meant. Hiccups is the only nonambiguous word listed and does not need clarification.

6. The answer E. [*I C 4, E 2 b, i (1)*] Any problem or symptom for which patients are currently being treated should be included in the HPI and have the seven parameters determined. Digoxin is a cardiac medication that cannot be forgotten and put in the PMH. Any cardiac symptom needs to be uncovered and reported in the HPI.

7. The answer is D. [*I D 1, 3 a–e*] A patient's response to illness is so varied that this information helps to personalize two people with the same diagnosis. The primary site of cancer and its treatment are important medical facts that are not relevant to the PP. The number of children and place of employment are part of the PP, but without more information, these facts do not give great insight.

8. The answer is B. [*I E 2 a (3), c, i, j (3), k*] Although childhood illnesses are part of the PMH, they are less relevant for an 85-year-old woman. Rarely can 85-year-old individuals remember when and what they had as a child. If a major disease has continued through adulthood, then this will be ascertained during the adult PMH. The patient's surgical history as well as medications, alcohol, and allergies are essential in treating the patient now.

9. The answer is A. [*I G 1 c, 2*] Occasional headache, knee stiffness, hay fever, and decreased hearing are fairly common maladies that occur in a 65-year-old man. Occasional chest pain, which may signal a cardiac problem, needs more clarification, including exploration by the seven parameters. Unless the clinician believes that the chest pain is totally benign, it should be discussed in the HPI.

10. The answer is D. [*I F 1 a, 2 a, b*] Although a traumatic death is important to a patient, it should not be part of the FH. It should be reported in the PP. The FH should give the clinician details about whether there are any familial or genetic diseases that may have an impact on the patient. The primary site of cancer, IDDM, hypertension, and the cause of renal failure are facts that the clinician should query in the FH.

11–15. The answers are: 11-D, 12-A, 13-E, 14-A, 15-C. [*I C 2 a, b, e, f*] The setting is the background in which a problem occurs. In this case, the pain begins while the patient does aerobics, which gives the clinician valuable information.

The length of time a symptom lasts is part of the chronology of a symptom. The chronology also includes previous episodes, duration, and any change in pattern. A pain that occurs nightly, two or three times a week for the past 3 weeks describes the chronology of the symptom.

The quality of a symptom is a description of the characteristics of the symptom. Descriptive words, such as dull, achy pressure, help to differentiate the pain. The quantity of a symptom rates the magnitude of the pain.

Aggravating factors are conditions that cause the symptom to continue to get worse. In this case, the aerobics (exercise), which increases the pain, is an aggravating factor.

4

Content Challenges of the Medical History

Judy Lewis, Eileen Storey,
Carrie S. Mukaida, Nancy A. Stilwell,
Carol A. Pfeiffer, Polly J. Macpherson

I. INTRODUCTION. This chapter deals with sensitive topics in the medical history about which information is difficult to obtain because of the clinician's lack of training or discomfort with the topic. Sections I–VII discuss areas that the authors feel should be included in every complete medical history—the sexual, substance use, occupational, nutritional, and mental health histories. Sections VIII–X cover the special histories required from patients with trauma, chronic disease, terminal illness, and acquired immune deficiency syndrome (AIDS).

II. SEXUAL HISTORY. A basic sexual history should be part of all medical histories as sexuality is an important element of the emotional and physical well-being of human beings throughout the life span. Detailed information should be collected if the patient presents with a specific concern related to sexuality, health risks related to sexual practices, or contraception and fertility issues.

    A. Placement in the structured interview. Appropriate places in which to discuss sexuality and sexual practices in the structured interview are reviewed below. If the topic does not arise spontaneously, the clinician must be sure that sexual information is obtained in every interview.

        1. Medical history
            a. The history of the present illness (HPI) provides an appropriate place for discussing the sexual history. In chronic disease, the physical limitations, depression of adjustment or loss, and medications may all have an effect on sexual functioning. When questions are asked in the context of an illness, they may be less threatening to patients who may be embarrassed or sensitive about discussing sexual issues.
            b. The past medical history (PMH) may provide a natural opportunity to ask about sexual functioning, particularly in the reproductive history or if there is a history of sexually transmitted disease (STD).

        2. Patient profile (PP). Taking a social history may provide an appropriate opportunity to ask about sex partners and marital or co-parenting relationships, since many other aspects of social interaction and emotional well-being are discussed in the PP.

        3. Review of systems (ROS). Although information about the genitourinary system is a part of the ROS, this is probably the least appropriate place in the interview to introduce the subject of sexuality because of the closed-ended nature of the questions.

    B. Format of questions. Interviewers often struggle for neutral terms and achievement of a comfort level in asking questions about sexuality that enable patients to respond freely and honestly. The discomfort of the clinician concerning the sexual history should diminish with time and experience. If a particular sexual preference or practice is unacceptable to the clinician or interferes with his or her ability to provide good care to the patient, the patient should be referred to another provider.

        1. Open-ended questions. All questions should be open-ended, such as, "Are you currently sexually active?" Assumptions about behavior can be avoided with this approach. It is very easy to inhibit the discussion of sex by making inappropriate assumptions about age, sex of partners, or type of sexual activity.

        2. Nonjudgmental attitudes. It is equally important that the clinician not pass judgment on the information provided by the patient, keeping in mind that there is a great variety of human sexual behavior. If risk behaviors are identified, they should not be addressed until a complete data base has been obtained.

3. Terminology. The terms describing sexual behavior have a direct impact on the quality and usefulness of the information collected. Neutrality and understandability are two critical elements to consider in selecting terminology.

   a. Neutrality. It is important for clinicians to use neutral terms in asking about sexual behavior; for example, using the patient's words to describe behavior, such as, "The patient reports multiple (or between 10 and 20) partners in the past year" is more appropriate than saying "The patient is promiscuous." In the first statement, there is no value judgment, and it is actually more accurate than the second statement because one person's definition of promiscuity may be very different from another's (e.g., more than one partner may be "promiscuous" to some people).

   b. Understandability. It is important that patients understand what is being said by the clinician, or they may be reluctant to participate in a discussion.

   (1) Clinicians should avoid street terms because it may indicate a lack of respect for the patient.

   (2) Pictures or anatomic charts may help to clarify behavior or terminology.

C. Specific content. The basic content of the sexual history is to discover whether a person is sexually active and satisfied with this part of his or her life, to identify any sexual problems or concerns, and to introduce the idea that sexuality is an acceptable issue for discussion in a health care setting. Basic questions should cover the following areas:

1. Level of sexual activity

   a. A simple inquiry as to whether or not the patient is currently sexually active is usually sufficient to determine the level of sexual activity.

   b. It may be necessary to be direct by asking, "Are you having sexual intercourse with anyone at this time?"

   c. The clinician may begin by asking whether the patient is in a relationship and then ask if it is a sexual relationship.

2. Satisfaction with sexual activity. It is important to determine if patients are happy with their current sexual activity level and if there have been any recent changes in interest in, or levels of, sexual activity.

3. Concerns about sexual issues. A simple follow-up question might be, "Do you have any questions or concerns about matters of sexuality?"

D. Screening purposes. There are specific questions about sexual behavior that clinicians should ask once they have established that a patient is or has been sexually active to screen for risk behaviors (i.e., STDs) and contraceptive practices. If risk behaviors or sexual dysfunction are identified, an extensive history should be completed to determine the appropriate management or therapy.

1. Number of sexual partners. Even if patients are married, it is important to know if they or their spouses have other sexual partners.

2. Gender preference. Heterosexuality should not be presumed, and inquiry should be made as to whether the patient has had sex with partners of the same sex, the opposite sex, or both sexes. If the patient seems surprised by the question, the clinician should indicate that it is a question asked of all patients because of the serious health implications for many sexual behaviors.

3. Prevention of STDs. If the patient is sexually active with more than one partner or is sexually active with a partner who has other partners, it is important to ask about the use of condoms for the prevention of STDs.

4. Contraceptive use. It is important to establish whether the patient is concerned about pregnancy. If the patient does not wish to become pregnant or does not wish his partner to become pregnant, the clinician should discuss contraceptive use.

III. SUBSTANCE USE HISTORY. The use of alcohol, tobacco, and other drugs is important information for the medical history as these substances can contribute to ill health or interfere with the effects of prescribed medication. Relatively large numbers of people use both legal and illegal substances. Recent studies of the American population indicate the following about the incidence and prevalence of substance intake: Average daily caffeine consumption is 200 mg, usually in the form of 2–3 cups of coffee; 30% of Americans smoke cigarettes; most people drink alcoholic beverages, and

5%–10% of the adult population suffer from alcoholism; 62 million Americans have tried marijuana, and 18.2 million are current users; 20 million Americans have tried cocaine, and 4 million use it regularly.

A. **Placement in the structured interview.** The appropriate place in the interview to ask questions about substance use is generally one of the following.

1. **PP.** Some clinicians include information about smoking, drinking, and drug use in the PP or social history when other health behaviors or the daily routine of the patient may be discussed. This may fit quite nicely with a discussion of diet, social activities, and exercise.

2. **ROS.** This is probably the least appropriate place to ask for a history of substance use because of the closed-ended nature of the questions, but it is sometimes used as a way of considering all other areas, which may contribute to the patient's general condition.

3. **HPI.** In many cases, the patient's chief complaint (CC) or presenting symptoms may be directly related to substance use (e.g., a cough in smokers or agitation and sleep loss in heavy coffee drinkers). When the patient presents with a symptom, which may be related to substance use, the HPI is the most appropriate place to collect this history.

4. **PMH.** When substance use is not related directly to the HPI, the PMH is probably the most appropriate place to ask questions about substance use. It makes it clear to the patient that these questions are basic elements of health and illness. This discussion can easily follow questions about the use of prescribed and over-the-counter medications.

B. **Format of questions.** Questions about substance use should be asked in a manner that does not presume normative behavior or judge that which is described. Clinicians must not project their subjective opinions about substance use in pursuing a complete and accurate history.

1. **Opened-ended questions,** such as, "Do you smoke?" "Many people today drink alcohol, do you?" or "I need to ask a few questions about drug and alcohol use to get as complete a history as possible." These approaches are less apt to offend patients who abstain from all use for religious or moral reasons. It is important for clinicians to be familiar with the makeup of their patient population in terms of general expectations about substance use.

2. **Nonjudgmental attitude.** The clinician must maintain neutrality in asking questions and listening to responses. While it may be appropriate to offer counseling for the health risks of certain behaviors, this should not be done until a complete data base has been developed.

3. **Use versus abuse.** It is important that clinicians do not describe casual users of illicit drugs as "drug addicts." Experimentation, occasional use, regular use, and addiction are useful distinctions. Perhaps the label "abuse" should be abandoned altogether and replaced with "use."

4. **Dependency.** It is important to explore the nature of the patient's use of the drug, the enjoyable effects (and the bad effects), circumstances of use (i.e., alone or with others), and the ability or willingness to stop. Psychological and physiological dependencies can be equally difficult to treat.

5. **Denial.** Patients with a substance dependency often try to minimize their use and their dependency. Most patients, however, if approached in a nonjudgmental and nonthreatening way will provide accurate information.

C. **Specific content.** The best approach is to start with the legal substances, such as caffeine, tobacco, and alcohol. Additional questions may cover other drugs, prescription drugs, and recreational drugs. It may be appropriate to ask specifically about marijuana and cocaine use in young adult and adolescent patients. Use of any substance should be explored with the same series of questions.

1. **Quantification.** Characterization of the health risks of and level of dependency on alcohol, caffeine, tobacco, and drug consumption is important.
   a. **Frequency.** How often and how long the patient has used the substance should be established.
   b. **Quantity.** How much the patient uses at each occasion must be determined.
   c. **Route of administration.** How the patient takes the drug (i.e., orally, inhalation, injection) is very important.

2. **Effect on other people.** To determine the effect of the drug behavior on other people, the clinician might ask, "Do your spouse or your fellow employees ever comment that you may be drinking too much?"

3. **Effect on the patient.** Questions should be posed about the effect of the substance on the patient, such as, "Do you become irritable after drinking four or five cups of coffee?"

D. **Screening purposes.** If the clinician feels that the patient has a problem with one or more of the substances he or she is using, then a detailed history must be obtained. If a serious dependency problem is identified, the patient should be referred to someone who has specific training in the treatment of drug and alcohol problems. Two commonly used inventories for alcohol-specific problems are described below.

1. **CAGE** is a simple four-item mnemonic.
   C—History of attempting to **cut down** on alcohol intake
   A—**Annoyance** over criticism about alcohol
   G—**Guilt** about drinking behavior
   E—Drinking in the morning to relieve withdrawal anxiety (**eye-opener**)

2. **MAST.** The Michigan Alcoholism Screening Test (Table 4-1) has been shown to be highly efficient in identifying alcoholic patients, particularly the following three questions:[1]
   a. "Has your family ever objected to your drinking?"
   b. "Did you ever think you drank too much at one time?"
   c. "Have others ever said you drink too much for your own good?"

IV. OCCUPATIONAL AND ENVIRONMENTAL HISTORY.
Occupational disease causes significant morbidity and mortality in the United States. Data are sparse, but crude national estimates indicate that 400,000 new cases of occupational disease occur each year, and 100,000 deaths each year are due to such disease. The primary care clinician plays an increasingly important role in the management of occupational illness. Essential to the clinician's recognition of these conditions is the occupational history.

A. **Placement in the structured interview.** The occupational history is an important part of the general medical history.

1. **Initial data** serve four purposes. For all patients, the occupational history is necessary to:
   a. Alert the clinician to **issues of importance to the present illness**. Recognition of occupational illness in a patient allows for:
      (1) Correct diagnosis and management
      (2) Prevention of disease in others
      (3) Appropriate compensation
      (4) Recognition of hazards not previously known
   b. Bring to light the **risk factors that require medical monitoring,** such as exposure to lead, cadmium, asbestos, or other known toxins
   c. **Provide data** for retrospective review for such efforts as case-control studies that seek to evaluate suspected hazards
   d. Facilitate compliance with **state recording requirements** for tumor registries, birth certificates, and death certificates

2. **Basic questions.** The occupational history can be readily incorporated into the general medical history by asking questions about the following six areas:
   a. Current occupation
   b. Employment status (i.e., working or retired)
   c. Jobs held longest
   d. Exposure to fumes, chemicals, dusts, loud noise, or radiation
   e. Hobbies
   f. Temporal relationship with work or other environments

B. **Possible occupational illness.** The general occupational history and medical history indicate when the clinician needs to pursue the possibility of an occupational or environmental illness.

1. Three circumstances prompt further investigation.
   a. A **temporal relationship** suggests an association with an exposure, that is, a change in job followed by the onset of symptoms or symptoms that occur only in a particular setting.

Table 4-1. Michigan Alcohol Screening Test (MAST)

Points	Questions
(0)	1. Do you enjoy a drink now and then?
(2)	2. Do you feel you are a normal drinker?*
(2)	3. Have you ever awakened the morning after some drinking the night before and found that you could not remember a part of the evening before?
(1)	4. Does your spouse (or parents) ever worry or complain about your drinking?
(2)	5. Can you stop drinking without a struggle after one or two drinks?*
(1)	6. Do you ever feel bad about your drinking?
(2)	7. Do friends and relatives think you are a normal drinker?*
(0)	8. Do you ever limit your drinking to certain times of the day or to certain places?
(2)	9. Are you always able to stop drinking when you want to?*
(4)	10. Have you ever attended a meeting of Alcoholics Anonymous (AA)?
(1)	11. Have you gotten into fights when drinking?
(2)	12. Has drinking ever created problems with you and your spouse?
(2)	13. Has your spouse (or other family member) ever gone to anyone for help about your drinking?
(2)	14. Have you ever lost friends or girl/boy friends because of drinking?
(2)	15. Have you ever gotten into trouble at work because of drinking?
(2)	16. Have you ever lost a job because of drinking?
(2)	17. Have you ever neglected your obligations, your family, or your work for 2 or more days because you were drinking?
(1)	18. Do you ever drink before noon?
(2)	19. Have you ever been told you have liver trouble? Cirrhosis?
(2)	20. After heavy drinking, have you ever: had delirium tremens (DTs); had severe shaking; heard voices; or seen things that weren't there?
(4)	21. Have you ever gone to anyone for help about your drinking?
(4)	22. Have you ever been in a hospital because of drinking?
(0)	23. (a) Have you ever been a patient in a psychiatric hospital or on a psychiatric ward of a general hospital?
(2)	(b) Was drinking part of the problem that resulted in hospitalization?
(0)	24. (a) Have you ever been seen at a psychiatric or mental health clinic or gone to any doctor, social worker, or clergyman for help with an emotional problem?
(2)	(b) Was drinking part of the problem?
(2)	25. Have you ever been arrested, even for a few hours, because of drunk behavior?
(2)	26. Have you ever been arrested for drunk driving?

Reprinted with permission from Barker LR, et al: *Principles of Ambulatory Medicine*, 2nd ed. Baltimore, Williams & Wilkins, 1986.

*Negative responses are "alcoholic" responses.

Scoring: A total of 4 or more points is presumptive evidence of alcoholism, while a 5-point total would make it extremely unlikely that the individual is not alcoholic. However, a positive response to 10, 23b, or 24b would be diagnostic; a positive response indicates alcoholism.

      b. Specific hazards are identified on screening questions.

      c. The **nature of the patient's medical condition** warrants consideration of occupational or environmental factors. Conditions that prompt further questions are listed in Table 4-2.

  2. Further investigation requires the following information:

      a. Types of jobs held by the patient

        (1) Place of employment

        (2) Dates of employment

        (3) Principal products

        (4) Job duties (routine and nonroutine)

        (5) Exposures

        (6) Use of protective equipment

      b. It should be determined if **co-workers are experiencing symptoms or illness**.

      c. Potential exposures at home, specifically pets, humidifiers, hobbies, work of family members, or neighborhood pollution, should also be noted.

  C. Further evaluation. With the data obtained thus far, the clinician can make a reasonable judgment about the need for further evaluation of an illness that may have been caused by or be related to exposures at work or elsewhere in the environment. Further evaluation might include **checking**

Table 4-2. Medical Conditions That Prompt Careful Review of Occupational History

Skin conditions	Liver disease
Respiratory disease	Neurologic disease/neuropsychiatric
Hearing loss	syndrome
Musculoskeletal problems	Cancer
Exacerbation of ischemic heart disease	Illness of unknown cause

appropriate references or **consulting with clinicians** who specialize in occupational disease diagnosis and management. Consultation is available through several sources.

1. Academic medical centers may have faculty in occupational medicine who can evaluate work-related conditions.

2. Specialists in occupational medicine can often be identified through the state chapter of the American College of Occupational Medicine or of the American Lung Association.

3. Some state health and labor departments have resources.

4. The National Institute for Occupational Safety and Health in Cincinnati can help with references and referrals.

V. DIETARY AND NUTRITIONAL HISTORY

A. Overview of *The Surgeon General's Report on Nutrition and Health*

1. Death and disability. Diet is implicated in the leading causes of death and disability in the United States, including coronary heart disease, cancer, stroke, diabetes mellitus, and atherosclerosis. Alcohol-related causes of death and disability include accidents, suicides, and chronic liver disease (including cirrhosis). These conditions account for almost 70% of the 2 million deaths annually.

2. Morbidity. Significant morbidity from diseases, such as hypertension, osteoporosis, dental caries, periodontal disease, and gastrointestinal disease, is also related to diet.

3. Public health policy recommendations
   a. Dietary guidance should be promoted through nutrition education for both consumers and health professionals and through improved food labeling.
   b. Nutrition programs and services are recommended to allow access to appropriate diets for all Americans, especially those with high-risk health problems.
   c. Research and surveillance are recommended in the following areas: the relationships between dietary factors and the prevention of chronic diseases, the nutritional needs of the elderly, and effective strategies for nutrition and health education.

4. Nutrients that are a health concern for many patients are discussed below.
   a. Fats and cholesterol
      (1) A reduction in fat intake to 30% of total calories is recommended, particularly limiting saturated fat intake (from fatty cuts of meat and whole milk dairy products).
      (2) Food preparation with little or no additional fats and oils is encouraged (i.e., broil, grill, roast, or boil rather than fry).
      (3) Cholesterol intake of 300 mg can be achieved with the consumption of 6–7 oz of animal protein foods a day and three to four egg yolks a week.
   b. Energy and weight control. Maintenance of a desirable body weight occurs when calorie intake is balanced by energy expenditure. Excess calories come from foods high in fats and oils, alcoholic beverages, sugars, and excessive portions.
   c. Complex carbohydrates and dietary fiber
      (1) Approximately 50%–60% of total calories should come from carbohydrates, predominantly starches.
      (2) A dietary fiber intake of 20–35 g/day can be achieved with four or more servings of vegetables and fruits and four or more servings of whole grain products.
   d. Sodium
      (1) Estimated safe and adequate sodium intake for adults is 1.1–3.3 g/day. The average sodium intake is 4–6 g/day.
      (2) Although only about 25% of individuals with hypertension are sodium sensitive, prudence is suggested in using sodium.

(3) Processed foods, including meals and snacks eaten out, provide about one-third of dietary sodium; another third is added by the consumer.

e. Alcohol. Consumption of up to two drinks a day is not associated with disease among healthy men and nonpregnant women. However, alcoholic beverages contribute "empty" calories and may replace other foods.

f. Calcium. A chronically low calcium intake, especially in adolescent and young adult women, may be associated with an increased risk for osteoporosis. Dairy products provide about 75% of dietary calcium. Therefore, a diet that does not include dairy products may be deficient in calcium.

g. Iron. Iron deficiency anemia is the most prevalent form of anemia in the United States. Children (especially in low income families), adolescents, and women of childbearing age are at high risk.

B. The role of the clinician is to identify patients at risk for malnutrition.

1. Primary malnutrition occurs when there are inadequacies, excesses, or imbalances in nutrient intake.

2. Secondary malnutrition occurs when disease and disability cause inadequate food intake, impaired absorption and utilization of nutrients, increased losses or excretion, or increased requirements of nutrients.

3. Risk factors for malnutrition, which may warrant further investigation or intervention, are listed below.

    a. Body weight less than or greater than 20% of ideal

        (1) The **1983 Metropolitan Height and Weight Tables** are widely used. The desirable weights represent those associated with lowest mortality among insurance policy holders. Best used as goals for healthy adults, these weights may not be appropriate for elderly or seriously ill individuals.

        (2) The **body mass index (BMI)** calculates a ratio of weight to height (kg/m^2). A BMI of 19–27 correlates with ideal body weight.

    b. Recent weight gain or loss of greater than 10%, which may signal the onset of obesity or of an eating disorder or catabolic condition

    c. Conditions that increase metabolic needs, including fever, infection, trauma, growth, malignancy, or burns

    d. Conditions that increase nutrient losses, including exudative enteropathies, vomiting, diarrhea, draining fistulas or abscesses, hemodialysis, or chronic blood loss

    e. Chronic diseases, such as diabetes mellitus, hyperlipidemia, or gastrointestinal disease

    f. Social or diet history that suggests an inability to obtain or ingest adequate amounts of food

    g. A diet or nutrition problem as perceived by the patient

4. Placement in the structured interview. Problems involving the patient's diet and nutrition status may be identified at each step of the medical history. A positive response to a nutrition-related inquiry may need in-depth questioning.

    a. The HPI gives the clinician the opportunity to ask about recent changes in weight, appetite, or food intake. It is also appropriate to ascertain whether these changes have occurred volitionally or as a consequence of a present illness, medication use, or psychosocial problem.

    b. The PMH may address the following issues:

        (1) Problems with adherence to a diet previously prescribed to treat a medical problem

        (2) Manifestation and treatment of food allergies or intolerances

        (3) Any self-imposed diet regimens (i.e., fad diets, alternative health care practices) that may have affected the patient's health

    c. A family history (FH) of disease (e.g., diabetes mellitus type II, hypercholesterolemia, breast or colon cancer), for which patients may have a genetic predisposition and which are also associated with nutrition risk factors, should signal the clinician to screen the patient's diet to offer advice about preventive health measures. For example, a 40-year-old woman with a FH of breast cancer and coronary heart disease would be a candidate for nutrition counseling for reduction of dietary fat intake.

    d. The PP may uncover life-style behaviors with effects on nutrition (Table 4-3). The clinician should inquire about the following:

        (1) Physical activity, exercise patterns, manual dexterity, or handicapping conditions, which may interfere with food shopping, preparation, or eating

Table 4-3. Factors That May Affect Nutritional Status

Socioeconomics and environment
    Finances
        Income (steadiness of employment)
        Use of public assistance programs (e.g., Food Stamps; Special
            Supplemental Foods Program for Women, Infants, and Children
            (WIC); Meals on Wheels; Congregate Meal Programs for Older
            Americans; School Lunch Programs)
    Cultural, ethnic, and religious food practices, preferences, and taboos
    Education and literacy level
    Food acquisition and preparation
        Availability of transportation for shopping
        Availability of food (markets, home-grown)
        Seasonal variations in availability of foods and effect on food costs
        Food storage and cooking facilities
        Meals and snacks eaten away from home (fast foods, restaurants)
        Use of prepared, frozen, canned, or commodity foods
Physical and psychological factors affecting food-related behavior
    Appetite (good, poor, changes)
    Perception of taste and smell
    Food allergies, intolerances, or aversions
    Unusual behavior: binging, vomiting, purging, pica, diuretic or laxative
        abuse, self-starvation or fasting, and "yo-yo" dieting
    Problems with eating, chewing, or swallowing; decreased salivary flow;
        and dental or oral health problems
    Psychological status (depression, anxiety, eating disorders, dementia)
    Physical activity and sleep patterns (type, duration, frequency)
    Physically handicapping conditions, which may affect ability to shop
        and cook
Other factors
    Use of prescription and over-the-counter medications (nutrient–drug
        interactions)
    Smoking, drug, or alcohol abuse
    Use of vitamins, minerals, or other food supplements (A megadose is 10
        times the RDA for the nutrient.)
    Use of home remedies or alternative treatments

    (2) Adequacy of financial resources and use of food assistance programs (e.g., Food Stamp
        Program; Meals on Wheels; Elderly Nutrition Program; Women, Infants and Children
        Supplemental Foods Program)
    (3) Frequency of meals and snacks eaten out
    (4) Use of food supplements and vitamin and mineral supplements
  e. The ROS should address the following:
    (1) Dental or oral problems, such as changes in taste (dysgeusia or hypogeusia), smell
        (anosmia), salivary secretion, mastication, or deglutition
    (2) Gastrointestinal problems, such as nausea, vomiting, constipation, diarrhea, or indi-
        gestion

5. Thorough nutrition assessment should be considered if there are several nutrition-related
  problems identified in the medical history. In addition, the assessment should consist of interpretation and consideration of the following:
  a. Physical examination
  b. Anthropometric data (i.e., height, weight, skinfold, and muscle circumference measure-
    ments)
  c. Biochemical data
  d. Dietary history and food intake data analysis
  e. Psychosocial data

6. Referral to a registered dietitian may be appropriate if an in-depth nutrition history is needed.

C. Assessing dietary intake in a clinical setting

1. **The 24-hour recall** is a simple, useful tool for gathering qualitative information about an individual's food intake as it relates to the daily routine. It gives the clinician a basis for identifying problem areas and for making specific suggestions for improvement. If the patient's diet is compared with the four basic food groups (Table 4-4), gross inadequacies or overconsumption of protein, iron, calcium, riboflavin, vitamins A and C, and calories can be detected.

   a. Clinicians should ask patients to report the amounts of all foods and beverages consumed in the previous 24-hour period, beginning in the morning. Clinicians can prompt patients by asking, "When did you eat again," "What did you eat next?" "How much did you eat or drink?"

   b. Clinicians should summarize the reported intake, asking if patients remember anything else.

   c. Clinicians should determine how the reported day might be different from a typical day and how weekend eating might change.

   d. **Sources of error** exist with the 24-hour recall when used for individual assessment.

      (1) Individuals may under- or overestimate or not remember accurately the amounts consumed.

      (2) The previous day's intake may be atypical.

      (3) Snacks and foods, such as sauces, gravies, salad dressing, and condiments, are difficult to quantitate.

Table 4-4. Diet Evaluation by Food Groups

Serving Size	No. Servings Eaten	Recommended No. Servings				
		Child	Adolescent	Adult	Pregnant Woman	Lactating Woman
Milk 1 cup milk, yogurt Calcium equivalent: 　1½ oz cheese 　1 cup pudding 　2 cups cottage cheese		3	4	2	4	4
Protein foods 2 oz meat, fish, or poultry Protein equivalent: 　2 eggs 　2 oz cheese 　½ cup cottage cheese 　1 cup cooked beans 　4 tbsp peanut butter		2	2	2	3	2
Grains		4	4	4	4	4
Vitamin A source ½ cup cooked or 1 cup 　raw dark green or 　orange vegetable 　or fruit		3/week	3/week	3/week	3/week	3/week
Vitamin C source ½ cup fruit or juice 　(citrus, tomato)		1	1	1	1	1
Other fruits and vegetables ½ cup cooked or 1 cup 　raw or 1 medium fruit		2	2	2	2	2
Fats and oils[*]		2	2	2	2	2
Miscellaneous[†] Candy, soft drinks, or 　sweets						

[*]Tablespoons
[†]High-calorie, low-nutrient foods

2. Food frequency questionnaire is a cross-check of an individual's intake to ascertain the frequency of intake of certain foods over a period of a week or a month. The food frequency questionnaire may be selective, probing about specific foods suspected of being deficient or excessive in the diet. A **food frequency checklist** is shown on the nutrition history worksheet illustrated in Figure 4-1. This questionnaire provides a qualitative assessment of an individual's intake, which can be corroborated with clinical and biochemical findings.

3. Food intake diary or record. Patients are asked to record their intake immediately after eating. Ways of estimating portions (i.e., household measures, size, volume) should be reviewed for quantitative accuracy. Records are usually kept for 3 days (2 weekdays and 1 weekend day) or for a week or more. The clinician can then review the records with the patient to clarify any questions about food preparation, ingredients, portion sizes, or unusual foods.

    a. The food intake record can be used to *quantitatively* estimate an individual's nutrient intake, using dietary analysis computer software. Such programs can average several days' intakes and compare nutrient intakes with the Recommended Dietary Allowances (RDAs).

        (1) The RDAs are developed and updated periodically to estimate the nutrient needs of healthy population groups, not individuals.

        (2) The RDAs include a "margin of safety" and, therefore, overestimate nutrient needs for many people. They do not take into account special nutrient needs of the sick or elderly.

        (3) Because standards for individual needs do not exist, the RDAs are frequently used to judge the adequacy of vitamin and mineral intake.

    b. Food intake records, along with other records (e.g., home glucose monitoring, symptoms of allergic or other untoward reactions to food) allow the patient to make more objective observations and help the clinician with problem identification and solution. In behavioral modification of eating habits, the food intake records are valuable self-monitoring tools.

VI. MENTAL HEALTH HISTORY.

VI. MENTAL HEALTH HISTORY. The mental health history is a brief exploration of the patient's past and current mental health status. It is *not* a mental status examination and involves no formal testing. The goals of the mental health history are to learn the patient's perception of his or her mental health and coping abilities, to assess a patient whose needs go beyond basic medical care, and to determine whether further evaluation or formal neuropsychological testing is appropriate.

A. Overview. Initially, the clinician must determine the patient's normal baseline, recent deviations from the baseline, and the parameters of each.

    1. Data should reflect the same parameters that are gathered for any physical symptom.

    2. Clinicians must determine the patient's perception of why a change has occurred; this often provides valuable information on the sources of the problem.

    3. It is essential to look for other sources of mood or behavioral changes, such as medications or underlying physical conditions.

B. Placement in the structured interview. There is no right or wrong place for the mental health history in the context of the whole interview.

    1. It may flow logically from the CC if the patient presents with an emotional problem (e.g., "I have been feeling so anxious lately").

    2. If emotional problems or previous psychiatric interventions are revealed in the PMH or the FH, the mental health history can logically proceed from here.

        a. The patient's cues usually signal an opening. Any sign of deep emotion or digression into significant life events offers both the chance to empathize with the patient and to collect the appropriate data.

        b. In relating the PMH, patients often associate health events with major life events, such as, "I had my heart attack in 1985, which was about 6 months after my wife died." To obtain a more complete mental health history, the clinician might respond, "That must have been a stressful time for you. How do you feel you are coping now?"

    3. When there is no obvious opening, it may be necessary to create a separate place for the mental health history. The transition could be handled with a comment, such as, "Now I would like to ask you some questions about your emotions or feelings and the ways in which you cope with the stresses in your life."

Nutrition Counseling Service | Patient information
University of Connecticut Health Center

NUTRITION HISTORY

Date _____ Diet ℞ _____ M.D. _____

Dx/problems _____

B/D _____ M F S M W D Sep. Ethnicity _____ Education _____ Occupation _____

Previous diets _____ Previous diet instructions _____

Height _____ Weight _____ Weight change _____ Activity _____

Medications _____ Condition of mouth _____

Significant lab data _____ Diet supplements _____

Food intolerances _____ Bowel function _____

Cooking facilities _____ OTC _____ Economic resources _____

Where meals eaten _____ Food preparation, meal planning, shopping _____

Other comments:

Estimated Intake	Type, Amount, Preparation	Daily	4–6x/ Week	2–3x/ Week	1x/ Week	24-hr Recall or Typical Day's Food Intake Pattern	Calories

Milk
  Whole
  Skim
  Yogurt							

Vegetables
  Green, yellow,
    raw, cooked							

Fruits, juices
  Citrus
  Other							

Starches
  Breads, cereals
  Rice, pasta
  Potatoes
  Crackers
  Chips, snacks
  Other							

Protein foods
  Meat, fish
  Poultry
  Cold cuts
  Eggs, cheese
  Organ meats
  Legumes
  Nuts
  Peanut butter							

Fats
  Butter, margarine
  Oil, lard
  Salt pork
  Cream
  Salad dressing							

Sweets
  Desserts
  Candy, jelly
  Syrup, honey
  Pastries							

Beverages
  Coffee, tea
  Soda
  Alcohol
  Other							

Salt Sugar							

Recommended Meal Pattern

	Amount	Calories	Carbohydrate	Protein	Fat
Milk					
Bread					
Fruit					
Vegetable					
Meat					
Fat					
Total					

Figure 4-1.

C. Components of the basic mental health history

1. **Changes in mood.** "How has your mood been lately?" "Is this different from usual?" "When did you notice changes?" "Can you describe the changes?" "What do you think might be causing this change?"

2. **Changes in eating.** "How has your appetite been?" "Has your weight changed during this time?"

3. **Changes in sleeping.** "How have you been sleeping lately?" "Have you noted any changes?"

4. **Changes in work habits or concentration.** "Have you noticed any changes in your ability to work or concentrate?"

D. Success in gathering data for a mental health history depends on the way in which it is approached. If the clinician is relaxed and comfortable, the patient is likely to follow his or her lead. The clinician can offer positive verbal and nonverbal reinforcement by using occasional comments, such as, "I see," or "I am following you," and by maintaining good eye contact and a comfortable body position (i.e., leaning forward to show interest or support), thereby giving consistent messages of caring and attention. Many different styles can succeed, but they usually include questions with the following characteristics:

1. Questions that will not arouse defensiveness (e.g., "How has your mood been?" versus "Are you feeling anxious?")

2. Questions that are open-ended rather than leading (e.g., "Have you noticed any changes in how you sleep?" versus "You haven't noticed any changes in how you sleep have you?")

3. Questions that cannot be perceived as judgmental or demeaning

4. Questions that move from the broad to the specific (i.e., general, open-ended questions first followed by specific questions only as necessary)

E. Indicators that a mental health history should be pursued. The following situations not only necessitate a mental health history but also should alert the clinician to the possibility that further mental health evaluation and treatment may be appropriate.

1. The patient indicates that his or her emotional or cognitive state is of serious concern (e.g., "I have been feeling so hopeless," or "I have been so worried").

2. The patient indicates that he or she has deep negative emotions about a physical condition (e.g., "I have found a lump and I am sure I am going to die").

3. The patient presents with symptoms that may be associated with an emotional issue (e.g., fatigue, weight loss). These symptoms must be carefully assessed since they may have either physical or psychological origins (e.g., cancer, anorexia, depression).

4. A FH of mental illness is revealed.

5. The patient describes or alludes to "difficult periods" or mental illness in the past.

6. The patient's living environment is a place of high stress or physical or emotional abuse.

7. Substance abuse is an issue for the patient or for someone with whom he or she lives.

8. The patient offers clues by what he or she fails to say rather than by information that is offered (e.g., reluctance to talk about the family or to respond to general questions about the past may indicate problems that he or she is not yet ready to discuss).

9. The patient's daily routine exceeds normal limits (e.g., the patient rarely leaves the house despite the absence of physical limitations, or the patient reports chronic fatigue that interferes with normal activities despite normal or extra hours of sleep).

10. If the clinician is concerned about suicide, the following information must also be ascertained:
    a. The patient should be asked directly whether he or she is thinking about suicide. A direct question is the best way to gather this information, and it will *not* cause harm to a patient who is not suicidal. Examples include, "I am worried that you might harm yourself. Have you thought about hurting yourself?" "You seem very upset. Are you thinking about suicide?"
    b. The patient should be asked whether he or she had ever considered or attempted suicide in the past, and if so, when and how.

    c. If the patient indicates that he or she is considering suicide, data on the plan, the availability of means, and the time frame must be obtained.

F. Denial. Sometimes, patients verbally deny any emotional or cognitive problems, despite the fact that they truly exist. While clinicians must guard against "looking for trouble" when it is not there, it is always preferable to search and find nothing than to neglect the search. The following are cues that must be pursued even though the patient may deny difficulties. Through careful questioning and exploration, the clinician should be able to obtain the information, be supportive and empathetic in eliciting problems, and possibly intervene before more serious problems arise.

  1. The clinician must question the patient's ability to cope with a serious illness or disability even though the patient denies a problem under the following circumstances:
    a. The severity of the illness is such that anyone would be expected to have difficulty adjusting.
    b. The illness adds to an already stressful, complicated living situation made so by economic, psychological, or social factors.
    c. The patient has a history of difficulty coping.
    d. The patient's support system is inadequate.

  2. When clinicians perceive signs or symptoms of emotional or cognitive dysfunction, they must assess these signs in the context of the patient, the illness, and the situation. The following descriptions are not exhaustive, and rarely is one of them alone sufficient to diagnose dysfunction. Observations must be incorporated along with data from the assessment to form a complete picture of the patient's mental and physical status.
    a. Affect (expression of emotion) seems inappropriate for the situation.
      (1) Affect seems blunted or flat—that is, the patient shows little or no emotion in a situation where it would be expected.
      (2) Affect seems exaggerated for the situation—that is, the patient shows extreme emotion in a situation that normally would not elicit such a response.
      (3) Affect is inappropriate—that is, the emotion shown is opposite of what is expected.
    b. There is evidence of a thought disorder or memory dysfunction.
      (1) An inability to engage in normal conversation is noted.
      (2) An inability to remember or sequence basic information is noted.
    c. Empirical observation suggests dysfunction—that is, extreme thinness or obesity, unexplained bruises, or unusual speech behavior.

VII. FAMILY VIOLENCE HISTORY. A major source of injury and psychosocial problems in family life is violent physical interaction. The cultural pattern of beating those who are the most loved is supported by a long tradition of discipline of children and wives. "Spare the rod and spoil the child" is a maxim for raising responsible adults. In colonial times, there were norms for the diameter of the stick that should be used to beat wives and children. In 20%–30% of American families, there are episodes of spousal or child abuse. With this hierarchical and patriarchal history, the potential for abuse as a cause of injury must be kept in mind in interviewing patients. It is not a necessary part of every interview, but since it is common and lethal, it must be included when there is an accident or injury to a child, an adult, or an elder.

A. Placement in the structured interview. There are many possibilities for the placement of questions about family violence. Since this interview is not done on every case, the questions should be organized to fit into the interview when suspicions of abuse are raised.

  1. HPI. In cases of accident and injury, the setting of the "symptom" is a basic parameter and should be explored in-depth.

  2. PMH. Physical abuse is usually an escalating problem so a patient with a new injury may have had many in the past. An attempt to document prior office or emergency room visits and other injuries may be helpful.

  3. FH. Patterns of physical abuse are taught to children by their parents. Thus, inquiries about patterns of interaction in the family of origin (birth) can give clues to the present situation.
    a. A woman whose mother was abused is more likely to be abused herself.
    b. A man whose mother was abused is more likely to abuse his wife.
    c. Parents who were abused as children are more likely to abuse their children.

4. **PP.** A thorough social history is probably the best source of data about the factors that are suggestive of family violence. By carefully covering social support, daily routines, family relationships, work history, and financial status, the clinician can gather most of the information needed to explore this sensitive issue. A question about how disagreements in the family are handled is a good introduction when a vulnerable child, spouse, or elder is in the household.

5. **ROS.** This is an inappropriate place for a family violence history since it consists of closed-ended questions and directed material.

B. **Format of questions.** The variability in norms surrounding the discipline of children makes it difficult to inquire about abuse. It is best to begin with open-ended questions that will elicit the patient's story about the cause of an injury or "accident." Judging the acts of the spouse or parent should be avoided in favor of empathic listening and nonjudgmental questions.

1. **Open-ended questions** can be used to begin an inquiry into the present illness, such as, "Could you tell me just what happened this morning when the injury occurred? I need to know just what happened when you fell down the stairs. Could you tell me the whole story?"

2. **Direct questions** that have a high information yield include: "How were you hurt?" "Has anything like this happened before?" "When did it first occur?" "How badly were you hurt in the past?" "Was a weapon used?" "Are there any weapons in the house?"

3. If the story of the accident sounds false in the HPI, the topic can be raised again in the PP with the following questions: "Who lives in the home?" "How are the relationships between you and those who live there?" "How old are the children?" "Has your wife/girlfriend/boyfriend/husband ever hurt them?" "What happens when one of you gets angry?"

C. **Indicators that an abuse history should be pursued**

1. **Imbalance of power between spouses or between parent and child.** Abuse is more likely in relationships where the power rests primarily with one individual. Women with little authority are more likely to be abused. Very young children are more likely to be victims as are elders with limited strength and resources.

2. **Social isolation.** People who are involved in the community are less likely to abuse or to be abused.

3. **Unemployment.** The loss of a job often precedes wife battering. The stress of losing income and having more unoccupied time at home increases the risk of family violence. Women with jobs outside the home are also at less risk for being victims.

4. **Poverty.** While there is spousal abuse in all social classes, the risks are higher where there are fewer resources and more stressors.

5. **New parents.** The arrival of an infant is a time of high stress, and both mother and child are at high risk of injury.

6. **Drug use.** Abusive mothers are more likely to be taking antidepressants and tranquilizers than nonabusing mothers. Alcohol and street drug use are risk factors for abuse as well. Often the escalating pattern of wife beating occurs in the context of binge drinking and the use of cocaine or heroin.

7. **Extrafamilial violence.** Men who are violent within the home are more likely to be violent outside the home.

VIII. **CHRONIC ILLNESS.** Chronic illnesses have increased in prevalence as infectious diseases have come under control and life expectancy has increased.

A. **Prevalence**

1. **Overall.** A national survey found that 50% of the civilian population had one or more chronic conditions.

2. **Effect on functioning**
   a. **Activity.** Twenty-five percent of individuals with chronic conditions experience some limitation of activities.
   b. **Mobility.** Ten percent of individuals with chronic conditions experience some limitations of mobility.

3. **Multiple conditions.** It is very common for individuals to have more than one chronic condition; the average number of chronic conditions is 2.2.

B. Characteristics of chronic illness

1. **Long-term.** While acute illnesses may span days or weeks, they have a discrete end point. Chronic illnesses are long-term by nature and often require continuous contact with one or even multiple clinicians.

2. **Uncertainty.** Chronic illnesses may have an unpredictable course.
   a. Prognosis is often variable.
   b. Flare-ups and remissions are episodic.
   c. Planning for activities of daily living (ADLs) and the future is often difficult.

3. **Emphasis on palliation.** Living with symptoms requires an emphasis on symptom management as a part of the overall treatment plan, including:
   a. **Level of pain and discomfort.** Some level of control over pain episodes or adapting movements to reduce discomfort should be identified.
   b. **Restricted activity.** New outlets for creativity, tension release, and increasing sense of self-worth should be identified.
   c. **Quality of functioning.** Physical adaptations in the home environment, which may increase independence in self-care activities, should be examined.

4. **Effect of multiple conditions.** A single chronic condition may result in others due to:
   a. Degenerative and systemic nature of chronic disease
   b. Greater susceptibility to other diseases
   c. Long-term exposure to the health care system, resulting in increased iatrogenic conditions

5. **Intrusiveness.** Treatment regimens and limitations on activity require a reorganization of the patient's life-style, including:
   a. **Household routines.** The allocation of household tasks (i.e., grocery shopping, cooking) must be assessed; for example, a male patient with multiple sclerosis might assume the cooking responsibilities as he becomes less able to work.
   b. **Work.** Chronic illness may result in loss of employment and considerable readjustment to finding a sense of self-worth with increasing dependency on others for economic support.
   c. **Social isolation.** Loss of mobility and limitations on the ability to work or engage in social activities outside the household may also result in social isolation, contributing to poor emotional adjustment.

6. **Need for ancillary services.** In addition to medical care, chronically ill patients often require the services of a variety of other professional supports, such as social work, psychiatry, special education, and occupational, physical and recreational therapy. Simply organizing a schedule for these services requires a great expenditure of energy, and conflicting therapeutic advice can be confusing and frustrating to the patient and family.

7. **Expense.** The expenses associated with chronic illness often place the patient and family under additional stress. The need for routine monitoring, management of crises, use of multiple drugs over a long period of time, extensive contact with the health care system, and social support services all contribute to a heavy financial toll. Learning about insurance coverage and sources of support through government and private organizations is often a full-time responsibility.

C. Placement in the structured interview

1. The appropriate place to discuss issues relating to chronic illness will quite naturally fit in the HPI. The chronic illness may be either the reason for seeking health care or related to the patient's present health problem.

2. The PMH is the other place in which discussion of a resolved chronic condition might occur.

D. Specific content.
Clinicians must consider the multiple problems of daily living experienced by chronically ill patients, irrespective of the presenting complaint. In the interview, it is important to remember that the patient is the "expert" in the experience of the illness and is often a source of critical information for the ongoing management of the condition. It is also important to include the following information:

1. **Prevention and management of crisis episodes.** It is important to determine the predictability of crisis episodes, early warning signs, and the ways in which the patient lessens their severity.

2. **Control of symptoms.** It is important to note how visible the symptoms are, how patients manage the symptoms, and how much the symptoms interfere with daily functioning.

3. **Carrying out prescribed regimens.** It is important to determine how patients feel about the prescribed management regimens, the problems encountered, and how these have been adapted.

4. **Dealing with social isolation.** All patients with chronic illness should be asked if they have limited their activities or interactions with others as a result of the condition, and if so, how they feel about these limitations.

5. **Adjustment to the disease over time.** The course of many chronic illnesses changes over time, and it is important to determine what these changes are and how the patient has dealt with them.

6. **Normalizing interactions and life-styles.** Clinicians should determine how patients view themselves in the context of the disease, what management strategies have been developed for dealing with their presentation to strangers and friends, and how the disease has affected their life-styles.

7. **Financial resources.** It is important to determine the type of insurance coverage the patient has and whether financial limitations have interfered with the patient's ability to follow recommended treatment.

8. **Impact on home and family.** Any psychological, marital, or family problem and its resolution should be recorded.

IX. TERMINALLY ILL PATIENTS

A. **Overview.** Gathering histories from terminally ill patients requires specialized knowledge, skills, and sensitivity because the situation is clinically and emotionally complex for the patient, the caregiver, and family members. Objectivity can be difficult to maintain, particularly because it is important to communicate a high degree of empathy throughout the history-gathering process. Encounters with terminally ill patients may bring to the forefront the clinician's personal attitudes about death and dying, including fears and a humbling reminder of one's own mortality. Interviewing sessions are of necessity quite brief; a full history is often gathered over a number of encounters, sometimes resulting in conflicting information. At times, family members or significant others become the only source of information. Natural impediments to full patient participation and cooperation, such as the presence of pain and general weakness, are often exacerbated in terminally ill patients.

B. **Perspectives.** Interviews with terminally ill patients involve emotionally laden issues that are colored by the personal feelings, fears, and experiences of all participants.

1. Terminally ill patients react not only to future losses but to all of their past and present losses as well. Fear and anxiety emerge along with a sense of guilt at leaving family members. Patients may also worry about their failure to have been a "good patient" and "please" the caregiver when treatment regimens do not have the desired results. In addition, a number of fears are common to terminally ill persons (IX E 1 c).

2. Family members are faced with many of the same fears as the patients but may experience additional guilt at "being spared" and remaining alive. The physical and emotional demands of caring for a terminally ill person are extensive.
   a. Family members may feel overwhelmed, resentful, and subsequently angry at both themselves for having these feelings and at the patient for "causing" the stress.
   b. Family members may feel helpless to respond to the patient's pain and other symptoms and resentful of the clinician and other caregivers for whom the patient may ask repeatedly.
   c. Family members often "empower" the clinician with magical health abilities and may frequently speak of their faith in a "miracle cure," thus putting unrealistic expectations upon the physician-patient relationship.
   d. Sudden shifts in roles and responsibilities among family members can generate stress and disorganization in the family unit.

3. Clinicians and other caregivers bring to the care of the terminally ill patient not only the objective and scientific perspective of the health care practitioner but also the subjective dimensions of their relationship with the patient, family members, and colleagues.

   a. Interviewers must be aware of their own beliefs and attitudes about death and dying and be able to recognize how these beliefs and values are manifested in their behavior, reactions, fears, and comfort level in interviewing terminally ill patients.

   b. The belief that caring can be successfully accomplished, without cure, must be developed.

   c. Interviewers must incorporate their personal belief systems into their professional roles and behaviors, while maintaining personal integrity and the ability to be genuine and empathetic.

C. Variables influencing behavior of participants. In addition to self-awareness, clinicians must also be informed about the patient's physical, emotional, and social situations. Many variables influence the behavior and management of terminally ill patients.

   1. Religious beliefs and practices address and proscribe very specific behaviors and responses around the issues of death, dying, the quality and quantity of life, the physical handling of the body and property of the deceased, and the "proper" roles for patient, family members, neighbors, and other community members. Formal membership in a religious organization is not directly related to the nature or degree of religious influence on a patient's behavior.

   2. Cultural and ethnic backgrounds provide guidelines for acceptable and "normal" responses to terminal illness, dying, and death. Cultural proscriptions also exist for attitudes toward pain, bodily functions, modesty, and funeral practices to name a few. Grief and mourning are also culturally determined.

   3. Age. Attitudes and understanding of death and dying and reactions to a terminal illness differ throughout the life span.

   a. The rudiments of the adult concept of death as final, inevitable, and universal may be found in even very young children.

   b. The seriousness and tension that envelop a family with a member who is terminally ill are certainly sensed and reacted to, if not fully understood, by even very young children.

   4. Past experiences and emotional ties with family members or loved friends, past experiences with loss other than death, such as divorce or a loss of job or home, also influence an individual's expectations and responses in the face of terminal illness.

   5. General mental health, intelligence level, and economic status have a profound influence not only on the patient's reaction but also on the family's ability to function.

   6. Specific life skills, such as planning, organizing, communication, and knowledge and ability to marshall community resources, determine the timing and type of intervention necessary from caregivers.

   7. The specific terminal illness and its expected course, including the likelihood of pain, various treatment regimens, time frames, and the circumstances of the death itself, are major determinants of the behaviors of all concerned. This information becomes the foundation upon which plans and responses to manage the terminally ill patient and their family are formulated.

D. Emotional aspects of death and dying. Elisabeth Kübler-Ross, M.D. (a Swiss psychiatrist), formulated a framework for understanding the emotional reactions of terminally ill patients. She conceptualized five "developmental stages" based upon her interviews with hundreds of dying adults and children who described their feelings, their fears, and their observations about the behavior and reactions of others involved in their care. The stages are somewhat arbitrarily designated and are not always readily observable in every individual. The order and intensity of each stage may also vary. Shifts may occur quickly and repeatedly among stages. The goal for the clinician is to determine what stage a person is experiencing. It is inappropriate to "help the patient move along" from one stage to another, as individuals progress at their own pace and order, some not "finishing" all stages before death occurs.

   1. Denial and isolation stage. Patients refuse to believe what is happening, believing that there has been a mistake and finding many examples of such mistakes, and may be reluctant to discuss illness, treatment plans, or alternatives. Patients feel removed, isolated, and separated from family, caregivers, friends, and even the "whole world." They may feel that they are different from everyone else.

2. **Anger stage.** Patients ask "Why me?" Resentment and blame are directed at family members, caregivers, or even God. Patients may envy others who they feel "deserve" this more than they do. Anger is strong and may be expressed as rage or extreme hostility. Verbal outlets and safe listening opportunities should be provided.

3. **Bargaining stage.** Patients practice good behavior in exchange for postponement of the inevitable. Goals are set, "if . . . , then . . ." situations are constructed. Even God may be approached as an agent for bargaining. Prior guilt-provoking incidents are examined, and opportunities for forgiveness may be requested to set the record straight, increasing the chances of successful bargaining.

4. **Depression stage**
   a. Reactive depression occurs when patients respond to the losses they are currently experiencing, such as loss of control of bodily functions and abilities. Reassuring patients that the loss is not all encompassing and that they are still attractive or capable is required; however, it is important to be realistic and truthful.
   b. Preparatory depression ("anticipatory stage") refers to a preparatory grief that is experienced by patients prior to the final departure from this world. Caregivers should express quiet understanding and empathy and avoid false cheerfulness. Giving "permission" to express sorrow and acceptance with minimal words is most effective at this stage. This is the time for patients to mourn all of their impending losses, just as family members will mourn the loss of the patients in a short time to come.

5. **Acceptance stage.** This stage is characterized by peacefulness, rest, and limited verbal and physical interactions. Patients withdraw, and their circle of interest diminishes dramatically. This behavior may look like "giving up," especially to family members who often have a difficult time during this stage. It is important to differentiate this stage from earlier expressions of anger and know when patients are asking for recognition from others of their own acceptance of the inevitable. Reassurances by and the physical presence of caregivers or family members are critical at this time.

E. **Interview with the terminally ill patient.** Clinicians must attend not only to the content of the interview but also must pay careful attention to their own attitudes and how they are being communicated during the session. Specific techniques that can be helpful when dealing with these patients are discussed below.

1. **Content.** Several areas of information, in addition to the general medical history, should be obtained directly from the patient. Family members or significant others may be interviewed as well, recognizing that a slightly different perspective may be obtained.
   a. **Patient's awareness.** It is important to determine the extent and accuracy of the patient's knowledge, understanding, and awareness of their impending death. This can be done by asking patients what they know about their condition and what they think or have been told about what to expect in the next few days, weeks, or months. Patients should be asked if they have known others with similar conditions and their outcomes. If patients do not express awareness of the terminal nature of their condition, it is inappropriate to inform them of the seriousness until more is known about their reactions or preferences.
   b. **Emotional perspective.** A description of the patient's past reactions to loss and his or her feelings about the current situation are useful to obtain. It is also instructive to determine what feelings patients have recently experienced and their reactions to these feelings. Reassurance is appropriate at this time if patients are experiencing typical reactions.
   c. **Needs, fears, and concerns.** It is crucial to ask periodically that patients name or describe their needs, fears, or concerns about the illness and the prognosis. The terminally ill person is typically concerned about one or more of the following (not necessarily in this order):
      (1) The ability to tolerate pain
      (2) A loss of personal dignity
      (3) Being abandoned physically or psychologically
      (4) Becoming a burden to loved ones and caregivers
      (5) Perceived reluctance of caregivers and family members to be honest
      (6) Exclusion from the decision-making process
   d. **Treatment preferences**
      (1) All responses of the health care team—from aggressive intervention to palliative measures—should be presented and understood as "treatment."

    (2) It is necessary to determine from patients what plans are currently in place and what options have been presented.

    (3) The patient's understanding of these options and their effects should be reviewed as well as the decision-making process and the role of the patient and family members in that process.

    (4) It is not uncommon for patients to express ambivalence about former choices, to revise treatment preferences, or to exclude or include family members in the decision-making process in the future.

  e. Life-style choices

    (1) Interviewers should have patients describe their preferences for the location and type of caregiving setting.

    (2) Patients should identify family members and significant others that they prefer to have involved.

    (3) Home care for the terminally ill is readily available and affordable in most communities in the United States today with formal home-based hospice programs in many. For patients without primary caregivers available in the home setting, hospitals and nursing homes are increasingly establishing palliative care capabilities. Free-standing specialized hospitals (hospices) are also available in some states.

2. Interviewers' attitudes and terminally ill patients. The attitudes of interviewers are important to ensure that interviews are successful. From the patient's perspective, the clinician's attitude is revealed in many little, seemingly insignificant comments and behaviors. Terminally ill patients are very sensitive to the quality and quantity of attention focused upon them, particularly fearing abandonment and believing that their care and comfort has a low priority in the health care arena. The medical history is an excellent opportunity to communicate to the patient genuine interest and a "lasting commitment through whatever lies ahead."

  a. Interviewers can demonstrate a compassionate attitude by explaining the reasons for questions and repeating explanations.

  b. Interviewers should assess the patient's willingness and ability to continue throughout a session (see IX A).

  c. Patients should be afforded ample opportunity to ask questions and clarify answers as the interview progresses, not just at the close.

  d. An unhurried pace coupled with focused attention will result in more fruitful interviews and will facilitate the establishment of an effective treatment relationship.

3. Techniques. Chapter 2, "Interviewing Skills," should be reviewed as the issues presented are equally if not more important in interviewing the terminally ill person. In addition, interviewers must remain flexible and be willing to divide the history-gathering process into several short sessions, repeating sections, and reviewing with patients their previous comments to assure the information gathered still pertains. Portable cassette tape recorders, journals, and use of family members or significant others as informants are often useful.

X. ACQUIRED IMMUNE DEFICIENCY SYNDROME (AIDS) AND HUMAN IMMUNODEFICIENCY VIRUS (HIV) INFECTION.

Infection with HIV and fear of being HIV-positive present a challenge for the clinician in interviewing patients. Issues relating to the major risk factors of sexual behavior and substance use are found in sections II and III, and those relating to the management of chronic disease and terminal illness are found in sections VIII and IX. This section will serve as an addendum to discuss other AIDS/HIV–specific issues.

A. Prevalence. The Centers for Disease Control (CDC) estimates that between 1 and 2 million people are infected with HIV and 150,000 cases of AIDS have been diagnosed. In some urban areas, AIDS has become the leading cause of death in the young adult age-group.

  1. While the disease in the United States was initially found in male homosexuals, spread through intravenous drug use has resulted in the infection of women and children.

    a. The rate of infection for women is presently 11% of the HIV-infected population.

    b. It is predicted that women's infection rates will be the same as men's by the year 2000.

    c. In 1991, AIDS will become the fifth leading cause of death in women.

  2. Because the infection may not be manifested in symptoms for up to 7–10 years and because risk behaviors have not been declining among all of the high-risk populations, it is likely that the rate of HIV infection will continue to increase.

B. Risk factors. HIV infection is spread through exposure to infected blood and body fluids (i.e., blood, semen, vaginal secretions), intravenous drug use, contact with blood products, and from mother to fetus and newborn child. HIV is not spread by kissing, touching, eating, or living with infected persons, nor is it passed on by the bite of insects or blood donation.

1. Testing of all blood donations for transfusion was initiated in the United States in 1985; however, there is still some concern that this may be a source of newly diagnosed infections because of the latency period of the virus.

2. Blood transfusions are still a major source of infection in developing countries.

C. Attitude of the interviewer. AIDS has received a great deal of media attention and generated much public concern because of its high fatality rate and the fact that socially unapproved behavior is a significant contributing factor to its spread. Thus, students may bring preconceived attitudes and fears with them to their first encounters with AIDS patients.

1. Students should be made aware of the fact that conducting a standard history and physical examination on an AIDS or HIV-positive patient poses no risk. Their feelings and fears about this issue should be addressed.

2. Since the 1950s and the advent of antibiotics, the infectious diseases to which health professionals are exposed have not been life-threatening. Thus, students, when confronted with AIDS, may realize for the first time that there *are* risks associated with being a clinician. This realization may force them to confront issues concerning their own mortality and responsibility.

D. Specific content of the interview. The specific content depends on whether the purpose of the interview is screening for risk behaviors, dealing with patients who are concerned that they might have HIV infection, or getting a history of the progression of the disease from someone who already has AIDS.

1. **Screening for risk behaviors.** This entails doing a complete sexual history (see II), a complete substance use history (see III), and a PMH for history of transfusions. Patients with any risk behaviors should be counseled on preventive measures.

2. **Patients concerned about HIV infection**
   a. Patients who express concern about the possibility of HIV infection should have a complete screening history and receive information about the use of condoms. When the screening history is positive for possible exposure to the virus, patients should be informed about anonymous confidential testing programs as well as the existence of excellent educational resources (e.g., pamphlets, video tapes) on preventing AIDS, many of which are available to clinicians for their patients.
   b. Patients who use intravenous drugs should be counseled on safe drug use practices and opportunities for rehabilitation and treatment.

3. **Patients with AIDS** should be interviewed following the guidelines for chronic illness (see VIII) and terminal illness (see IX). With the advent of AZT (Zidovudine), prophylactic treatment of *Pneumocystis carinii* pneumonia, and other new treatments currently evolving, AIDS may become more of a chronic illness.
   a. **Survival.** Clinicians should provide care to AIDS patients that gives them hope.
      (1) Without treatment, studies have demonstrated that there are long-term survivors of the disease.
      (2) Approximately 10% of AIDS patients survive 3 or more years after the diagnosis.
      (3) There are reports of patients surviving 10 years after diagnosis.
   b. **Social isolation.** There is considerable stigma associated with AIDS, and newly diagnosed patients may not feel comfortable sharing their diagnosis with friends and co-workers as this information can result in discrimination in employment and housing and rejection by family and friends. These aspects of the disease require an even more sensitive approach to interviewing patients with AIDS.

REFERENCES

Andreoli TE, et al: Acquired immunodeficiency syndrome. In *Cecil Essentials of Medicine.* Edited by Andreoli TE, et al. Philadelphia, WB Saunders, 1990 pp 620–626

Callen, M: *Surviving AIDS.* New York, Harper Collins Publishers, 1990

Karan, L: AIDS prevention and chemical treatment needs of women and their children. *J Psychoactive Drugs* 21:395–399, 1989

Kübler-Ross E: *On Death and Dying.* New York, Macmillan, 1969

Levy BS, Wegman DH (eds): *Occupational Health: Recognition and Prevention of Work-Related Diseases.* Boston, Little, Brown, 1988

Proctor NH, Hughes JP, Fischman ML: *Chemical Hazards of the Workplace.* Philadelphia, JB Lippincott, 1988

Rom WN (ed): *Environmental and Occupational Medicine.* Boston, Little, Brown, 1983

Rosenstock L, Cullen MR: *Clinical Occupational Medicine.* Philadelphia, WB Saunders, 1986

Strauss AL, et al: *Chronic Illness and the Quality of Life,* 2nd ed. St. Louis, CV Mosby, 1984

Whitfield CL, Davis JE, Barker LR: Alcoholism. In *Principles of Ambulatory Medicine.* Edited by Barker LR, Burton JR, Ziene P. Baltimore, Williams & Wilkins, 1982

Zenz C (ed): *Occupational Medicine: Principles and Practical Applications.* Chicago, Year Book, 1987

STUDY QUESTIONS

Directions: Each of the numbered items or incomplete statements in this section is followed by answers or by completions of the statement. Select the **one** lettered answer or completion that is **best** in each case.

1. The most commonly used substance in the United States currently is

(A) nicotine
(B) marijuana
(C) alcohol
(D) caffeine
(E) cocaine

2. A 24-hour recall of food intake may be taken as part of the medical history for all of the following purposes EXCEPT to

(A) qualitatively evaluate the patient's usual food intake
(B) screen a patient's diet for consumption of problem nutrients
(C) prescribe a diet for a specified condition
(D) calculate the patient's caloric needs
(E) give advice about making specific changes in diet

3. Questions from other parts of the history overlap with those covered for a patient concerned about getting AIDS or with transmission of HIV infection with the exception of

(A) sexual history
(B) substance use history
(C) FH
(D) PMH
(E) nutrition history

Directions: Each item below contains four suggested answers of which **one or more** is correct. Choose the answer

A	if **1, 2, and 3** are correct
B	if **1 and 3** are correct
C	if **2 and 4** are correct
D	if **4** is correct
E	if **1, 2, 3, and 4** are correct

4. Clinicians should determine the number of sexual partners of their patients in which of the following circumstances?

(1) When patients present with an STD
(2) When patients are concerned about contraceptives
(3) When patients bring it up
(4) When patients are concerned about AIDS

5. When patients indicate a change in sleeping patterns, clinicians must obtain information about

(1) use of medications
(2) the patient's beliefs about the change
(3) changes in the patient's work
(4) changes in the ability to concentrate

6. The mental health history should be pursued when the

(1) patient's story provides an opening
(2) patient has a family member present
(3) patient's CC indicates anxiety
(4) patient returns for a second visit

7. The process of taking a mental health history is most successful when the clinician

(1) asks specific questions first
(2) offers reinforcing feedback
(3) avoids sensitive areas
(4) remains nonjudgmental

8. Behaviors that suggest emotional dysfunction include which of the following?

(1) Crying when presented with a diagnosis of a serious illness

(2) Major weight gain in the absence of physical pathology

(3) Anxiety about impending surgery

(4) Blunted affect in the course of a major illness

9. Which of the following variables have the least influence on the behavior of a terminally ill person in terms of his or her reaction to the prognosis?

(1) Age, social and religious background, and ethnicity

(2) Financial status, employment history, and family relationships

(3) Economic status, mental and emotional health, and intelligence

(4) Sex, marital status, and educational level

Directions: The group of items in this section consists of lettered options followed by a set of numbered items. For each item, select the **one** lettered option that is most closely associated with it. Each lettered option may be selected once, more than once, or not at all.

Questions 10–14

Mrs. Q, a 75-year-old terminally ill woman with no known living relatives and few visitors, has frequently expressed her desire to speak with her clinician to discuss her "future plans." She had been afforded this opportunity at least once a week over the past month during the course of morning rounds to little avail. The clinician has spent 10 minutes with her on various occasions, yet she still complains that nobody will listen to her and nobody cares about helping her with "her plans." She keeps lists of her questions on small scraps of paper, scattered among her few belongings.

Upon interview regarding these complaints and her plans, she is vague, sometimes contradicts her most recently stated desires, claiming she never said that. Her questions and comments "tumble out of her." She rarely waits for a full answer and seems not to be listening to the explanation anyway. She often asks for more information about her prognosis and her future. She is experiencing "a little pain, once in a while." She is reported to be tolerating food and liquids well but is not sleeping well, preferring to take short cat naps throughout the day and evening. At night she is restless and is sometimes observed quietly crying to herself. The nursing staff reports that she is generally very communicative, asks lots of difficult questions, which they are unable or unwilling to answer, referring her instead to her clinician.

The clinician wants to engage in more "productive" sessions with Mrs. Q to become better informed about her desires and to be able to formulate an appropriate plan with her. Select the order in which each strategy should be undertaken by the clinician so as to result in a more positive and productive physician-patient relationship.

(A) Review the details of the patient's illness in a language she can understand

(B) Set up a social service consult to explore possible family ties and resources

(C) Schedule a frequent number of short sessions with the patient to discuss agreed upon topics for each session

(D) Access in more detail the patient's reported experiences of pain, and treat these pain episodes if appropriate

(E) Determine the patient's understanding and perception of her illness, its course, and her expectations for the future

10. Step 1

11. Step 2

12. Step 3

13. Step 4

14. Step 5

ANSWERS AND EXPLANATIONS

1. The answer is D. [*III*] Caffeine has the broadest base of users and the highest average daily consumption. History of use is important as a prelude to asking about other more sensitive substances as well as for its own impact on health. Excessive consumption of caffeine can cause sleeplessness, agitation, and tremors and may interact with some medications.

2. The answer is C. [*V C 1*] A diet prescribed to treat a specified condition is based on currently accepted, medically therapeutic interventions for the diagnosis. The 24-hour recall is one of several tools used in taking the diet history component of the nutrition assessment. The 24-hour recall is frequently used as a basis for diet planning and instruction for nutrition intervention.

3. The answer is E. [*X D 1*] A screening for risk factors includes sexual behavior, substance use, FH of the disease (primarily for young children), and PMH of transfusions. Nutrition is not a major area of risk for HIV infection, while it does play a significant role in the management of HIV-infected patients.

4. The answer is E (all). [*II A, D*] Clinicians should determine the number of sexual partners of all sexually active patients. Screening sexual history questions should be asked in all complete histories as well as in histories of patients who express concern about contraception and STDs.

5. The answer is E (all). [*VI A 1–3, C 1–4*] A change in sleeping patterns is a symptom that may be indicative of physical problems, emotional problems, or both. Some prescription and over-the-counter medications may cause insomnia (e.g., asthma medications) while others cause sleepiness (e.g., some antihypertensives, antihistamines). Changes in sleep patterns can cause emotional or cognitive changes while stressful life events or simple environmental changes (e.g., shift in working hours) can influence sleep patterns. Therefore, it is important to ask the patient what he or she thinks may be causing the change. All of the data must be gathered in an attempt to determine causality and to identify the underlying problem.

6. The answer is B (1, 3). [*VI B 1–3*] The mental health history, a brief exploration of a patient's past and current mental status, may be put in a number of places in the structured interview. It may flow logically from the CC if the patient presents with an emotional problem, or it may fit in the PMH if previous psychiatric interventions are revealed here. It may also be necessary to create a separate place for the mental health history if no obvious opening presents.

7. The answer is C (2, 4). [*VI D 1–4*] Success in gathering a mental health history depends on the way in which it is taken. Open-ended, nonjudgmental questions that move from general areas to specific areas (only as necessary) are usually successful in encouraging patients to discuss their mental health history. Reinforcing feedback lets patients know that the clinician is comfortable hearing what they have to say and encourages them to continue. In dealing with sensitive material, patients are likely to be keenly aware of interpersonal cues and may stop abruptly if they feel judged or labeled. Asking broad, open-ended questions lets the patient guide the content; reinforcement and a nonjudgmental attitude encourage more detail in sensitive areas.

8. The answer is C (2, 4). [*VI F 2 a–c*] Behaviors that suggest emotional dysfunction include weight gain in the absence of physical pathology or a blunted or flat affect in a situation where emotion would be expected. When clinicians perceive signs or symptoms of emotional or cognitive dysfunction, they must assess these signs in the context of the patient, the illness, and the situation.

9. The answer is D (4). [*IX C 1–7*] The least influential variables have to do with sex, marital status, and educational level. Gender differences in responding to a terminal illness have not been consistently demonstrated. Single and married persons express similar responses and experience similar stages and behaviors. Educational level may influence the ability of a person to express verbally what he or she is experiencing, but it has not been shown to be a major determinant of an individual's reactions and behavior in the face of a terminal illness.

10–14. The answers are: 10-D, 11-C, 12-E, 13-A, 14-B. [*IX A–C*] The first step is to make a determination of the extent and pattern of the patient's pain and to treat it aggressively if needed. Other issues and topics, which depend on the patient's cooperation and participation, cannot be successfully undertaken until her pain is addressed. The second step should be to reassure the patient of the clinician's continued involvement by scheduling a frequent number of short sessions and to elicit from the patient her priorities for topics to be addressed, some of which may have little to do with clinical medicine but have a lot to do with her fears and concerns. After determining the patient's perceptions of her illness as a third step by giving her control over what will be the most important dialogues between the clinician and patient, the details of the illness can be reviewed as step 4. Because a referral to a social service agency may be perceived by the patient as an attempt by the clinician to ignore her pleas to establish a close relationship, it should be considered after more productive tasks are undertaken as step 5.

5
Difficult Dyads: Challenges in the Medical Interview

Carol A. Pfeiffer

I. OVERVIEW

A. Model. A useful model for examining some of the sources of conflict and misunderstanding in the interaction between the patient and the clinician has been proposed by Mishler.

1. **Voice of medicine.** The voice of medicine represents the clinician's world view, which is primarily based on an **objective interpretation of events,** using logic and rationality to interpret human experience. The methods and ideology are based on the scientific method, and the language is technical. This voice has had a very powerful impact on our ability to understand and treat disease.

2. **Voice of the lifeworld.** The voice of the lifeworld reflects the commonsense world of the lay person. It is a **subjective interpretation of events** that interrelates social and psychological events with physical events. It uses the everyday language of the patient. This voice must be heard to foster a therapeutic relationship between the patient and clinician.

B. Student clinician

1. **Goals.** The goal of the student clinician who is learning clinical skills is to acquire the voice of medicine. The goal of the faculty preceptor is to teach that voice.

2. **Translation from the voice of the lifeworld to the voice of medicine.** In taking a history, medical interviewers typically translate the patient's words; for example, a patient may say "Since I have been married . . . ," but the interviewer translates this statement to "Four years ago . . ." to obtain a correct chronological sequence; however, in translating the patient's words, the interviewer is not considering the importance of the marriage in the etiology of the problem—that is, the real cause of the symptom that began when the patient was married may be social and not physical. The translation from the voice of the lifeworld to the voice of medicine may cause the interviewer to lose important information.

3. **Lack of experience.** The student comes to medicine entrenched in the voice of the lifeworld. While the student is learning the voice of medicine, he or she must also listen to and learn about the everyday experiences of people with medical problems. Student clinicians are typically young adults whose stage in the life cycle means that they have had relatively little experience with the lifeworld, especially of patients who are old and sick. Death and disability have not been part of their daily routines. While students learn the seven parameters of an illness and the relevant review of symptoms, they must also learn how the pathophysiology of a particular disease affects the patient's physical and psychological function.
   a. **Disease,** the physical process that leads to symptoms, is the primary concern of the voice of medicine.
   b. **Illness,** the impact of the disease on the functioning of the individual, is the data source of the voice of the lifeworld.

4. **Challenges.** A serious challenge to the student, who has the authority of the white coat but not the knowledge to go with it, is to balance the need to know the voice of medicine with the need to learn about the lifeworld. It is tempting to focus on the voice of medicine and to ignore the voice of the lifeworld. This is also the source of many of the problems of difficult interviews.

C. Patient

1. **Acute versus chronic problems**
   a. **Acute problems.** When the patient brings an acute problem to the clinician, the voice of medicine usually works well. The objective, rational approach to a problem of brief duration leads to either effective treatment or cure via the "tincture of time." For example, a patient with shortness of breath due to a pneumonia that can be treated effectively with antibiotics is an easy problem. The clinician or patient may be frustrated by some aspect of the regimen or the symptoms, but the patient is soon well, and both parties are satisfied.
   b. **Chronic problems** create more difficulties because a history of frustrating diagnosis and management gives both the patient and provider low expectations as they seek a satisfactory resolution. For example, the patient with shortness of breath due to emphysema is a challenge. The disease may be treated but not cured, and its natural history is a downhill course with increasing disability. The frustration of the patient and the clinician may parallel each other and lead to difficult interactions. In this situation, it is important for the clinician to listen to the voice of the lifeworld in planning treatment with the patient.

2. **Folk beliefs.** The patient's view of health and illness is based on ethnic and cultural background, social class, and education. Each can be a serious barrier to communication in the clinical encounter. For example, unproven remedies abound for the care of chronic diseases, especially those with periods of exacerbation and remission. The patient with rheumatoid arthritis who spends large sums of money to sit in cool, damp caves that are supposed to cure arthritis (although the caves are purportedly filled with radon gas) is very frustrating to the clinician. Clinicians may be able to help patients avoid such treatments if they are careful to inquire about the patient's level of frustration in dealing with the disease, including which remedies the patient has tried and which have been successful.

3. **Personal biography.** The patient also brings his or her individual characteristics to the encounter. Past encounters with the health care system shape current patient behaviors. Patients also present particular personality characteristics, which are more or less difficult for clinicians. For example, most clinicians can remember a time when they interpreted a set of common symptoms to mean that they had a serious chronic or fatal disease. An experienced provider knows that common symptoms usually mean common problems, but the medical student's personal encounter with pathophysiology in the classroom makes him or her a difficult patient.

D. Encounter

1. **Match.** The difficulty of the interview depends greatly on the match between the clinician and the patient. The more disparate the cultural and linguistic backgrounds of clinician and patient, the greater the probability of a difficult encounter. The presence of a chronic health problem or overidentification of the clinician with the patient may also increase the probability of difficulty; for example, an Iranian medical student with a turban and beard who interviews an elderly French Canadian is apt to experience problems even if both speak fluent English.

2. **Power issues.** The model of physician–patient interaction held by both participants in the encounter is important.
   a. **Clinician dominance.** The clinician controls the topics of conversation and opens and closes all new topics because he or she has specialized knowledge. This is appropriate in acute and critical care situations where the patient cannot easily respond (e.g., the accident victim in the emergency room), but in chronic and non–life-threatening situations, this dominance creates difficulties for physician–patient interaction.
   b. **Mutual participation.** The flow of the interview is set by both clinician and patient; new topics are introduced by both. This model is especially useful in chronic illness and preventive care. The novice, however, may have difficulty sharing control while collecting the information required by the preceptor's voice of medicine. For example, an adult male with a long history of rheumatoid arthritis has experienced a flare-up in his disease. Usual tactics for controlling the flare-up have not worked. The clinician is aware of a new treatment method that could help the patient, but it may have severe side effects. In such circumstances, the mutual participation model, where the decision to try or not try the new regimen is made by both, is likely to lead to a better outcome.

II. STRATEGIES FOR THE MANAGEMENT OF SPECIFIC PROBLEMS
A. Cultural differences
1. Problems
a. Ethnicity
(1) **Impact on verbal communication.** If the patient and the clinician do not share a common language, the difficulties are obvious, and an interpreter is necessary. When they do speak the same language, but its roots are in very different ethnic traditions, the problems remain, and interpretation may still be necessary. For example, a white middle class student is the clinician for a lower class black woman with an 8-month-old child with an ear infection. The mother tells the student with a smile on her face that this is a really "bad baby." The student becomes concerned about the possibility of child abuse because of the mother's peculiar affect as she describes her child in this negative way. However, if the student clarifies the mother's perception by asking her to describe the baby's bad behavior, he or she will learn that the child's active, exploring, curious behavior is described as "bad," but it is seen as evidence of a child with great promise in coping with the world.

(2) **Impact on nonverbal communication.** The correct distance for an encounter, the frequency and duration of eye contact, the appropriate posture, and the amount of touching may vary enormously with different ethnic groups and may create serious problems in the clinical interview. These issues are further complicated by the fact that they are not easy to observe. For example, when a student from Egypt interviews a bachelor from New England, the student sits very close to make "comfortable" eye contact. When the New Englander moves away, the student moves even closer. The patient becomes even more uncomfortable because the interviewer is so close and is unable to share relevant information.

b. Class or education
(1) **Vocabulary.** The clinician's use of jargon or multisyllabic words is confusing to most patients, especially those with little education who are less able to interpret the clinician, thereby limiting physician-patient communication. For example, a mother who never graduated from high school is interviewed by a student with little skill in knowing when he is talking beyond an individual's comprehension. He views the mother as a "poor historian" with a limited grasp of her child's medical problems. The student has very little data about the child's present illness or past medical history largely because he has asked about the radiation (four syllables) and intensity (four syllables) of the child's pain, the dates of immunizations (five syllables), the length of gestation (medical terminology), and the onset of the symptom. The student should have asked the following questions: When did the pain begin? How bad was it? How did you know? Did it go anywhere? Was your infant born on time or early? Has your infant had her shots? These questions would have resulted in more data and a better relationship with the patient.

(2) **Respect and familiarity.** Clinicians are more comfortable and less formal with members of their own social class; in return, patients ask more questions, are more confident, and give more information. Many clinicians have poor opinions of patients' abilities and look with favor only on those who are clean, articulate, and cooperative. Preceptors may foster this bias in teaching clinical medicine by using private floors to give the student the perceived advantage of talking with middle class individuals who are viewed as easier patients.

2. Strategies for coping
a. Interviewing skills.
The most basic strategy for dealing with difficult interviews is to use the skills outlined in Chapter 2 for developing rapport with patients. Using open-ended questions and allowing uninterrupted talk by the patient encourage the patient to participate in the interview. The cohesiveness of the interview can be strengthened by the use of transitions that explain to the patient the clinician's thought process. Summary statements can give the patient assurance that he or she has been heard. Researchers have contrasted directive and mutual participation interviewing styles.
(1) In the **directive style,** the clinician asks mostly closed-ended questions, starts all new topics of conversation, and interrupts frequently. The directive style does allow the clinician to obtain more details, but the level of detail does not result in a better written history or oral case presentation.

(2) In the **mutual participation style,** there is a much higher percentage of open-ended questions, new topics are introduced by both patient and clinician, and there are fewer clinician interruptions. Patients are more satisfied with the mutual participation encounter.

b. Cultural learning. If clinicians deal routinely with patients of a particular class or ethnic background, it is essential that they learn about that culture's views of health and illness to enhance their ability to hear the voice of the lifeworld as expressed in that culture and to understand the views of the cause and cure of disease. For example, Hispanic culture divides disease and treatment into the categories of hot and cold, and it is important to treat a "hot" disease with a "cold" treatment and vice versa. In osteoarthritis, where both a heating pad and an ice pack are useful short-term pain relievers, it is important to know the quality of the disease in the culture and to match the treatment to the cultural perception.

c. Using an interpreter. When the language barrier requires the use of an interpreter, triangular communication can be enhanced in the following ways:

(1) The clinician should acknowledge the language difficulty and let the patient know that a challenge in understanding and knowing each other is anticipated.

(2) Eye contact should be maintained with the patient, and he or she should be addressed even though the translator is speaking.

(3) Forms can be completed in advance by the interpreter and the patient to cover some areas of the history, allowing the clinician to limit the focus of the interaction.

(4) The clinician should learn the language of the patient population with whom he or she will be working. If the clinician is not interested in learning another language, then a colleague with whom the patients can communicate directly should be sought.

(5) The clinician should be cautious in the use of touch and the interpretation of body language since these are affected by cultural norms. It is important to learn what is expected by the other culture and then make use of it.

B. Overinvolvement

1. Problems

a. Seduction. Many medical students have difficulty dealing with the potential sexual stimulation involved in doing a physical examination and in gathering a sexual history. Many students also feel that they do not have the right to ask intimate questions and examine breasts and genitalia; however, these issues pass with experience and practice. Seductive behavior between clinicians and patients is an infrequent but serious problem. For example, a medical student who finds one of her patients very attractive has difficulty pursuing the sexual history and fails to learn of his homosexual behavior. This failure to gather data limits the ways in which the student can organize the patient's symptoms.

b. Identification. The clinician may confuse his or her needs with the patient's needs. Students may have great difficulty if a patient has a serious medical problem and is close to them in age, reminds them of a relative, or has the same medical problem as a family member. For example, a student whose mother has recently been diagnosed with multiple sclerosis is assigned to interview a patient who has had a long, troubled course with multiple sclerosis. She is so overcome by the patient's disability and her fears for her mother's future that she cannot interview the patient adequately. The patient does not understand why the medical student is so distant from her and so rejecting.

c. Dependence. Patients who view themselves as deprived and neglected individuals may elicit strong reactions from students whose self-image is based on strong needs to care. Many clinicians have great difficulty saying "no" to patients and attempt to be all things to their dependent patients. The very real dependence of those who are very sick may frighten both the patient and the novice clinician and lead to overinvolvement. For example, a student interviews a patient with severe complications from diabetes and forms a good relationship with him. The next week the student is working on the same floor and is able to visit the patient again. The patient has a grievance with the hospital, which the student legitimates, and gradually this becomes a major preoccupation for the student.

2. Strategies

a. Role definition. Whenever the student becomes overinvolved with a patient, part of the solution is to develop a clear set of boundaries. An understanding of the professional role and its obligations and limits is crucial. It is wise to discuss a patient who elicits sexual feelings or identification with a preceptor or mentor who can help the novice clinician to understand the patterns of difficulty and strategies for finding solutions. Too intense involvement and availability can limit the patient's ability to find his or her own solutions.

b. **Self-knowledge.** Students bring their own issues about health and illness and their own history of relationships to the medical interview. Understanding why certain circumstances are particularly difficult can help the student anticipate problems and then solve them. For example, the student whose father had a myocardial infarction and bypass surgery should anticipate that patients with the same problems will elicit a much stronger reaction than those who have other problems.

c. **Identifying the issue.** In working with a patient, it is often valuable for the clinician to acknowledge his or her own problems if they relate to those of the patient. For example, a student who has had a miscarriage and is working with a patient who just had a spontaneous abortion may find herself overinvolved in the patient's response. It may be wise for her to acknowledge the pain of her own loss and, at the same time, allow the patient to have a very different emotional response.

d. **Acknowledging the patient's needs.** This is particularly important with dependency needs, which have a basis in the patient's loss of function. It is also critical for clinicians to appreciate the patient's psychological needs while setting limits for themselves as the provider. For example, if a student interrupts a visit to interview a patient, it is important to establish whether the visitor and patient welcome the interruption or if this is a unique opportunity for the visitor and patient to visit. If the patient's needs are assessed before the encounter, the chances of success are enhanced.

e. **Acknowledging the clinician's needs.** People choose medicine for many reasons, some of which have to do with being needed by those in very difficult circumstances. The struggle to become a clinician and the desire to be a perfectionist in patient care may turn this desire into a real dislike for patients. A preventive strategy here is in setting boundaries on one's availability, especially with those who are looking for overinvolved relationships. For example, a mother who lacks confidence in her own parenting skills may continuously phone the clinician or visit the office about problems that are of little significance. While the clinician may expect this behavior in a new parent, the continuation of this behavior is of little value to the mother's confidence or the child's well-being. Clear boundaries about calling and about the duration of the consultation can limit this behavior and aid the mother's confidence.

C. **Negative emotions.** "To be put off by the difficult or provocative or uncooperative patient is to fail to understand the nature of hopelessness and the diversity of potentially adaptive responses to such feelings" [Meyer Ben Feival].

1. **Problems**
    a. **Anger and hostility.** Difficult situations produce strong emotions and are part of the grief reaction to the loss of health and the fear and loss of control that are part of being ill. For example, a 40-year-old man with severe heart disease whose activities of daily living are sharply curtailed may become very angry as the student documents the items in the patient profile. This patient obviously finds it very stressful to report the loss of valued work activities, relationships, and energy.
    b. **Dislikes.** Patients lament the fact that they cannot find a clinician who is perfect. Clinicians often prefer clean, neat, cooperative patients who have "interesting" diseases and those whose behavior is not the cause of their disease. Dislike of alcohol- or drug-dependent patients, and smokers who suffer the consequences of their behavior may result. For example, a patient presents reluctantly to the clinician with little clear information about her problems. She is articulate, clean, and neat but not cooperative. The discrepancy between expectations of good communication and a reliable historian with the reality of scanty data leaves the clinician dissatisfied with the clinical encounter.
    c. **Anxiety.** Virtually every patient is anxious because of either the setting of the clinician's office or fear about a symptom. Although some level of anxiety is protective for the patient, it can interfere dramatically with the patient's ability to give information and to hear the advice and explanations of the clinician. In the extreme, anxiety becomes denial, and the patient may not be willing to describe serious symptoms or to take important steps in treating them. For example, a patient has decided that his stomach pain is cancer. He fears having this confirmed by a clinician and avoids medical care until a family member takes over. His ability to communicate the history of the present illness is very limited by his fear of the diagnosis. His level of denial is such that he can only describe symptoms if they are extracted from him.

2. Strategies

a. Confronting the emotion

(1) If the anger, dislike, anxiety, or hostility originates with the clinician, the first step is to recognize the emotion and attempt to control it by discussing the difficult situations with preceptors and colleagues to learn which situations and patients are likely to produce negative emotions. Confronting the emotion and finding its source can help clinicians to deal more positively with patients.

(2) When the negative emotion originates with the patient, similar strategies can be employed. The first step is to identify the anxiety or hostility perceived in the patient and allow the emotion to be expressed. Confront the emotion directly, then ask open-ended questions, and use the other techniques of active listening to help the patient explore the underlying reasons for these feelings. When individuals are given permission to tell their story and express their uncomfortable feelings, they may then be free to behave in unexpectedly positive ways.

b. Empathizing with the circumstances

(1) Many groups of patients are routinely ridiculed by the housestaff and the attending clinicians as a means of expressing their sense of futility in dealing with difficult patients in difficult circumstances. Other patients fall into social categories that are seen as deviant by the larger culture (e.g., welfare mothers, homosexuals), and it is not easy to avoid prejudice and negative emotions in dealing with these individuals. Understanding oneself and accepting one's frailties without denying them is part of the clinician's role.

(2) As a patient's negative emotions are expressed, the clinician can empathize with the particular circumstances and apologize if he or she is directly responsible for a delay or error in care. In circumstances where third parties are the focus of the bad feeling, it is unwise to blame them or apologize for them. Rather, the clinician should acknowledge the patient's feelings and empathize with his or her discomfort.

c. Working on solutions

(1) Problem-solving for the clinician who has strong negative emotions toward patients centers on supervision from preceptors and colleagues to learn interviewing techniques that will allow him or her to develop better rapport with individuals and their circumstances. It also involves making working conditions better so that difficult people and circumstances are not seen in times of exhaustion. It also means acknowledging the hierarchical nature of our society where the poor are also more likely to be sick and working for changes in that system. For student clinicians who are habitually negative toward a large proportion of their patients, referral for psychological or psychiatric care is appropriate; self-referral is the most effective means of changing behavior. Medicine is definitely not a good career choice for students who are routinely anxious, hostile, or angry with patients.

(2) Having explored the patient's emotions, the clinician is now in a position to help the patient solve the problems.

(a) For the patient who is anxious about a physical symptom, the medical history, physical examination, tests, diagnosis, and management plan may deal with the anxiety in a very therapeutic way.

(b) For the patient who dislikes the clinician, an opportunity to explore that emotion and some empathy for the lack of mutual caring may in fact change the emotion enough for care to proceed. If that is not the case, the clinician can offer to refer the patient.

(c) For the angry, hostile patient, it is sometimes enough to be heard; having stated the emotion, the patient may be more able to develop possible solutions, and the clinician can certainly help with the problem-solving process of generating alternatives and then choosing among them.

(d) In instances where patients are chronically angry and hostile, more sophisticated management is required. Referral to psychiatric care is appropriate. Patients do not have an option of leaving the sick role by selecting another career, so those for whom being a patient is a serious burden remain members of a difficult dyad.

D. Difficult situations

1. Problems

a. Psychological or psychogenic problems. The voice of medicine has developed a mind–

body split. The psychological and physical distress of those with well-understood organic problems is accepted and respected. Patients with "real" disease (that which can be diagnosed and whose pathophysiology is understood) are the deserving ill who merit our sympathy and support. Those patients who do not have a clear organic basis for their physical symptoms are highly suspect both to themselves and to their caretakers. A "diagnosis" can be a welcome prize and vindication to a patient who has had a long course of unexplained symptoms even if the natural history of the newly labeled disease is one of disability and death.

    b. **Sad or crying patients.** A normal response to disease is sadness. As the patient mourns a loss or suffers with pain, tears are an expected means of expression. Sharing such emotions with, and being comforted by, the clinician is part of a therapeutic relationship.

2. **Strategies**
    a. **Learning psychosocial medicine.** With the psychogenic patient, a careful medical history and workup are important, but they must be limited, and the clinician must also explore and understand psychosocial medicine as it relates to the patient. If the clinician accepts the cultural bias that discredits the somatizing patient, then he or she cannot expect the patient to accept the basis for his or her symptoms as psychological. Understanding the mind–body connection can help both the patient and clinician if the stigma of having a psychological or social basis for physical problems can be limited.
    b. **Listening skills.** The sad or crying patient can benefit from the clinician's ability to listen. It is tempting to deal with the openly grieving patient by quickly changing the subject or trying to cheer up the patient. This allows the clinician to avoid the unpleasant emotion but also lays the groundwork for future difficult encounters. A more effective strategy is to ask the patient to discuss his or her feelings of sadness. If the patient cannot discuss them presently, the clinician must return to the subject later in the interaction. If the patient is openly weeping, a tissue is the best response and then a gentle open inquiry as to the source of the tears. Staying with the patient while he or she expresses strong feelings is hard work, but it is usually beneficial to the patient. It is not necessary to have solutions to impossible problems; it can be enough to be present while people share their pain, fears, and hurt.
    c. **Referral to a resource network.** Many of the problems that clinicians and patients face cannot be solved. Clinicians typically prefer problems that they can fix, and patients would obviously prefer to have curable diseases. In the face of the realities of living and dying, clinicians need to learn what they can and cannot handle. This can guide them in the choice of a specialty and help them identify the referral networks that will benefit their patients. For example, the student who is anxious whenever he examines a patient under 12 years of age should avoid pediatrics. The pediatrician with a patient who has an overanxious father needs to know of community resources that teach parenting skills. The student who becomes hostile and angry when seeing patients with cancer should avoid oncology. The oncologist needs a nurse and social worker who can also be available to patients who are in distress.

REFERENCES

Billings JA, Stoeckle JD: *The Clinical Encounter: A Guide to the Medical Interview and Case Presentation.* Chicago, Year Book, 1989

Fisher S: *In the Patient's Best Interest: Women and the Politics of Medical Decisions.* New Brunswick, NJ, Rutgers University Press, 1986

Freeling P, Harris CM: *The Doctor–Patient Relationship,* 3rd ed. New York, Churchill Livingstone, 1984

Henderson G: *Physician–Patient Communication: Readings and Recommendations.* Chicago, Charles C Thomas, 1981

King M, Novick L, Citrenbaum C: *Irresistible Communication: Creative Skills for the Health Professional.* Philadelphia, WB Saunders, 1983

Lipp MR: *Respectful Treatment: A Practical Handbook of Patient Care,* 2nd ed. New York, Elsevier, 1986

Mishler EG: *The Discourse of Medicine: Dialectics of Medical Interviews.* Norwood, NJ, Ablex Publishing Corporation, 1984

Mizrahi T: *Getting Rid of Patients: Contradictions in the Socialization of Physicians.* New Brunswick, NJ, Rutgers University Press, 1986

Pendleton D, Hasler J: *Doctor–Patient Communication.* New York, Academic Press, 1983

Todd AD: *Intimate Adversaries: Cultural Conflict Between Doctors and Woman Patients.* Philadelphia, University of Pennsylvania Press, 1989

West C: *Routine Complications: Trouble with Talk Between Doctors and Patients.* Bloomington, Indiana University Press, 1984

Zola IK: *Socio-Medical Inquiries: Recollections, Reflections, and Recommendations.* Philadelphia, Temple University Press, 1983

STUDY QUESTIONS

Directions: Each of the numbered items or incomplete statements in this section is followed by answers or by completions of the statement. Select the **one** lettered answer or completion that is **best** in each case.

1. Which of the following statements best characterizes the voice of medicine?

(A) It is an objective interpretation of events
(B) It is a reflection of the patient's story
(C) It is a subjective interpretation of events
(D) It is a means of sharing control with the patient
(E) It uses everyday language

2. All of the following statements characterize the voice of the lifeworld EXCEPT that

(A) it is a subjective interpretation of events
(B) it is the patient's story
(C) it is best elicited with specific orderly questions
(D) it is best heard with few interruptions
(E) it is told in everyday language

3. Which of the following statements concerning clinicians who use a directive interviewing style is true?

(A) They gather more specific facts
(B) They have a better rapport with their patients
(C) They can more effectively present the patient's case
(D) They use a less technical vocabulary
(E) They are less likely to have difficult patients

Directions: The group of items in this section consists of lettered options followed by a set of numbered items. For each item, select the **one** lettered option that is most closely associated with it. Each lettered option may be selected once, more than once, or not at all.

Questions 4–10

For each quote or concept listed below, select the "voice" that it most accurately represents.

(A) Voice of the lifeworld
(B) Voice of medicine
(C) Both
(D) Neither

4. "I never sleep a wink"

5. "I used to sleep 8 hours every night, but now I only sleep 2"

6. "There was just a teaspoon of blood, but it terrified me"

7. Mutual participation style

8. Physician dominance style

9. Illness

10. Disease

ANSWERS AND EXPLANATIONS

1. The answer is A. [*I A 1, 2*] The voice of medicine is an objective view of the patient's medical problem. It is a translation of the patient's subjective story by the clinician using logic, rationality, and a technical vocabulary.

2. The answer is C. [*I A 1, 2*] The voice of the lifeworld is the subjective story of the patient that is told in everyday language and is best elicited by open-ended questions that allow the patient to speak with few interruptions. This voice must be heard to foster a therapeutic relationship.

3. The answer is A. [*I A 1; II A 2 a (1)*] The directive interviewing style does allow the clinician to gather more specific facts, but it does not foster a better relationship with patients or result in a more comprehensive view of the patient as revealed in the case presentation. In the directive interviewing style, the clinician asks mostly closed-ended questions, starts all topics of conversation, and interrupts frequently.

4–10. The answers are: 4-A, 5-B, 6-C, 7-C, 8-B, 9-A, 10-B. [*I A 1, 2, B 3 a, b, D 2 a, b*] The voice of the lifeworld can be translated from ordinary speech, such as, "I never sleep a wink," to the voice of medicine, which is very precise, as in "I used to sleep 8 hours but now only sleep 2." The voices are combined in statements such as, "There was just a teaspoon of blood, but it terrified me," which include both the specific information of the voice of medicine and the subjective patient response. The mutual participation style makes use of both voices. The voice of medicine is consistent with physician dominance. Illness is the patient's experience and reflects the voice of the lifeworld. Disease, which focuses on the pathophysiology, is the voice of medicine.

6
The Physical Examination

Anthony J. Ardolino

I. INTRODUCTION. The physical examination is performed in a number of clinical situations, including the office, emergency room, and hospital settings. The purpose of the physical examination is also varied. It may be performed in response to specific symptoms or to detect asymptomatic disease. This variety necessitates modification of technique.

Section II of this chapter is concerned with the choreography of the physical examination, which is applicable to all physical examinations. Section III concerns the regional approach to the comprehensive examination, which is a thorough examination performed for patients admitted to a hospital or for patients visiting a clinician for the first time. Section IV concerns the periodic health examination, which is a modification of a comprehensive physical with special emphasis on health maintenance, disease prevention, and identification of asymptomatic disease. Section V concerns directed examinations, which are further modifications of the complete examination, occurring in outpatient and emergency room settings where a more focused, time-limited examination is required.

II. CHOREOGRAPHY OF THE PHYSICAL EXAMINATION. The physical examination is conducted in a logical, flowing manner.

A. Approach to the patient

1. **Introduction.** The examiner should provide the patient with his or her **name** and **title** (e.g., clinician, resident, or medical student) and begin the examination by **shaking hands**. Shaking hands is a socially acceptable way to initiate patient contact and is followed logically by examination of the hands and skin.

2. **Hand washing.** The examiner's hands should be washed **before every examination,** preferably in view of the patient.

3. **Explanation.** Each component of the examination should be explained to prepare the patient for anticipated maneuvers and discomfort.

B. Position of the examiner. Traditionally, the clinician is **on the right side of the patient** during the examination. While this is more conventional than truly essential, remaining in one position allows a more efficient examination and consistency of technique from patient to patient. Examining from the right is easier for right-handed individuals; left-handed examiners may find that some components of the physical are better performed from the left. In all cases, the examiner should be comfortably stationed in relation to the patient.

C. Position of the patient

1. **Ambulatory patients on examining tables.** Patients should be seated comfortably at the end of the examining table with their legs hanging freely. As the examination progresses, patients are aided into the supine position with the footrest pulled out to support the legs. Certain examinations require that the backrest be adjusted from supine to various heights.

2. **Patients in hospital beds.** The bed should be adjusted to the appropriate height for the examiner to perform each maneuver comfortably. The degree of illness or medical devices (e.g., intravenous lines or respirators) may necessitate alterations in the usual examination procedure. Special attention to patient comfort is essential.

D. Flow of the examination

1. Ambulatory patients

    a. With the patient seated, the hands and the exposed **skin** on the forearms are examined initially. The **vital signs** are then taken. A **systematic regional approach** is then followed. The **head, eyes, ears, nose, mouth, throat, neck, thorax, lungs,** and the **axillae** are examined in order. In female patients, the first portion of the **breast examination** is performed at this time.

    b. With the patient in the supine position, the **breast examination** is completed on female patients. The **cardiovascular examination** begins in the supine position and may necessitate additional maneuvering (e.g., raising the backrest to 30°–45° or left lateral decubitus). The examination then proceeds down the body to include the **abdomen,** the **inguinal area,** the **extremities,** and the **musculoskeletal examination.** The **neurologic examination** is then initiated.

    c. With the patient standing, the back and its range of motion, gait, cerebellar function (Romberg), and the male genitalia are examined.

    d. The rectal examination in men and the **pelvic examination** in women are best performed as the final components of the examination.

2. Hospitalized patients. Patients in hospital beds or stretchers may necessitate alterations in the maneuvers or sequence used in the examination, usually due to the severity of their illness. For further detail, refer to Chapter 7 III.

III. REGIONAL APPROACH TO THE COMPREHENSIVE EXAMINATION

A. General appearance. The first observations made in the physical examination are those of the patient's overall condition. These should include objective descriptions of specific information, including the following:

1. Demographic data, including the patient's **age, sex,** and **race** are noted. If the patient appears significantly younger or older than the stated age, this should be recorded.

2. Level of consciousness may be described as **alert, somnolent, stuporous,** or **comatose.**

3. Level of distress is an important component. Descriptive terms such as "resting comfortably," "in no apparent pain," or "in acute distress" are used to reflect this.

4. Patient affect should be noted. Acceptable terms are "flat," "appropriate," or "anxious."

5. Other readily apparent observations about the patient's physical condition are often included at this time, even if they are organ-specific. Examples include:

    a. "The patient is in marked respiratory distress."

    b. "The patient walked in without assistance."

    c. "The patient was brought in via stretcher and is unable to sit or stand."

B. Statistics and vital signs

1. Height is measured with patient standing in stocking feet. While one recorded height is sufficient in young adults, elderly patients should be measured periodically to monitor shortening from vertebral disc space narrowing or compression fractures.

2. Weight should be measured and recorded at all encounters. The pattern of weight gain or loss can be an important indicator of wellness and disease. Medication dosage is often weight-dependent.

3. Body temperature is easily measured with electronic or mercury thermometers.

    a. Rectal temperature is preferable to **oral temperature.** It is a more accurate reflection of core temperature and is less affected by technique (e.g., mouth breathing and ingested liquids can alter oral measurements).

    b. Electronic thermometers in common use do not record temperatures below 94° F. If hypothermia is suspected, special thermometers must be employed.

4. Pulse. The **radial artery pulse** is taken for a full **60 seconds** to determine the patient's heart rate. The examiner places his or her second and third fingers firmly over the patient's radial artery. Certain clinical situations, such as an irregular heart beat, necessitate that the examiner listen simultaneously to the heart with a stethoscope to confirm the actual heart rate.

    a. Rhythm of the heartbeat is recorded as **regular** or **irregular**.

    b. Normal pulse rate for an adult is between 60 and 100 beats a minute.

        (1) Tachycardia is a pulse rate greater than 100.

        (2) Bradycardia is a rate below 60.

5. Respiratory rate. The patient's breaths are counted for a full minute. The examiner should make these observations as discreetly as possible, since self-consciousness may lead the patient to hyperventilate.

    a. Rhythm of the **respiratory pattern** is noted. Common abnormalities include:

        (1) Cheyne-Stokes respiration (a regularly irregular sine wave-like pattern of respirations)

        (2) Biot's respiration (an irregularly irregular pattern)

        (3) Apnea (a prolonged period without respiratory efforts)

    b. Normal respiratory rate for adults is 12–16 breaths a minute. **Tachypnea** refers to a rate in excess of normal, and **bradypnea** to rates below normal.

6. Blood pressure is accurately determined using a **sphygmomanometer** (blood pressure cuff) and a **stethoscope**. The cuff is wrapped firmly around the upper arm, 1 cm above the antecubital fossa. The stethoscope is placed over the brachial artery. The cuff is inflated until the radial pulse, as determined by palpation, is lost. The cuff is gradually deflated, while auscultating with the stethoscope. The initial sound appreciated is **systole,** and the pressure at which all sounds cease is **diastole**.

    a. Normal blood pressure is from 100–140 systolic and from 60–90 diastolic for adults. Blood pressure greater than 140/90 is considered in the **hypertensive range**.

    b. Cuff size should be appropriate for the patient's arm. The cuff must be large enough for the cuff bladder to encircle two-thirds of the arm. A cuff that is too small yields a falsely elevated blood pressure, and conversely, a cuff too large records a falsely low blood pressure. Blood pressure determinations are usually done in both arms with the patient sitting comfortably.

    c. Measuring orthostatics. Many clinical situations, such as gastrointestinal bleeding or a history of syncope, require that the examiner measure the blood pressure in the supine and standing positions. These are called postural or orthostatic blood pressure readings and should be accompanied by a pulse rate determination in each position.

    d. Pulsus paradoxus. Normal systolic blood pressure falls 3–5 mm Hg with inspiration. An exaggeration in this physiologic response is referred to as pulsus paradoxus, occurring in many disease states (e.g., cardiac tamponade, asthma, obstructive pulmonary disease, constrictive pericarditis).

        (1) The examiner should determine carefully the highest pressure (systole) where sounds are audible only in expiration.

        (2) The column of mercury is slowly lowered to a point where sounds are audible in both inspiration and expiration.

        (3) The gap between the two measurements is the pulsus paradoxus. A gap of 10 mm or greater is considered pathologic.

C. Skin examination begins with the hands and forearms. The rest of the integument is exposed at the time that each section of the body is examined (e.g., skin of the back is viewed along with the chest and lung examination).

    1. By inspection the examiner assesses:

        a. Color and **pigmentation**

        b. Hair distribution

        c. Lesions. Each lesion is described by its **color, size, shape, distribution,** and **epidermal integrity**.

    2. By palpation the examiner determines:

        a. Surface moisture (from dry to diaphoretic)

        b. Temperature

        c. Texture

        d. Turgor or resiliency, which is determined by gently pinching the skin between thumb and forefinger

        e. Elasticity, which may be assessed concurrently

        f. Lesions, which are palpated for firmness and assessed to be raised or flat

D. Hands and nails

    1. Dorsal and palmer surfaces of each hand should be observed with attention to **color, muscular integrity, joint deformities,** and **skin lesions**.

2. Finger nails are observed for **color** and **deformities**. **Vascular integrity** is assessed by gently compressing the nail and releasing, then noting the rapidity of capillary filling.

E. Head

1. Inspection

   a. Shape and **contour** of the head are assessed with attention to **symmetry** and bony **deformities**.

   b. The **scalp** is examined for skin lesions.

   c. Hair distribution is noted with reference to areas of hair loss (alopecia).

   d. The skin over each mastoid process is inspected for ecchymoses **(Battle's sign)**.

2. Palpation

   a. The **scalp** is palpated to assess for tenderness and masses, and if there is suspected trauma, to detect depressed fractures.

   b. The examiner may gently tug on a few hairs to determine ease of hair removal.

F. Eyes

1. Conjunctiva and sclerae

   a. The lower conjunctiva is inspected by gently retracting the lower eyelid and having the patient look upward.

   b. The upper conjunctiva is visible only by retracting the upper eyelid, usually employing a sterile swab-handle as a fulcrum placed on the outer portion of the lid.

   c. Sclerae. The **color** and **vascular pattern** are noted. **Hemorrhages, pigmented lesions,** and **exudates** are noted, if present.

2. Pupils

   a. Pupillary size in room light is recorded in millimeters.

   b. Pupillary light reflexes are assessed as follows: The examiner holds a penlight at the right temple and shines it tangentially on the right eye, assuring that the light does not illuminate the left eye (Figure 6-1). The pupil being illuminated should constrict directly to the light, while the contralateral pupil constricts consensually. This is then repeated on the left side.

   c. Accommodation. The patient is asked to focus on an object in the distance, then to refocus on another object closer (e.g., the wall and then the examiner's finger). The pupils should constrict and the eyes converge.

3. Extraocular movements are tested by observing eye orientation at rest and the degree of movement of each eye.

   a. The patient is asked to follow the examiner's finger as it is moved in **eight cardinal directions** in front of the patient (Figure 6-2). The patient's head should remain stationary.

   b. Nystagmus, or involuntary rapid movements of the eyeball, in any direction should be recorded.

   c. Conjugate eye movement is coordinated by six muscles controlled by three cranial nerves. The examiner observes for dysconjugate or nonparallel eye movement and determines which muscle and nerve are affected.

   (1) CN VI supplies the lateral rectus muscles, moving each eye outward in a horizontal plane.

   (2) CN IV enervates the superior oblique muscles, which control medial, downward movement for each eye.

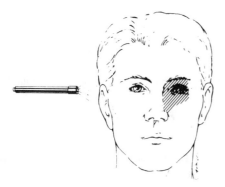

Figure 6-1. Pupillary reflexes. The penlight is held to the side so as to cast a shadow over the left eye. The right pupil should constrict *directly* to the light, and the left pupil should constrict *consensually*. This is repeated with the penlight held to the left side.

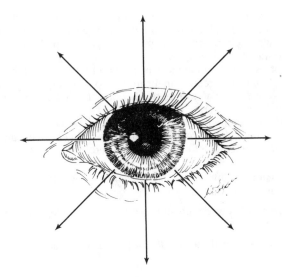

Figure 6-2. Extraocular movements. The patient is directed to gaze successively in all eight directions with the examiner returning to the midpoint after each direction.

      (3) CN III supplies the remaining four muscles, controlling all other movements.

  4. Visual fields are roughly assessed by determining the patient's peripheral vision in each quadrant.
    a. The examiner is positioned 1–2 feet directly in front of the patient. The examiner should cover one eye and use him- or herself as a control for the field of vision.
    b. The patient is asked to cover one eye and stare at the examiner's uncovered eye with the other.
    c. Held equidistant from the patient, the examiner's hand is slowly brought from the periphery until it is visible to the patient. This is repeated in all four quadrants.

  5. Visual acuity
    a. Distance vision is assessed by using a standard eye chart with the patient standing 20 feet away.
    b. Close vision is tested using a standardized reading chart or any text.

  6. Ophthalmoscopic examination
    a. With the ophthalmoscope held 2–3 feet away from the patient, the examiner looks for a **red reflex** emanating from each pupil, which suggests retinal integrity.
    b. With the ophthalmoscope held a few inches from the patient's eye, the examiner focuses on the **cornea, anterior chamber, iris, posterior chamber,** and **retina**.
    c. Funduscopic examination is a careful observation of the **optic disc, retinal arteries** and **veins,** and the **macula**. Arteriolar changes, hemorrhages, microaneurysms, and exudates are noted if present.

G. Ears

  1. The pinnae, or outer ear, is examined by **observation** and **palpation** for epidermal lesions or subcutaneous masses.

  2. Otoscopic examination
    a. The examiner grasps the pinnae and gently retracts it up and back, while introducing the otoscope into the **canal**. The canal is assessed for mucosal integrity, discharge, cerumen, and foreign bodies.
    b. Tympanic membrane (TM) is **inspected**.
      (1) Normal membrane should be opalescent with the distant end of the **malleus,** the **umbo,** clearly visible. Anterior and inferior to the umbo is found a **light reflex,** indicative of a normal TM orientation.
      (2) Abnormalities include perforations, bulging, or retraction of the membrane, opacity of the TM, visible fluid behind the TM, or vascular hyperemia.

3. **Hearing acuity** is grossly assessed by responses to whispered words spoken one foot from the patient's ear. Acuity to high-pitched sounds can be roughly tested with a watch tic or by rubbing the patient's hair between the examiner's fingers. Formal audiology testing is required for precise recording of hearing acuity.

   a. **Weber test.** A 128 Hz tuning fork is placed in the center of the forehead. The vibratory sensation should be perceived in the midline or diffusely. The sound lateralizes toward an ear with a **conductive abnormality** (e.g., otitis media) and away from an ear with a **sensory–neural deficit**.

   b. **Rinne test.** The tuning fork is struck and placed on the right mastoid process (measuring bone conduction), then directly in front of the right ear. The **"air" conduction** should be louder than **bone conduction**. This is repeated for the left ear.

H. **Nose.** A **nasal speculum** is introduced into each nostril with observation made regarding the mucosa, airway patency, and discharge.

   1. **The nasal septum** is viewed with attention to mucosal integrity, septal deviation, and perforations.

   2. **The turbinates** are viewed specifically for polyps, vascular lesions, or masses.

I. **Mouth**

   1. **Inspection**
      a. The patient is asked to open his or her mouth. A tongue blade is used to systematically expose the **gingiva, buccal mucosa,** and the **inferior aspects of the tongue**. Observations are made regarding **color, pigmentary changes,** and **mucosal lesions** of each structure.
      b. The general repair and absence of **teeth** should be recorded.
      c. Normal structures, including **Stensen's ducts, Wharton's ducts,** anterior and posterior **tonsillary pillars,** and the **tonsils** are identified.
      d. When the patient is asked to protract the tongue and say "aaah," the **uvula** should rise and fall in a midline position.

   2. **Palpation.** The examiner introduces a gloved hand to palpate the tongue, area beneath the tongue, and buccal mucosa with attention to masses and tenderness.

J. **Neck**

   1. **Inspection.** The examiner inspects the neck for **symmetry,** visible **masses,** and for the **normal lordotic curvature** of the cervical spine.

   2. **Range of motion** is tested by asking the patient to move the head as far as possible to the left, right, backward, and forward. The chin should reach the chest on full forward flexion.

   3. **Palpation**
      a. **Lymph nodes.** Palpation of submental, submandibular, preauricular, posterior auricular, occipital, anterior cervical, posterior cervical, supraclavicular, and infraclavicular lymph nodes is done (Figure 6-3). Palpable nodes are categorized by **size, shape, consistency** (i.e., soft, firm, or hard), **mobility,** and **tenderness**.
      b. **The carotid artery pulse** is palpated along the medial edge of the sternocleidomastoid muscle. The strength of all arterial pulses are recorded using a "plus" system: $2+/2$ = normal; $1+/2$ = diminished pulse; $0+/2$ = no palpable pulse (Table 6-1A).

   4. **Auscultation**
      a. **The carotid artery** is auscultated using the diaphragm of the stethoscope, and the presence or absence of a **bruit** is recorded.
      b. **Thyroid gland.** The examiner auscultates with the stethoscope over the thyroid gland, listening for a **vascular "hum."**

   5. **Thyroid gland**
      a. **Inspection.** The gland may be visible in thin patients or if enlarged.
      b. **Palpation.** The preferred method of palpating the thyroid gland is to have the examiner stand to the side or behind the patient and reach both hands around the neck with fingers forward. The patient is asked to swallow while the examiner feels the gland slide upward beneath his or her fingers. A sip of water helps the patient swallow. Parameters recorded are the **size, symmetry, consistency,** and the presence of **nodules** or **masses**.

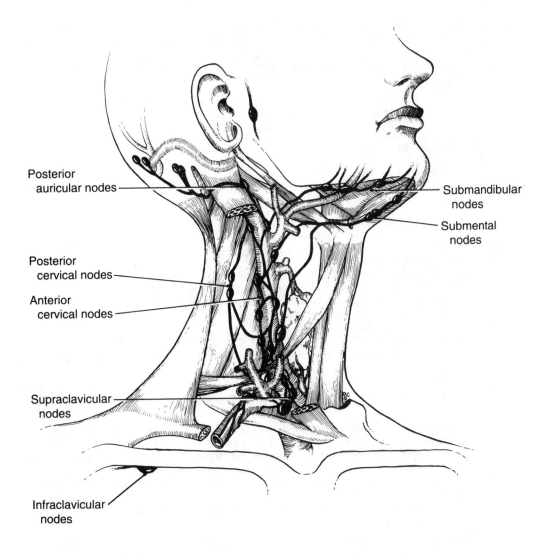

Posterior auricular nodes

Submandibular nodes

Submental nodes

Posterior cervical nodes

Anterior cervical nodes

Supraclavicular nodes

Infraclavicular nodes

Figure 6-3. Lymph nodes of the head and neck.

K. Chest and lungs

1. Inspection
   a. **The chest wall** is inspected for **symmetry** and **contour**.
   b. **The anterior-to-posterior (AP) diameter** is compared to the lateral dimension (AP should be less than lateral).
   c. **The thoracic spine** is inspected for scoliosis and exaggerated kyphosis.
   d. **The respiratory effort** is inspected, including:
      (1) Overall **ease** or **difficulty** of respiration
      (2) **Paradoxical diaphragmatic movement** (normal: diaphragm down with inspiration; abnormal: diaphragm up with inspiration)
      (3) **Use of accessory muscles,** such as trapezius, strap muscles, or sternocleidomastoids
      (4) **Intercostal muscle retractions** (abnormal)

2. Palpation
   a. **Chest wall exertion** is tested by placing the examiner's hands on the lower posterior chest wall bilaterally and asking the patient to take a deep breath. **Symmetry of movement** is noted.
   b. **Spine.** The examiner lightly **raps the vertebral processes** from the cervical to sacral spine to assess tenderness.

Table 6-1. Grading Systems Used in the Physical Examination

A. Arterial Pulses

  2 + /2 = normal strength   1 + /2 = diminished   0 + /2 = absent pulse

---

B. Cardiac Murmurs

1 + /6 = faintly audible	4 + /6 = murmur plus palpable thrill
2 + /6 = clearly audible	5 + /6 = murmur heard throughout precordium
3 + /6 = loud	6 + /6 = audible with stethoscope held off of the chest wall

---

C. Deep Tendon Reflexes

  0 + = absent
  1 + = diminished
  2 + = normal
  3 + = normal brisk
  4 + = hyperactive
  clonus = sustained reflex activity

D. Muscle Strength

  5 + /5 = normal muscle strength
  4 + /5 = slightly diminished strength
  3 + /5 = diminished strength with some movement against gravity
  2 + /5 = very diminished strength with no movement against gravity
  1 + /5 = muscle tone without movement
  0 + /5 = absent muscle strength

---

   c. Posterior **costovertebral angles** are **percussed** lightly with the side of a closed fist to elicit possible tenderness, implying renal or perirenal inflammation.
   d. **Tactile fremitus** is assessed with both hands held firmly on the chest wall, asking the patient to repeat resonating phrases, such as "99" or "blue moon."

 3. **Percussion**
   a. **Technique.** The examiner places the distal interphalangeal joint of the middle finger of the nondominant hand firmly upon the chest wall and briskly raps the joint with the flexed index finger of the dominant hand. The examiner percusses all lung fields systematically, moving from left to right to compare corresponding lung segments.
   b. **Terminology.** Acceptable terms are **dull, flat, resonant, hyperresonant,** and **tympanitic**.
   c. **Diaphragmatic excursion** is determined by percussing the location of the diaphragm posteriorly at rest and then at full inspiration. Normal excursion is 2–4 cm.

 4. **Auscultation**
   a. **Technique.** The diaphragm of the stethoscope is pressed firmly to the chest wall in the intercostal areas. All lung zones are auscultated, again moving back and forth to test for symmetry. A full examination must include auscultating anteriorly, especially at the apices and lower over the right middle lobe and lingula.
   b. **Terminology**
     (1) **Normal breath sounds** are described as **vesicular**.
     (2) **Abnormal,** or **adventitious,** sounds include:
        (a) **Crackles,** which are fine high-pitched sounds (qualitatively like hair being rubbed between two fingers), usually on inspiration
        (b) **Wheezes,** which are high-pitched sounds on expiration or inspiration
        (c) **Rhonchi,** which are coarse, variable sounds with inspiration and expiration
   c. **Vocal fremitus** is elicited by asking the patient to whisper the number "99" and assessing uniformity of sound transmission in all zones.
   d. **Egophony** ("E–A change") is tested by auscultation while the patient says a prolonged "EEEE. . . ." A solid or liquid mass will alter the transmission of the sound to an "AAAA . . ." sound.

 L. Cardiovascular examination

 1. **Arterial system.** Each artery is examined in a regional manner (e.g., carotids as part of the neck examination and renals with the abdominal examination). **Arterial insufficiency** in the extremities is indirectly assessed by noting **hair loss, skin integrity** and **ulceration, color** (red vs. cyanotic), and **capillary filling** of the nail beds.

    a. Palpation. The carotid, radial, femoral, popliteal, posterior tibial, and dorsalis pedis arteries are palpated bilaterally. A $2+/2$ system is used to record strength: $2+/2$ = normal; $1+/2$ = diminished; $0+/2$ = absent pulse (see Table 6-1A).

    b. Auscultation. The stethoscope is used to auscultate the carotid, femoral, and renal arteries to assess for bruits.

2. Venous system

    a. Inspection. Central venous pressure (CVP) can be roughly measured. The patient is placed in a recumbent position at a 30°–45° angle. A light shone tangentially over the internal jugular vein is used to identify the meniscus of the venous blood column. The vertical height of the meniscus above the manubrium is measured in centimeters. This measurement is added to 5 cm (the manubrium is considered to be a constant 5 cm above the right atrium in all positions), and the total is the CVP **(normal range: 5–8 cm H_2O).**

    b. Palpation. Superficial veins of the arms and legs, and the **deep veins** in the thigh and popliteal area, should be palpated. Pain, tenderness or palpable firmness (cords) implies thrombotic or septic phlebitis. **Homans' sign** is pain in the calf upon flexing of the leg at the ankle and is purported to show venous thrombosis. Teaching of this sign is entrenched in medical history, although its sensitivity and specificity are so poor that it has little if any clinical usefulness. Indirect measures of peripheral venous insufficiency include **edema, superficial varicose veins, skin ulceration,** and a **violaceous color** change.

3. Cardiac examination should begin with the patient supine.

    a. Palpation

        (1) Point of maximal impulse (PMI) of the apex of the heart

            (a) Normal location is approximately the 4th or 5th intercostal space in the midclavicular line.

            (b) The PMI should occupy a 1–2 cm area and be brisk and tapping in quality.

            (c) Lateral displacement or dispersement of the PMI suggests left ventricular hypertrophy.

            (d) Medial displacement, implying a vertical orientation of the heart, is seen in chronic obstructive pulmonary disease.

        (2) Precordium. The side of the examiner's hand should be placed firmly on the chest wall over the heart.

            (a) A **right ventricular heave** is appreciated over the right sternal border.

            (b) A **left ventricular lift** is palpable from the left sternal border laterally.

        (3) Over murmur. If a murmur is auscultated (see III L 3 b (4), d), the chest wall over the murmur should be palpated. A palpable murmur is called a **thrill.**

    b. Auscultation with the diaphragm, to detect high-pitched sounds, is done by pressing the stethoscope firmly to the chest wall. At least four discrete areas must be auscultated—the **2nd intercostal space on the right** and on the **left,** at the **lower left sternal border,** and at the **apex** of the heart (over the PMI).

        (1) S_1 (closure of the mitral and tricuspid valves) is best appreciated at the lower left sternal border, and its intensity and quality are recorded.

        (2) S_2 (aortic and pulmonic valve closure). The intensity, quality, and physiologic splitting of S_2 are best appreciated at the 2nd intercostal space on the left.

        (3) High-pitched **clicks** and **opening snaps** are characterized by their relation to S_1 and S_2, and the location of maximum intensity.

        (4) Murmurs are characterized by the following:

            (a) Loudness (see Table 6-1B)

            (b) Relationship to S_1 and S_2 (Table 6-2)

            (c) Location of **maximum intensity** on chest wall

            (d) Quality of sound (e.g., "blowing," "harsh," or "rumbling")

            (e) Radiation, or transmission of the murmur to the carotid arteries, the left axilla, or to the back

            (f) Change in intensity and **quality** with various maneuvers

        (5) A pericardial **rub** is described by its relation to the cardiac cycle (systole and diastole) and location on the chest wall.

    c. Auscultation with the bell of the stethoscope detects low-pitched sounds. The bell must be held lightly on the chest wall to maximize the transmission of low-pitched sound.

        (1) An S_3 **gallop** is heard in mid-diastole at the apex of the heart. An S_3 is normal in children and adolescents and abnormal in older adults (implying left ventricular dysfunction).

Table 6-2. Timing of Cardiac Murmurs

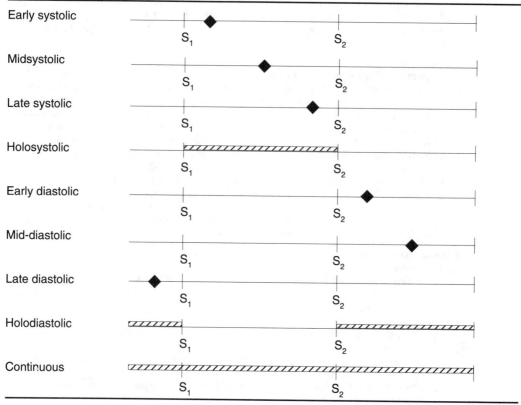

(2) An **S_4 gallop** is a presystolic sound heard best at the left lower sternal border. It reflects atrial contraction into a stiffened ventricle, seen in hypertension or as a normal finding in older adults.

(3) The **diastolic rumble** of the **mitral stenosis** murmur is best appreciated with the bell at the apex and with the patient supine or in a left lateral decubitus position.

d. **Cardiac maneuvers.** To appreciate or accentuate certain heart murmurs, various maneuvers are employed.

(1) The patient is placed in a **sitting position** with legs dangling. This intensifies the click/murmur of mitral valve prolapse and the murmur of subaortic stenosis and decreases the intensity of other murmurs.

(2) The heart is auscultated with the patient **standing**. This yields comparable results to the sitting position.

(3) The patient **sits, leans forward,** and is asked to **exhale** and **not breathe**. The examiner listens with the diaphragm in the left 2nd intercostal space. This maximizes the appreciation of an aortic insufficiency murmur.

(4) The patient is asked to **grasp the examiner's hand** and to squeeze. This accentuates regurgitant murmurs more than stenotic ones.

(5) The patient takes slow deep breaths. **Inspiration** increases the intensity of right heart murmurs, while decreasing left heart murmurs. **Expiration** accentuates left-sided murmurs.

(6) The patient is rolled partially onto his or her left side, into a left **lateral decubitus position**. Mitral stenosis, an S_3, and an S_4 can be heard in this position.

(7) The **Valsalva maneuver** intensifies mitral valve prolapse and subaortic stenosis. The patient is asked to hold his or her breath and to bear down against an open glottis.

M. Breast and pelvic examinations. See Chapter 7.

N. Axillary node examination

1. Both axillae should be palpated with the patient's arm held in a relaxed position, the examiner advances his or her fingers as far into the axillae as possible.

2. Four areas are palpated: along the chest wall medially, along the inner aspects of the anterior and posterior deltoid muscle, and laterally along the humeral head.

3. Lymphadenopathy is characterized by size, consistency, mobility, and tenderness.

O. Abdominal examination

1. **Inspection** of the abdomen includes the following:
   a. **Contour.** Acceptable terms are flat, distended, scaphoid, and protuberant.
   b. **Venous pattern.** If visible at all, this pattern extends from the groin upward. Abnormal spoke-like radiation of veins from the umbilicus is called a **caput medusa.**
   c. **Skin changes.** Refer to section on skin (III C).
   d. **Hernias.** Localized protuberance of abdominal contents occur in several areas. These are referred to as umbilical hernias, spigelian hernias (at the lateral rectus border), and inguinal hernias (direct and indirect). A femoral hernia is palpable below the inguinal ligament in the left or right anterior thigh. An incisional hernia can be seen in previous surgical scars. (For the technique of hernia examination, see Chapter 7 II C 2 c).

2. **Auscultation** should be done **before palpation** or **percussion** so as not to alter peristaltic pattern, using the diaphragm of the stethoscope. All four quadrants of the abdomen should be auscultated for regional patterns of bowel sounds.
   a. **Bowel sounds** are recorded as absent, hypoactive, normoactive, or hyperactive. Additional descriptive and qualitative terms such as "rushes," "tinkles," or "gurgles" are often used. Bowel sounds are considered "absent" only after a full 2 minutes of auscultation.
   b. **Arterial pulses.** While technically part of the cardiovascular examination, renal and femoral pulses are auscultated at this time.
      (1) **Renal artery.** The examiner listens 1 cm up from the umbilicus and 1 cm to the left and right of the midline to assess renal artery **bruits.**
      (2) **Femoral artery.** The examiner listens over the palpable femoral artery pulse bilaterally for bruits.

3. **Palpation** is done with the balls of the fingers.
   a. **Light palpation** is used to assess superficial **masses** or **tenderness** in all areas of the abdomen.
      (1) The examiner assesses the degree of **tenseness of the abdominal wall,** ranging from flaccid to hard.
      (2) A tense abdomen is further defined as revealing **voluntary** or **involuntary guarding,** based on an assessment of the patient's volitional contribution.
   b. **Deep palpation** to all areas follows, again feeling for **masses** or **tenderness.**
   c. The examiner palpates the **liver edge** by curling his or her fingers over the right anterior costal border (Figure 6-4A) and asking the patient to inhale deeply. A flattened diaphragm or an enlarged liver will place the liver edge below the costal margin (recorded in centimeters or finger-breadths below the margin). The liver edge is described as **smooth** or **nodular** and **tender** or **nontender.**
   d. The **spleen** is palpable only if enlarged. The technique requires practice (see Figure 6-4B).
      (1) The examiner's fingers are placed laterally to the outside edge of the rectus muscle, 2–3 cm below the left costal margin.
      (2) The patient is asked to take a deep breath and exhale. During expiration, the examiner advances his or her fingers moderately deep as the abdominal muscles relax.
      (3) With the fingers held steady, the patient takes a second deep breath, and the examiner appreciates the firm spleen moving caudally and striking the fingers.
      (4) A useful maneuver is asking the patient to rotate moderately to the right (right lateral decubitus), which is best done by having the patient place his hand beneath his left buttock.
   e. The **abdominal aortic pulse** is palpated in the midline. The transverse width of the pulse is estimated. A widened palpable pulse implies an **aneurysmal dilatation of the aorta**.
   f. Any **visible hernia** is palpated to evaluate for **tenderness** or **reducibility.**

4. **Percussion**
   a. **Light percussion** is useful to assess **tenderness.**

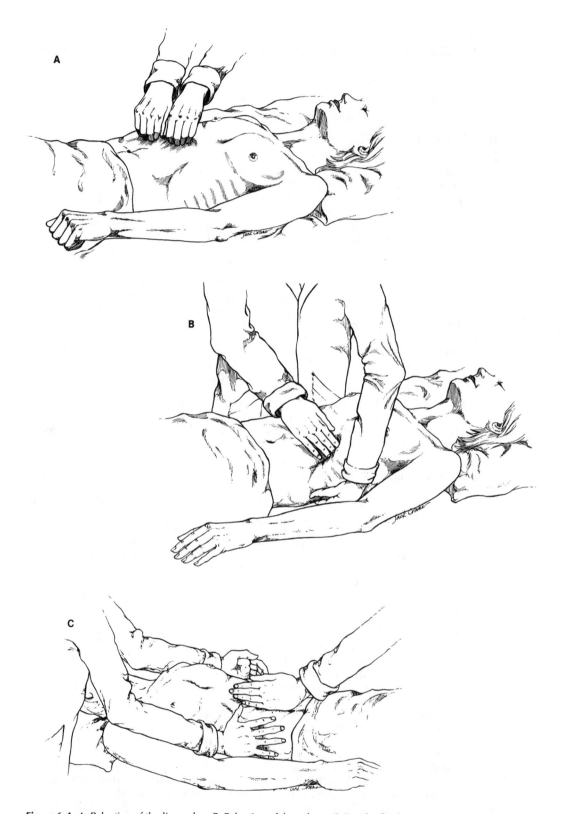

Figure 6-4. *A,* Palpation of the liver edge. *B,* Palpation of the spleen. *C,* Test for fluid wave. Examiner taps left flank while feeling at the right flank for a fluid wave.

    b. The **liver span** is determined by percussing in the midclavicular line from the chest down to the abdomen. The upper and lower edges should be clearly distinguishable from contiguous lung and abdominal structures. The span is recorded in centimeters (normal is 8–12 cm for adults).

    c. The upper edge of the **bladder** can be appreciated by percussion, especially if full or distended.

    d. The **stomach air bubble** is percussed as a tympanitic area in the left upper quadrant. Increased bowel gas will produce a more diffusely tympanitic abdomen.

    e. Percussion is a useful technique to detect an **enlarged spleen,** which may not be palpable. The examiner percusses laterally in the left upper quadrant, while the patient takes slow, deep breaths. A change in pitch is appreciated (from resonant to dull) as the solid spleen glides downward beneath the examiner's fingers on inspiration.

5. Additional maneuvers

    a. Rebound tenderness should be tested in patients with abdominal pain. The examiner compresses the abdomen with the fingers and quickly withdraws the hand. A positive finding is pain, often remote from the area palpated that is worsened upon the rapid withdrawal of the examiner's hand. A positive finding implies peritoneal inflammation, but this is of questionable validity.

    b. Ascitic fluid within the abdominal cavity is detectable by specific testing. The methods include:

        (1) Shifting dullness. The right side of the abdomen is percussed to establish a level of dullness at the flank. The patient is then rolled into the right lateral decubitus position, and percussion is repeated. In the presence of fluid, the level of dullness will "shift" upward on the abdominal wall.

        (2) Fluid wave. The patient or an assistant is asked to hold the edge of his or her hand firmly in the midline of the abdomen. The examiner briskly taps one side of the abdomen while feeling the other side with his or her hand. Ascites will be felt as a "fluid wave" transmitted from side to side (see Figure 6-4C).

    c. Murphy's sign is elicited by a thumb pressed firmly in the right upper quadrant in the midclavicular line 2 cm below the costal margin. A positive sign is pain on deep inspiration and implies gallbladder inflammation or irritation.

P. Male genitalia (see Chapter 7 II C)

Q. Rectal examination (see Chapter 7 II C)

R. Musculoskeletal examination

    1. The musculature of the upper and lower extremities is inspected with reference to size, contour, and symmetry. Muscle strength is conventionally tested as part of the neurologic examination (see III T).

    2. All joints are inspected for deformities, edema, erythema, or warmth.

    3. Passive **range of motion** is tested by the examiner actively moving each joint in all possible directions with only the patient's "passive" cooperation. The extent of movement is recorded. Restriction is recorded by degrees of movement (e.g., knee flexion restricted to 120°).

S. Back examination

    1. Inspection

        a. The entire back is **inspected for contour**.

        (1) Normal cervical and lumbar lordosis is noted.

        (2) Abnormal thoracic kyphosis and scoliosis are described by degree of deformity.

        b. Back range-of-motion is assessed with the patient standing. Flexion, extension, hyperextension, and lateral and rotary (twist) mobility are passively tested.

    2. Palpation

        a. The **sacral area** is palpated for edema, especially in bedridden patients.

        b. The **entire spine** is percussed to test for tenderness.

T. Neurologic examination

    1. Mental status examination. Orientation is tested in reference to **person** ("What is your name?"), **place** ("Where are we now?"), and **time** (day, date, month, and year). For a more detailed mental status examination, see Chapter 7 V.

2. **Cranial nerves** are formally tested in a rapid but thorough fashion.
   a. **CN I.** When indicated, the sense of smell is tested, using a common substance, such as soap. Caustic liquids, such as alcohol, may stimulate pain fibers and are not a true test of smell sensation.
   b. **CN II.** This nerve is tested in the eye examination.
   c. **CN III.** Pupillary responses and extraocular movements are tested in the eye examination (see III F 3 c).
   d. **CN IV and VI.** For extraocular movements, see III F.
   e. **CN V**
      (1) **Sensory.** Pinprick and light touch sensations are tested bilaterally for all three nerve branches: the ophthalmic, maxillary, and mandibular branches.
      (2) **Motor.** The muscles of mastication are palpated while the patient chews and are compared bilaterally.
   f. **CN VII.** The facial musculature is tested by the following:
      (1) The patient is asked to raise both eyebrows, and movement is assessed for symmetry.
      (2) The patient is asked to clench the eyes shut, and the examiner attempts to open each eye by retracting the lower lid.
      (3) The patient is asked to smile naturally and then to grimace and is observed for symmetry.
   g. **CN VIII.** See III G 3.
   h. **CN IX and X**
      (1) These are indirectly tested by a history of normal swallowing and phonation.
      (2) Directly, the movement of the uvula is observed during the mouth examination.
      (3) The gag reflex is elicited by pressing a tongue blade to the base of the tongue or to the posterior pharynx.
   i. **CN XI**
      (1) The sternocleidomastoid muscle strength is tested by having the patient turn his or her head to one side, and forcibly turning the head back to midline against the examiner's hand. This should be repeated on the opposite side.
      (2) Trapezius muscle strength is tested by asking the patient to shrug shoulders against resistance of examiner's hands.
   j. **CN XII**
      (1) The tongue is projected out and directed to the left and to the right.
      (2) The patient is asked to press his or her tongue into one cheek and then the other while the examiner feels from outside the mouth, assessing for strength in each direction.

3. **Muscle strength**
   a. Each muscle group must be tested individually and compared in strength to its contralateral counterpart.
   b. Muscle groups to be tested include: shoulder (flexion, extension, abduction, and adduction); biceps, triceps, and wrist (flexion and extension); interosseous muscles in the hand and grip strength; hips (flexion and extension); quadriceps, hamstrings, and ankle (flexion and extension); and toe (flexion and extension).
   c. This technique is best accomplished with the patient supine. The examiner provides active resistance against the patient's movements.
   d. Strength is recorded using a 5 + system (see Table 6-1D).

4. **Sensory examination**
   a. **Light touch** is tested by using a fluffed cotton swab, which is brushed lightly against the skin.
      (1) The face (CN V), forearms, arms, legs, and feet should be tested.
      (2) The examiner asks the patient to compare the sensation from one side to another on comparable sites.
   b. **Pain sensation** is tested in the same distribution and manner as light touch.
      (1) A broken tongue blade or cotton swab stick are suitably sharp objects to test for pain perception.
      (2) To minimize spread of blood-borne infection (e.g., hepatitis or human immunodeficiency virus), a pin or needle should not be used.
   c. **Vibratory sensation** is tested using a 128 Hz tuning fork.
      (1) The fork is struck, and the base is held to various joints, such as the elbow, knuckles of the hand, knee, ankle, and great toe.
      (2) The patient is asked to compare sensation from left to right.

(3) As a more quantitative technique, the examiner places his or her finger beneath the joint being tested and asks the patient to state when the sensation ceases. With the examiner serving as a control, mild deficits can be identified.

d. **Joint position sense** is tested in the thumb and great toe bilaterally with the patient's eyes closed. The examiner grasps the digit on the sides, moves the joint up and down, and then asks the patient to state where the joint has come to rest (i.e., up, middle, or down).

5. **Deep tendon reflexes** are tested using a rubber hammer, struck briskly against a tendon or muscle sheath. Reflexes can be suppressed by a tense or anxious patient. Isometric exercises, such as a hand grasp, can be used to override this and increase the reflex response. The examiner should note the extent and rapidity of the contraction and relaxation of the muscle and not the jerking of its attendant joint. The grading system is found in Table 6-1C. The following reflexes are tested:

a. **Biceps reflex** is tested with the arm held at approximately 90°. The examiner moderately compresses the biceps tendon with his or her thumb and strikes the thumb with the hammer.

b. **Triceps reflex** is also tested with the arm at 90°. The tendon insertion just above the elbow is struck.

c. The **brachioradialis** muscle head is struck just below the elbow.

d. The patellar tendon is struck just below the patella. The leg should be in a relaxed position.

e. The ankle jerk is elicited by striking the Achilles tendon sharply, while the foot is held by the examiner in a flexed position.

6. **Cerebellar examination**

a. **Rapid alternating movements.** The patient is asked to slap his or her thigh as rapidly as possible, while alternating from palmar to dorsal surface. Rapidity and coordination of movement are reported.

b. **Finger-to-nose.** The examiner holds an index finger in front of the patient and asks the patient to alternately touch the finger and his or her own nose. The examiner moves his or her finger three dimensionally in front of the patient to assess spatial orientation. Accuracy of movement is recorded. The test is done bilaterally.

c. **Heel-to-shin.** The patient places the heel of one leg on the shin of the other, then draws the heel up and down the tibia. If the patient is unable to retain heel on shin accurately, the test is considered positive.

d. **Romberg reflex.** The patient is asked to stand with hands held slightly out at the sides and then to close his or her eyes. The examiner should be prepared to support the patient if he or she loses balance. Inability to balance with eyes open and closed is suggestive of cerebellar dysfunction, while losing balance only with eyes closed is more indicative of posterior column disease.

7. **Abnormal reflexes**

a. **The Babinski reflex** tests the integrity of the pyramidal tract (Figure 6-5).

(1) The sole of each foot is stroked with a blunt object (e.g., tongue blade or base of a reflex hammer).

(2) The stroke begins at the lateral heel, up along the lateral plantar surface of the foot, and then in the medial direction along the metatarsal heads.

(3) The examiner watches the great toe for its initial movement.

(4) The **normal movement,** or a **negative Babinski reflex,** is an initial downward reflex of the great toe.

(5) An **abnormal movement,** or **positive Babinski reflex,** is an upward deflection of the great toe.

(6) Fanning or withdrawal of the other toes is irrelevant.

b. **Chaddock reflex** (performed only if the Babinski reflex is equivocal)

(1) This reflex also tests the integrity of the pyramidal system.

(2) The dorsal lateral surface of the foot is stroked with a blunt object.

(3) A positive, abnormal sign is dorsiflexion of the great toe.

c. **Oppenheim test**

(1) This test is equivalent to Babinski in implication and interpretation.

(2) The examiner rubs firmly along the tibia from knee to ankle and observes the great toe movement.

d. **Hoffmann's reflex**

(1) This tests the pyramidal track in the upper extremity.

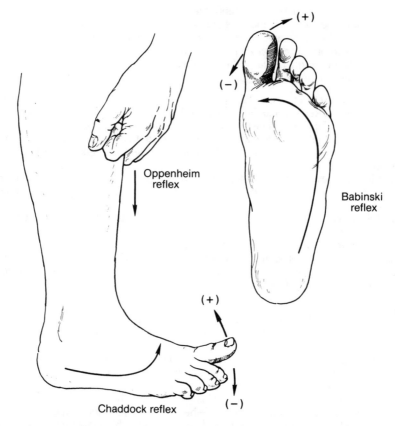

Figure 6-5. Babinski reflex, Oppenheim reflex, and Chaddock reflex.

(2) The middle finger is extended, and the nail is rapidly flicked by the examiner to hyperextend it.

(3) The thumb is observed; inward movement is normal (negative Hoffmann's sign), and outward movement is abnormal.

e. Frontal release signs are a group of primitive reflexes that are normal in infancy but whose presence in an adult imply frontal lobe disease. They include:

(1) Grasp reflex is a grasping movement of the patient's hand as the examiner draws his or her finger along the palm.

(2) Palmomental reflex is elicited by drawing a finger through the patient's palm (from thumb toward fifth finger) and observing a contraction of the mentalis muscle of the chin.

(3) Snout reflex is tested by gently tapping the middle portion of the patient's upper lip and observing for a puckering or snouting of the mouth.

(4) Glabellar reflex is elicited by tapping the midforehead with the finger. A normal response is a few blinks, then cessation of blinking. An abnormal sign is continued blinking with repeated tapping.

(5) Rooting reflex is tested by stroking the cheek from the mouth laterally and watching for a retraction of the mouth or turning of the head toward the stroke.

8. Gait

a. The patient is asked to walk back and forth in usual gait, while the examiner inspects coordination, fluidity, and symmetry of movement.

b. The patient is asked to walk on toes to test for coordination and peripheral muscle strength.

c. Heel-walk is similarly tested.

d. Tandem walk with one foot placed directly in front of the other tests strength and cerebellar function.

IV. SCREENING, OR PERIODIC EXAMINATION. A history and a physical examination make up this "routine physical," which is performed for a healthy, asymptomatic adult. The concept of this examination has been well-established for over 50 years. Its purpose, frequency, emphasis, and inclusion of various tests are discussed as follows:

A. Purpose. These routine, comprehensive examinations fulfill many explicit and implicit functions, simultaneously.

1. **Detecting asymptomatic disease.** Many diseases can be controlled or cured if they are discovered early; for example:
   a. Hypertension
   b. Anemia
   c. Certain cancers (e.g., breast, cervical, endometrial, prostate)

2. **Establishing rapport** between the patient and clinician (see Chapter 2). The patient's health care beliefs and baseline responses to symptoms (from stoic to histrionic) can be determined.

3. **Establishing "normal" physical criteria** for the patient with which subsequent symptomatic episodes can be compared.

4. **Identifying and modifying health risks** to promote wellness, such as:
   a. Smoking habits, alcohol use, and sexual behavior
   b. Diet and exercise

5. **Expanding the "clean bill of health"** to include a more active participation of clinician and patient in disease prevention.

B. Age-dependent frequency of periodic examinations. While different schedules are proposed by different groups, a reasonable schedule is as follows:

1. A complete examination should be performed first in early adulthood (age 18–20 years) and then every 5 years until age 40.

2. Since many diseases become more prevalent with age, the interval should be shortened to every 2–3 years from 40–65 years of age.

3. After 65 years of age, patients should be examined every year for life.

C. Physical aspect of the periodic examination. Special emphasis should be placed on **seven areas**. (Examination of these areas may be required more frequently than routinely scheduled periodic examinations.)

1. **Blood pressure.** Early detection and treatment of hypertension has been shown to **reduce risks** of **stroke, congestive heart failure,** and **renal disease**. Early hypertension is invariably asymptomatic.

2. **Hearing.** Detection of subclinical hearing loss can lead to risk modification (i.e., reducing occupational exposure) and, therefore, slowing of disease progression.

3. **Vision.** Problems with vision are common and, in most instances, easily corrected. For example, tonometry can detect asymptomatic glaucoma and is useful as a screening test in subgroups of patients.

4. **Teeth and gingivae.** Early treatment of caries and gingivitis as well as preventive care are highly effective.

5. **Breasts.** Early detection and treatment of breast cancer, particularly in asymptomatic women, has been shown to significantly improve morbidity and mortality.
   a. A complete examination is recommended every 2–3 years for all women under age 40 and yearly thereafter.
   b. A mammogram is recommended yearly in women over age 40.
   c. The examination should be coupled with self-examination instruction.

6. **Pelvic examination (including a Pap smear)**
   a. Both cervical and endometrial cancers are common, easily treated, and potentially curable when detected early.
   b. Schedules for frequency of examinations vary from yearly by the American College of Obstetricians and Gynecologists (ACOG) to every 2–3 years by the American Cancer Society (ACS).

7. **Rectum (including stool guaiac)**
   a. **Routine yearly rectal examinations** are recommended in all patients over age 40 to detect rectal masses and prostatic nodules.
   b. **Stool guaiac test** for occult blood is recommended as a screening procedure for colorectal cancer.
   c. Although controversial, **routine flexible sigmoidoscopy** is advocated by some at intervals of every 3–5 years after two negative examinations 1 year apart for asymptomatic patients over age 40.

D. **Inclusion of various tests.** There are very limited recommendations for screening blood tests at the time of the periodic examination.

   1. A **lipid profile** (e.g., serum cholesterol, triglycerides, high-density lipoprotein [HDL]) is the only laboratory value that is uniformly advocated.

   2. **Serum hemoglobin and hematocrit** should be obtained in a menstruating female.

   3. **Thyroid function** studies in women over age 60 are advocated by some clinicians.

   4. **Routine chest x-ray** should not be included.

V. PROBLEM-ORIENTED PHYSICAL EXAMINATION

A. **Components of a directed examination.** A complete physical examination is performed for a periodic health assessment or upon admission to a hospital, but many clinical encounters demand a more focused examination.

   1. **Clinical setting.** Most routine office visits, emergency room visits, and other situations requiring efficiency necessitate a directed examination.

   2. **Organ system focus.** The physical examination should be directed at the organ systems suggested by the chief complaint and the history of the present illness. The examiner must make a prioritized problem list and decide which components of the physical examination to include. The examination should be complete enough to encompass the major systems suggested by the history but not too exhaustive as to be inefficient. This requires skill in medical decision-making, creating a differential diagnosis, and assigning a probability to each disorder.

   3. **Associated organ systems.** Complete vital signs should be a part of every physical examination, regardless of symptoms. Other more remote components of the physical examination need to be included if they are particularly clinically important (e.g., peripheral pulses in a patient with abdominal pain to exclude a dissecting aortic aneurysm).

B. **Clinical examples**

   1. In the evaluation of a patient with shortness of breath, particular attention should be given to vital signs, neck veins, a thorough chest, lung and cardiac examination, and to the extremities (e.g., clubbing, cyanosis, edema).

   2. A history of a headache and stiff neck should generate an examination focused on vital signs, eye and funduscopic examination, neck range of motion, and a thorough neurologic examination.

C. **Limitations of the directed physical examination.** The directed examination is useful to confirm clinical suspicions derived from the medical history. It is by design not comprehensive, making its negative predictive value or ability to exclude disease relatively poor. In a focused examination that fails to identify positive findings, the examiner must reassess the patient's symptoms and redirect the examination.

REFERENCES

Bates B: *A Guide to Physical Examination and History Taking,* 5th ed. Philadelphia, JB Lippincott, 1987

Judge RD, Zvidens GD, Fitzgerald FT: *Clinical Diagnosis: A Psychological Approach,* 5th ed. Boston, Little, Brown, 1989

United States Preventive Services Task Force: *Guide to Clinical Preventive Services.* Baltimore, Williams & Wilkins, 1989

STUDY QUESTIONS

Directions: Each of the numbered items or incomplete statements in this section is followed by answers or by completions of the statement. Select the **one** lettered answer or completion that is **best** in each case.

1. The patient should be in a seated position for which of the following components of the examination?

(A) Auscultation of the heart with the bell of the stethoscope
(B) Examination of the male genitalia
(C) Inspection of the female breast
(D) Palpation of the abdomen
(E) Percussion of the abdomen

2. A patient is brought to the emergency room in January after being found comatose in a snow bank. An electronic thermometer records a rectal temperature of 94° F. Which of the following statements about this patient's temperature is true?

(A) An oral thermometer would measure core body temperature more accurately
(B) A mercury thermometer would be less accurate than an electronic thermometer
(C) The temperature should be confirmed with an oral temperature reading
(D) The true temperature may actually be above 94° F
(E) A special probe should be used in cases of potential hypothermia

3. A 75-year-old man presents for a complete physical examination. Detailed inspection of the skin includes a description of all of the following EXCEPT

(A) skin color
(B) hair distribution
(C) skin turgor
(D) skin lesions
(E) abnormal pigmentation

4. All of the following statements are true regarding the thyroid examination EXCEPT

(A) a gland that is palpable is abnormal
(B) the preferred position is for the examiner to reach both hands around the neck with the fingers forward
(C) upon swallowing, the gland should slide upward
(D) a vascular hum heard with the stethoscope implies hyperactivity of the gland
(E) a normal gland may be visible by inspection

5. An 18-year-old patient with a long history of asthma presents to an emergency room in marked respiratory distress. All of the following physical findings are likely to be present EXCEPT

(A) the diaphragm moves upward with inspiration
(B) the respiratory rate is 16
(C) the patient uses the trapezius muscles on inspiration
(D) intercostal muscle retractions are noted
(E) the patient is cyanotic

6. A patient presents with a history of an irregular heart beat. All of the following procedures are correct EXCEPT

(A) the radial pulse should be palpated for 30 seconds
(B) the stethoscope should be used to auscultate the apex of the heart
(C) the radial pulse rate should be contrasted to the apical heart rate
(D) the carotid pulse can be palpated and used to replace the radial pulse
(E) a complete cardiac examination should be performed

7. All of the following findings support venous disease in the lower extremities EXCEPT

(A) pale cool extremities bilaterally
(B) a deep purple color
(C) bilateral edema to the knees
(D) bilateral tibial ulcers
(E) a palpable cord in the right popliteal fossa

8. In what order should the abdominal examination sequence proceed?

(A) Inspection, auscultation, palpation, percussion
(B) Inspection, palpation, auscultation, percussion
(C) Inspection, palpation, percussion, auscultation
(D) Inspection, percussion, auscultation, palpation
(E) Palpation, auscultation, inspection, percussion

9. The effectiveness of the spleen examination is improved by all of the following factors EXCEPT

(A) a thin patient
(B) asking the patient to take slow deep breaths
(C) advancing the examiners fingers on expiration
(D) asking the patient to roll on the left lateral decubitus
(E) asking the patient to place his or her left hand under the left buttocks

10. Tests of cerebellar function include all the following EXCEPT

(A) rapid alternating movements
(B) finger-to-nose
(C) heel-to-chin
(D) Romberg reflex
(E) deep tendon reflexes

11. A 30-year-old asymptomatic woman presents for a routine physical examination. A comprehensive periodic health evaluation for this patient should include all of the following EXCEPT

(A) a blood pressure recording
(B) a complete breast examination
(C) a pelvic examination and Pap smear
(D) a flexible sigmoidoscopy
(E) counseling on smoking and alcohol use

12. All of the following statements are true concerning a directed physical examination EXCEPT

(A) the vital signs should be included
(B) the organ systems examined are determined by the chief complaint and the history of the present illness
(C) it is an effective way to exclude disease
(D) the examiner should make a differential diagnosis and examine the patient in a prioritized manner
(E) if positive findings are not found, the examiner should reassess symptoms and redirect the examination

ANSWERS AND EXPLANATIONS

1. The answer is C. [*II D 1 a–d*] The breast examination begins in the seated position to inspect for symmetry and retractions. The bell of the stethoscope is used to listen for an S_3, S_4, and a mitral stenosis murmur. All of these are best done in the supine or left lateral decubitus position. The male genital examination should be done in the standing position to detect hernias. The entire abdominal examination is done in the supine position to decrease muscle tone and maximize access to the abdominal contents.

2. The answer is E. [*III B 3*] Electronic or mercury thermometers are equally effective in measuring temperature, but the preferred method of measuring core body temperature is a rectal thermometer. The limitation of an electronic thermometer is that it does not record temperatures below 94° F. Therefore, a special probe must be used in cases of suspected hypothermia as the true temperature of the patient described in the question may be below 94° F.

3. The answer is C. [*III C 1, 2*] Skin turgor is determined by palpation. Turgor is determined by gently compressing the skin between the thumb and forefinger and releasing. Skin color, hair distribution, abnormal pigmentation and the presence or absence of skin lesions are all determined by inspection.

4. The answer is A. [*III J 4 b, 5 a, b*] A normal gland may be visible and sometimes palpable, especially in thin patients. The preferred position for examination is with the examiner in the back or on the side of the patient. Normal glands should slide upward upon swallowing. In hyperthyroidism, a vascular hum can be heard, implying increased vascular blood flow.

5. The answer is B. [*III K 1*] A young patient in respiratory distress should have a respiratory rate far higher than 16. All other physical symptoms described are consistent with someone in respiratory distress. Trapezius and intercostal muscles are recruited to aid respiration when the patient has a respiratory compromise. Cyanosis is a physical sign, indicating lack of oxygenation.

6. The answer is A. [*III L 1, 3*] Patients with an irregularly irregular heart beat require a thorough cardiovascular evaluation, including a complete cardiac examination. Either the radial pulse or the carotid pulse can be palpated for a minimum of 60 seconds. This should be contrasted to the apical heart rate as heard by auscultation with the stethoscope, since some arrhythmias present with a pulse deficit as recorded peripherally.

7. The answer is A. [*III L 1, 2*] Pale cool extremities suggest arterial insufficiency. Venous insufficiency presents with edema, a violaceous hue, and in severe cases, with skin ulceration. A deep venous thrombosis is suggested by a palpable cord in the popliteal area.

8. The answer is A. [*III O 1–4*] A careful detailed inspection should be the first component of every examination. The examination sequence for the abdominal examination differs from that of the chest or cardiac examination. Auscultation must come before palpation and percussion. Palpation and percussion may alter bowel sounds (i.e., decrease or increase their intensity). Auscultating first gives a more accurate representation of true bowel sounds.

9. The answer is D. [*III O 3 d*] Even normal spleens may be palpable in a thin patient. The technique of the examination is to have the patient take slow deep breaths and advancing fingers on expiration. The spleen becomes easier to palpate if the patient rolls to the right lateral decubitus position or places his or her left hand under the left buttock.

10. The answer is E. [*III T 6*] Careful examination of cerebellar function includes testing arms, legs, and gait. Rapid alternating movements and finger-to-nose both test upper extremity coordination. Heel-to-chin measures lower extremity cerebellar function. Romberg reflex and gait test overall cerebellar function. Deep tendon reflexes do not test cerebellar functions.

11. The answer is D. [*IV A, C*] The purpose of a comprehensive periodic health examination is to detect asymptomatic diseases for which the patient is at high risk as well as providing an opportunity for health risk identification and counseling. Blood pressure recording is recommended for all age-groups. A menstruating female should have a yearly breast examination and a biannual pelvic examination and Pap smear. Counseling on health risk, such as smoking and alcohol use, are crucial. While the recommendation for flexible sigmoidoscopy is controversial, the asymptomatic patients should not begin routine sigmoidoscopies until age 40 or 50.

12. The answer is C. [*V C*] The directed physical examination is designed to maximize efficiency. Vital signs are a crucial component of every examination. The examiner must determine which organs to examine based on the chief complaint and the history of the present illness. After making a differential diagnosis, the organ systems suggested by the differential should be examined. If positive findings are not found, the process must begin again. This is a very poor method to exclude disease, since it is not inclusive by nature.

7
Special Problems with the Physical Examination

Linnie Newman, Janice L. Willms
Henry Schneiderman, Anthony J. Ardolino

I. INTRODUCTION. In the course of mastering the conduct of a physical examination, the clinician will encounter circumstances under which special maneuvers, particular sensitivities, or patient disabilities require unique attention or deviation from the ordinary routine. This chapter considers three special problems in the physical examination: examining parts of the body that are not normally exposed to strangers (e.g., the breast, genital, and rectal regions), examining impaired individuals (e.g., physically disabled, mentally impaired, and bedridden patients), and using the mental status examination.

II. BREAST AND GENITAL EXAMINATIONS

A. Breast examination

1. **Overview.** For many women, the breast examination is as intrusive as the pelvic examination. Clinicians must be sensitive to these feelings and help their patients maintain control and modesty.
   a. **History.** The clinician should obtain a history of breast disease, breast cancer risk factors, and patient concerns before beginning the examination.
   b. **Content of examination.** The examination consists of inspection and palpation of the breasts and nipples and palpation of the axillae.
   c. **Placement in sequence.** In the course of a complete physical examination, the breast inspection most logically comes at the end of the sitting pulmonary examination; the palpation comes at the beginning of the supine examination. (See Chapter 6 II D for a discussion of ''sequencing.'')

2. **Inspection** of the breasts is done with the patient seated. The patient is asked to take her arms out of the gown and expose both breasts.
   a. **With arms raised.** The patient is asked to raise both arms over her head, enabling the examiner to inspect the breasts for:
      (1) **Symmetrical elevation**
      (2) The presence or absence of **skin retraction**
      (3) **Position** and **movement** of the **nipples** and **areolae**
   b. **With hands on hips.** The patient is asked to place her hands on her hips and press down. This tenses the pectoralis muscles and accentuates abnormal attachments of skin and glandular tissue to the underlying muscle fascia, enabling the clinician to inspect for:
      (1) **Symmetry of elevation** of the breasts as the muscles are contracted
      (2) **Dimpling of the skin** or asymmetric ''**tugging**'' at the **nipples**

3. **Palpation**
   a. **Positioning the patient.** The intent is to spread the breast tissue over the greatest chest wall area. Palpation is best done with the patient in a supine position.
      (1) **Each breast is palpated individually.** The breast being examined must be fully exposed; however, the other breast may be covered by the patient's gown.
      (2) The arm on the side that is being examined is raised and placed under the patient's head.
      (3) If the breasts are large, the examination is facilitated by placing a pillow or folded towel under the shoulder on the side to be examined.
      (4) The examiner may remain on the patient's right side for examination of both breasts.

    b. Technique of palpation. Important considerations for adequate palpation of the breast include:

        (1) A system that guarantees that all portions of the breast are palpated thoroughly. The examiner must keep in mind that breast tissue may extend high into the anterior axillary line and palpation should include the ''tail'' of the breast (Figure 7-1A).

        (2) The use of the palmar surfaces of the fingers rather than the fingertips to avoid ''jumping'' over tissue irregularities

        (3) Warm and gentle hands

    c. Three modes of palpation

        (1) Spokes. With this system, the breast is palpated from the nipple outward in the pattern of the spokes of a wheel (Figure 7-1B).

        (2) Spiral (concentric circle). Beginning with the areola, the palpation is conducted in an ever enlarging spiral until the entire breast, including the tail, has been examined (Figure 7-1C).

        (3) Quadrants. This method, appropriate only with relatively small breasts, divides the area to be examined into quadrants, each of which is palpated systematically. Again, it is important to extend the examination of the upper outer quadrant cephalad until breast tissue is no longer felt (Figure 7-1D).

4. Examination of the nipples. The **subareolar** areas, including nipples, are usually examined independently of the remainder of the breast.

    a. Subareolar tissue. After completion of the palpation of the peripheral glandular tissue, the subareolar tissue is palpated by gentle downward pressure, appreciating the slight depression under the areola in which the lacteal ducts collect as they enter the nipple.

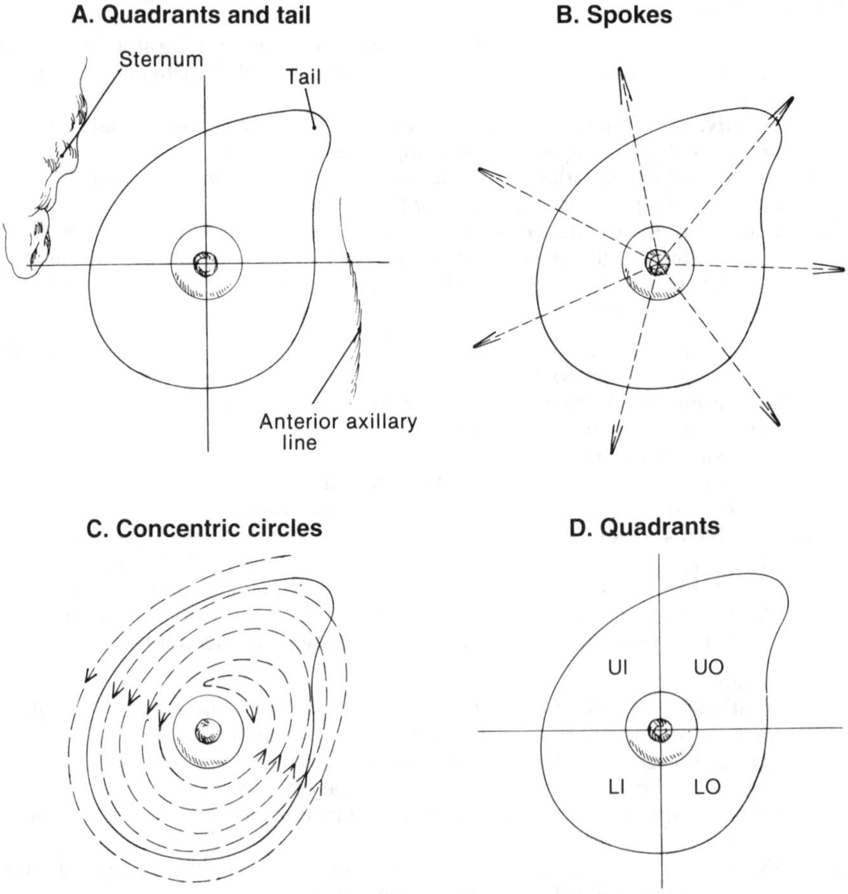

A. Quadrants and tail

Sternum

Tail

Anterior axillary line

B. Spokes

C. Concentric circles

D. Quadrants

UI | UO

LI | LO

Figure 7-1. Techniques of breast palpation. *A,* Quadrants and tail (left breast); *B,* spokes; *C,* concentric circles; and *D,* quadrants.

   b. Subnipple tissue. The examination must include the tissue directly beneath the nipple itself.

   c. Nipple secretion. The final step in the nipple examination is an attempt to express secretion.

     (1) The base of the nipple is secured between the examiner's index and middle fingers, and with a milking motion, the fingers compress the areola and nipple proximally to distally.

     (2) This compression along the course of the ductile tissue will bring any secretions in the terminal ducts to the surface of the nipple (Figure 7-2).

     (3) A gentle, continuous, milking motion provides the most information with the least discomfort to the patient.

5. Axillary examination (see Chapter 6 III N) is usually conducted before the patient is placed in the supine position. It is intended not only as a part of the breast examination but is necessary to determine the status of the lymph nodes.

6. Teaching breast self-examination. It is the examiner's responsibility to determine if the patient has been adequately trained in self-examination by asking the patient to demonstrate her technique.

   a. Observation. The patient should know how to observe her breasts for symmetry of movement (see II A 2) while facing a mirror.

   b. Palpation. Self-palpation should follow one of the three modes described in II A 3 c.

   c. Timing of self-examination. The patient should be reminded to do the examination monthly at the end of a menstrual period if she is still menstruating.

   d. Regions of abnormality. If the examiner has discovered variations of normal or fibrocystic changes in the patient's breast, the patient should be made aware of these areas.

   e. Reporting changes. The patient should be asked to demonstrate that she can locate cysts or cords and instructed as to what she should report in the way of changes.

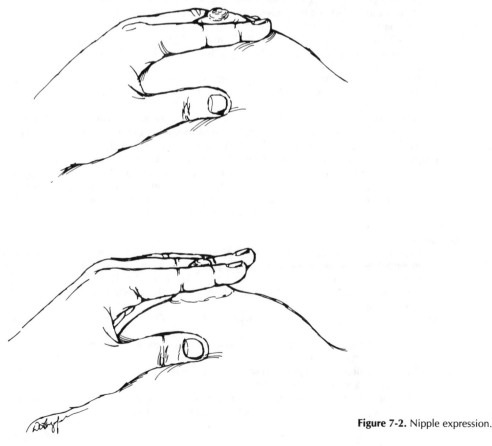

Figure 7-2. Nipple expression.

    f. Patient's questions. Any questions the patient may have regarding the conduct of her self-examination should be answered, and she should be provided with, or referred to, the excellent publications of the American Cancer Society on breast self-examination.

  7. Male breast examination. Dangerous disease of the male breast is rare. Transient enlargement is occasionally seen in adolescent boys. Breast tissue develops in adult men in the presence of high blood estrogen levels, such as those accompanying cirrhosis of the liver or exogenous estrogen treatment for prostatic cancer.

    a. When **inspection** of the anterior chest wall reveals **visible breast tissue,** the male breast should be palpated as described in II A 3.

    b. In the case of normal-appearing nipples **without visible breast tissue,** time should be taken to **palpate** the **areola** with gentle downward pressure.

B. Female pelvic examination

  1. Introduction. Both the patient and the clinician bring certain feelings and concerns to the pelvic examination. The woman brings her own past experience and experiences related to her by other women. Although some women say the pelvic examination is painful, more often they express a sense of embarrassment, vulnerability, and lack of control.

    Student clinicians are concerned about hurting the patient, being inept, and not recognizing pathology. Performing the pelvic examination may make the student feel that he or she is invading the patient's privacy. It may also induce feelings of embarrassment, fears of sexual arousal or revulsion, or a disruption of the physician–patient relationship. Clinicians need to be aware of their own feelings and deal with them in a constructive manner so that they do not interfere with the effective conduct of the examination.

  2. General approach

    a. Principles and preparation

      (1) Before beginning the pelvic examination, unless a complete physical is indicated, the clinician should check the patient's blood pressure and do heart, lung, breast, and abdominal examinations.

      (2) Even if the patient voided before the history and physical examination, the clinician should give her the opportunity to empty her bladder before beginning the pelvic examination.

      (3) The pelvic examination should be performed at the end of the physical examination. It is common courtesy that the woman be allowed to dress before a final discussion with the clinician.

      (4) In the hospital, if the pelvic examination is deferred for any reason, it is the clinician's responsibility to see that the patient has an examination before leaving the hospital if she has not been examined within an appropriate time period.

    b. Equipment. It is essential to have all necessary equipment ready before the patient is positioned, including a lamp, cotton swabs or a Cytobrush, fixative, nonsterile gloves, wooden spatula, water-soluble lubricant, speculum, slides for Pap smear, stirrup pads, hand-held mirror, pencil, and Hemoccult card. This includes duplicates of everything so that the clinician or chaperon does not need to delay the examination while the patient is in the lithotomy position.

    c. Language

      (1) Jargon. The clinician should use language appropriate to the woman's education and medical knowledge and avoid medical jargon. From talking with the patient during the history, the clinician should have a basis from which to start. The clinician should define medical terms [e.g., uterus (womb)] until he or she is sure that the patient understands what is being said.

      (2) Words to avoid. There are certain words, which may have a negative connotation for the patient.

        (a) Poor choice: "I am going to stick the speculum into you." **Alternative:** "I am going to insert the speculum."

        (b) Poor choice: "I am going to scrape some cells for the Pap smear. **Alternative:** "I am going to do the Pap test now."

        (c) Poor choice: "Let me know if the examination causes you any pain." **Alternative:** "If for any reason you want me to stop, let me know."

      (d) Poor choice: "Relax." **Alternative:** No words are necessary. The clinician pro-
motes relaxation by establishing rapport, maintaining eye contact, and keeping
the patient informed about what is to be done next.

   (3) Talk before touching. The clinician should always tell the patient what will happen
before the fact. There should be an explanation of an entire section (e.g., "The next
part of the examination is the bimanual. I will be inserting two fingers into your vagina
and placing the other hand on your abdomen to feel your uterus (womb) and ovaries.
The lubricant may feel cool.") There should also be a statement before each maneuver
(e.g., "I am now going to insert my fingers").

d. Positioning

   (1) Sitting up. The patient should be given the option to sit up (at an angle of approximately 40°) during the examination (Figure 7-3). This position is generally more comfortable for the woman, allows physician–patient eye contact during the examination,
and lets the woman use a mirror if she wishes to watch the examination.

   (2) Stirrups. The stirrups need to be positioned appropriately to the height of the woman.
The clinician should remember to lock the stirrups.

   (3) Stirrup pads. Metal stirrups are very cold and uncomfortable. Covering them is a simple procedure that will be appreciated by the patients.

   (4) Positioning in lithotomy. During positioning, it is less intrusive for the patient to touch
the clinician rather than vice versa. The clinician may ask the patient to put her feet
in the stirrups, then slide down until she feels the clinician's hand. At this point, the
clinician should put his other hand where he wants the patient's knees and ask,
"Please extend your knees so that they touch my hands."

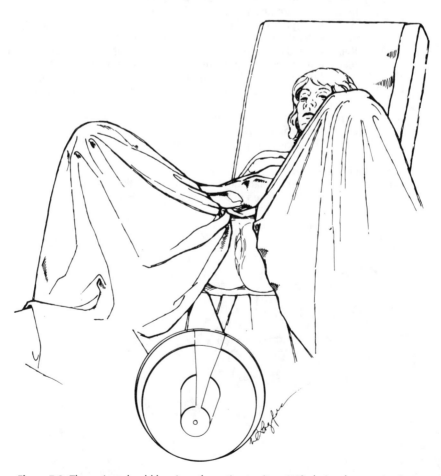

Figure 7-3. The patient should be given the option to sit up (40°) during the examination.

(5) **Draping.** The clinician (unless the woman requests otherwise) should cover the woman's legs with the drape and then make a well with the drape above the knees. As Figure 7-4 illustrates, this gives the clinician good visualization of the external genitalia, permits eye contact with the patient, and provides for some degree of modesty for the patient.

3. **Steps of the examination**
   a. **External examination**
      (1) **Explain procedure.** The clinician tells the woman that she will feel the clinician's hands as the external genitalia are examined.
      (2) **Offer mirror.** The clinician may offer a hand mirror to the patient so she can visualize the examination. If the patient accepts the mirror, the clinician should point out each structure as it is examined.
      (3) **Inspection and palpation** (Figure 7-5)
          (a) **Mons pubis.** The clinician inspects for normal, triangular hair distribution and for any infestations.
          (b) **Clitoris.** Without touching the clitoris or the hood, the clinician places an index finger on either side of the hood and slides it upward. This will expose the clitoris so that it may be inspected for color, malformations, and skin lesions.
          (c) **Labia minora and majora.** The clinician inspects and palpates the labia minora and majora for any excoriations, nodules, or other abnormalities.
          (d) **Urethral orifice.** The urethral meatus is inspected for discharge. If secretion is seen, the clinician should milk the urethra and culture the discharge.
          (e) **Skene's glands.** Skene's glands are located at 2:00 and 10:00. Unless infected, these glands are rarely visible or palpable.
          (f) **Bartholin's glands.** Bartholin's glands are located at 5:00 and 7:00. They, like Skene's glands, are apparent only if cystic or infected.
          (g) **Rectocele and cystocele.** One of the easiest ways to check for rectocele and cystocele is to observe for any bulging or dribbling of urine while the patient bears down. Unless the patient is over 40 years old or has given symptoms suggestive of either problem during the history, this part of the examination may be eliminated.
          (h) **Perineum.** The clinician should inspect the entire perineum for skin lesions or other abnormalities.
          (i) **Anus.** The anus is inspected for hemorrhoids, warts, lacerations, fissures, or fistulae.
   b. **Speculum examination**
      (1) **Preparation.** The clinician should explain that for the next part of the examination, the speculum will be inserted in the vagina to do a Pap smear.

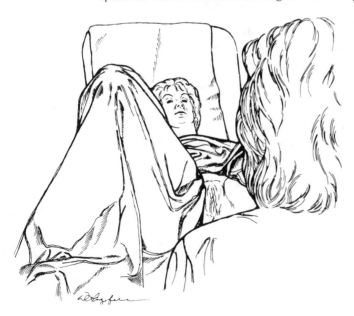

Figure 7-4. The patient illustrated is draped correctly, giving the clinician good visualization of the external genitalia and eye contact with the patient while providing the patient with some degree of modesty.

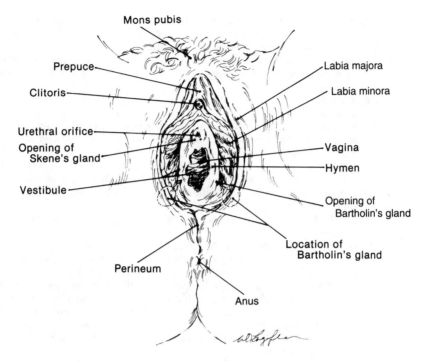

Figure 7-5. Anatomy of external female genitalia. The labia are separated for visualization of the structures between them.

(2) **Use of the speculum.** The clinician should demonstrate how the speculum is opened, especially noting the sound made by a plastic speculum.

(3) **Insertion of speculum**

(a) The clinician places the index finger of the nondominant hand into the inferior introitus. This involuntary muscle may be pressed gently down, which facilitates relaxation for insertion of the speculum.

(b) With the water-lubricated speculum between the second and third fingers of the dominant hand, the clinician gently inserts the speculum at a 45° angle, following the path of the vagina until there is slight resistance. Usually the full length of the speculum is admitted.

(c) After reminding the patient about the sounds of the speculum as it opens, the clinician widens the blades slowly.

(d) If the cervix is not visible, the clinician may maneuver the speculum until the cervix falls into view.

(e) If the cervix does not appear, the clinician removes the speculum partially and angles it more posteriorly.

(f) An alternative is to place a nonlubricated finger inside the vagina to find the exact position of the cervix before inserting the speculum.

(4) **Pap smear**

(a) **Obtaining samples**

(i) **Endocervical junction.** This specimen is obtained by twirling a saline-soaked cotton swab or the plastic Cytobrush 360° in the endocervical canal.

(ii) **Cervical.** This specimen is obtained by a 360° sweep of the cervix with a sampling spatula.

(iii) **Vaginal pool.** A cotton swab dipped in the posterior fornix obtains this sample.

(b) **Preparing slides.** Each sample is smeared on an appropriately labeled glass slide and fixed immediately with spray.

(5) **Cultures.** Once the Pap smear is done, the clinician may do any cultures indicated by the history or examination.

(6) **Mirror.** The clinician may offer a mirror to the patient at this time and help her adjust it so that she can see her cervix.

(7) Vaginal walls. If a plastic speculum is used, the clinician can inspect the vaginal walls directly for color and lesions. If a metal speculum is used, the clinician must inspect the vaginal walls as the speculum is removed.

(8) Removal of speculum. The blades of the speculum are curved. In order not to trap the cervix, the clinician must remove the speculum approximately halfway before allowing the blades to close.

c. **Bimanual examination**

  (1) Preparation

    (a) Explain procedure. The clinician should explain that two fingers will be inserted inside the vagina and that one hand will be on the patient's lower abdomen to feel the uterus and ovaries.

    (b) Gloves. The glove on the dominant hand is lubricated with a water-soluble lubricant. The nondominant glove (abdominal hand) should be removed.

    (c) Examiner position. The bimanual examination is done with the clinician standing.

  (2) Examining the uterus

    (a) Cervix. The clinician palpates the cervix, checking for consistency, pain, or irregularities.

    (b) Fundus. To examine the uterus, the clinician places the fingers under the cervix and elevates it with a pumping motion. The abdominal hand should press firmly inward at the pubic hair line (for a nonpregnant uterus).

      (i) If the uterus is **anteverted,** the fundus will rise against the abdominal hand. Once the fundus is located, the abdominal hand maintains pressure so that the uterus is immobilized. The internal fingers reach behind and on each side of the cervix and palpate the posterior uterus for size, shape, and consistency.

      (ii) If the uterus is **retroverted,** it is palpated from the rectum.

  (3) Examining the ovaries

    (a) Without removing the vaginal hand, the clinician places two internal fingers deep in the lateral fornix, pushing them up against the abdominal fingers near the iliac crest.

    (b) To palpate the ovary, the abdominal fingers must meet so that the ovary is felt as it "escapes" to one side or the other.

    (c) To accomplish this, the clinician begins moving the abdominal fingers first, parallel to the inguinal ligament in a smooth, firm motion.

    (d) As these fingers meet the internal fingers, the latter curl downward without coming out of the vagina. This maneuver may be repeated until the ovary is felt, and then performed for the opposite ovary.

    (e) Ovaries are not always palpable; however, the clinician must be confident that the technique was correct before assuming that this is the case.

    (f) If the patient is obese or extremely tense and the clinician feels that this has interfered with the examination, this observation should be documented.

d. **Rectovaginal examination**

  (1) Preparation

    (a) Explain procedure. The clinician should remind the patient that this is the last part of the examination and that it will accomplish the three objectives listed below. To achieve these three goals, the clinician tells the patient that one finger will enter the rectum and one finger will be inserted into the vagina to:

      (i) Allow palpation of the remainder of the uterus

      (ii) Allow palpation of the septum between the vagina and rectum

      (iii) Check for any polyps or hemorrhoids in the rectum

    (b) Give instructions. The clinician tells the patient to bear down as though she were having a bowel movement when she feels the clinician's finger at her anus. The patient must be reassured that she will not have a bowel movement, but that this maneuver will make it easier for the finger to enter the rectum.

    (c) Clinician's preparation. The clinician should always change gloves before beginning the rectal examination. No contaminant, such as blood or vaginal pathogens, should be introduced into the rectum. The clinician must liberally lubricate both rectal and vaginal fingers and should be seated during insertion for good visualization. The examiner should then stand to get sufficient leverage for the examination.

  (2) Examination

    (a) Insertion of fingers. While seated, the clinician repeats instructions to the patient, places the middle finger at the anus, and then gently inserts the finger anteriorly. Once the rectal finger is inserted, the index finger should enter the vagina.

    (b) Rectovaginal septum. The rectal and vaginal fingers are approximated across the septum and moved against one another in scissor fashion. The normal septum should be thin enough that the fingers feel as though they are touching.

    (c) Posterior surface of uterus. With the dominant foot on the step of the examination table for better leverage, the rectal finger sweeps the posterior surface of the uterus, checking for size, shape, consistency, and mobility. This is the best position from which to palpate a retroverted uterus.

    (d) Rectal examination. The clinician now removes the vaginal finger and sweeps the rectum 180° in one direction and then 180° in the other. Once the rectal finger is removed, the clinician places a small amount of stool on a Hemoccult card for later occult blood testing.

e. Closure

    (1) Assist patient. It is difficult for the most agile person to get up from the lithotomy position. The clinician should suggest to the patient that she push back before trying to sit up and then help her as she does so. A cloth should be provided for the patient to remove lubricant from the perineum.

    (2) Final interview. The clinician should not discuss any part of the examination or give any directions until the patient is dressed and comfortable. Then the final discussion and patient education can be done under optimal conditions.

C. Male genital and rectal examination

1. Overview. Many students are apprehensive about the male genital examination. In addition to concerns about their own inexperience, they worry about patient reaction and the possibility of penile erection. If the examination is conducted professionally, the patient's concerns are largely alleviated. Erection may occur as a normal reaction to manipulation of the penis. Should this happen, it is up to the examiner to reassure the patient that this is not unusual and allow the patient time if he requests it before completing the examination.

    a. Sequence. The genital and rectal examinations are usually done at the end of the physical examination.

    b. Patient position. The genital examination is best done with the patient standing to facilitate adequate hernia and scrotal examination. If the patient is unable to stand, the examination may be done with him supine; however, an adequate hernia examination cannot be achieved under this circumstance.

    c. Examiner position. The examiner is seated in front of the patient with the patient's gown raised to expose the genitals.

    d. Gloves. Gloves should always be worn for this examination. Not only are gloves in the examiner's best interest, but they also provide a modicum of professional distance to the procedure. (For area anatomy, see Figure 7-6.)

2. Steps of the examination

    a. Penis

        (1) Skin. Note the pigmentation of the skin of the penile shaft and any lesions that may be present. Remember to inspect the ventral and dorsal skin.

        (2) Prepuce. If the patient is uncircumcised, retract, or ask the patient to retract, the foreskin.

        (3) Glans. Inspect the glans on all surfaces for skin lesions and hygiene.

        (4) Urethral meatus. Note the position of the meatus relative to the tip of the glans. Compress the glans gently between index finger and thumb. This will allow the meatus to open for better inspection and permit the expression of secretions if discharge is present. This is the appropriate time to take urethral cultures if they are indicated by the history or examination. Replace the foreskin.

    b. Scrotum

        (1) Inspection. Note the contour of the scrotal sac and all surfaces for lumps, ulcerations, inflammation, or asymmetry. Always lift the scrotal sac to see the underside.

        (2) Palpation

            (a) Testicles. Gently palpate each testicle between thumb and forefinger, noting size, consistency, shape, and presence of irregularities or tenderness. Pressure on the testicle normally produces a deep visceral sensation.

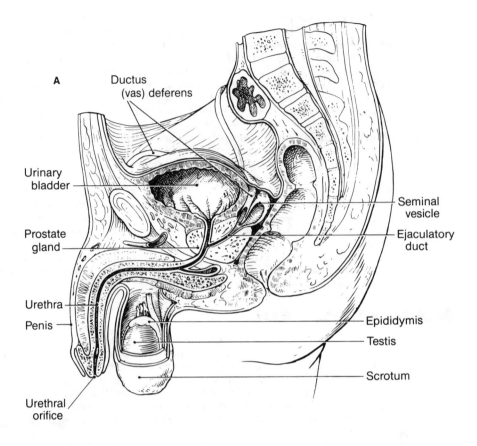

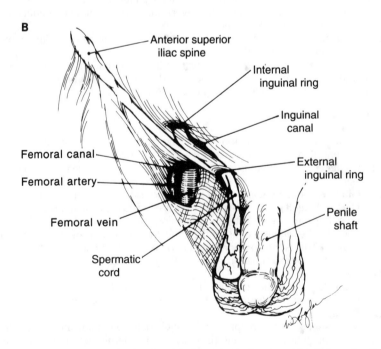

Figure 7-6. Anatomy of the male genitalia. *A,* Sagittal male pelvis; *B,* frontal surface.

(b) **Epididymis.** In the same manner, locate and palpate the epididymis. It should be clearly discernable from the superior–posterior pole of each testicle. Compare the two sides for size and tenderness.

(c) **Vas deferens and cord structures.** Locate each spermatic cord with its vas deferens, and palpate it between your thumb and fingers along its course from epididymis to superficial inguinal ring. Again compare the two sides for symmetry and both cords for swelling or tenderness.

c. **Inguinal (hernia) examination**

   (1) **Inspection.** Visualize the inguinal area for bulges; ask the patient to cough or bear down for this inspection.

   (2) **Palpation.** This is a two-step procedure, first for location of any direct inguinal hernia, and secondly to determine the status of the inguinal ring through which an indirect hernia may present. (Figure 7-7 illustrates the inguinal anatomy pertinent to the two presentations.)

      (a) **Direct hernia.** Locate the **pubic tubercle.** The bulge of a direct inguinal hernia may sometimes be appreciated immediately lateral to this structure. By placing the palmar surface of the index finger in this location and asking the patient to cough or bear down, a direct hernia will pulse against the finger. The direct inguinal hernia is relatively infrequent in adults, so some examiners choose to eliminate this step.

      (b) **Indirect hernia**

         (i) Beginning well down on the lateral scrotal sac, the index or middle finger is gently inserted alongside the cord structures, invaginating scrotal skin as the finger is moved up the inguinal canal.

         (ii) With the palmar surface of the finger against the abdominal wall, the external inguinal ring may be felt as a depression above the inguinal ligament and 2–3 cm lateral to the pubic tubercle.

         (iii) If the patient is asked to cough with the examiner's finger in the canal, a soft bulge descending along the canal against the examiner's fingertip is suggestive of an indirect hernia.

      (c) **Femoral hernia.** This hernia is rare and is commoner in women than men. It presents as a bulge below the inguinal ligament in the femoral triangle.

d. **Teaching the genital self-examination.** It is the clinician's responsibility to encourage regular self-examination of the penis and scrotal structures.

   (1) **Inspection.** The man may accomplish the inspection of the skin of the penis and scrotum in the same systematic fashion used by the clinician.

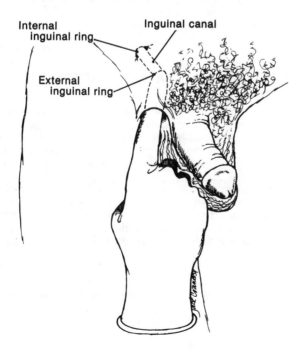

Internal inguinal ring

Inguinal canal

External inguinal ring

Figure 7-7. Hernia examination.

(2) **Palpation.** The testicles and cord structures may be palpated with the patient standing or lying down, since hernia examination is not an effective self-examination procedure.

(3) **Observation of self-examination.** The clinician should observe the patient doing his self-examination and explain the normal anatomy or any variations of normal that may be present. Careful instruction about changes that should be reported to a clinician enables most men to discover testicular masses or epididymal inflammation before they become symptomatic.

3. **Rectal and prostate examination.** This is usually the final step in the physical examination of the male patient.

   a. **Patient position.** This examination may be done in one of three positions: **left lateral decubitus, knee–chest,** or **standing** and **bent over the examining table**.

   b. **Examiner position.** Regardless of patient position, the examiner must position him- or herself at the back of the patient, facing the buttocks.

   c. **Gloves and lubricant.** Both hands should be gloved for this examination to facilitate careful inspection of the perianal area. For the rectal examination, the examining finger should be generously lubricated with a water-soluble gel.

   d. **Steps of the examination**

      (1) **Inspection.** Holding the buttocks apart, the clinician carefully inspects the perianal area for signs of skin disease, tags, hemorrhoids, fissures, or fistulas.

      (2) **Insertion of finger.** A well-lubricated index finger of the dominant hand is placed against the anus, and the patient is asked to bear down. The relaxation of the sphincter, resulting from the Valsalva maneuver, facilitates insertion of the finger beyond the sphincter. If the patient is then instructed to tighten the sphincter muscle, the examiner can note **sphincter tone**.

      (3) **Palpation of rectal vault.** The examining finger may be introduced 3–6 cm into the rectum. The hand is then rotated so that the palmar surface of the finger can negotiate a 360° sweep of the rectal wall, noting masses, irregularities of mucosa, or areas of tenderness.

      (4) **Palpation of the prostate gland.** The prostate is felt through the ventral rectal wall, in the midline, approximately 3 cm beyond the anal verge. The **posterior lateral lobes** and the **median sulcus** can usually be defined. The surface of the gland is firm, smooth, and normally bulges less than 1 cm into the rectal vault. Note the shape, size, consistency, and regularity of the palpable surface of the gland (Figure 7-8).

   e. **Closure.** Since the rectal examination usually completes the physical examination, the patient may now be given the privacy to dress or replace his hospital gown. Discussion of the examiner's assessment of the examination may then take place.

III. EXAMINATION OF THE BEDRIDDEN AND THE DISABLED* PATIENT

A. **Time.** There is a critical need for sufficient time to examine these individuals properly, as many aspects of the examination are time-consuming (e.g., removing the shirt from a wheelchair-bound paraplegic to auscultate the posterior thorax). If a half-hour is time enough for a third-year medical student to examine a routine patient, it may take this same student a full hour to examine an individual with disabling cerebral palsy with its attendant slow speech and contracted joints.

1. **Prioritization** is vital when the clinician must work around external time limits. The clinician is well advised to select in advance those portions of the examination that must be completed by the end of the encounter and to perform them first. For example, in a physically robust but mentally retarded child with epilepsy, the neurologic and mental status examinations, screening tests of hearing and vision,[†] and monitoring for physical signs of anticonvulsant side

---

*Some organizations of individuals with various sorts of physical or other difficulties prefer the words "challenge" or "challenged" to "disability" or "disabled."

[†]This is vital because any input deficit—typically of sight or hearing—will sharply increase the isolation of a retarded person.

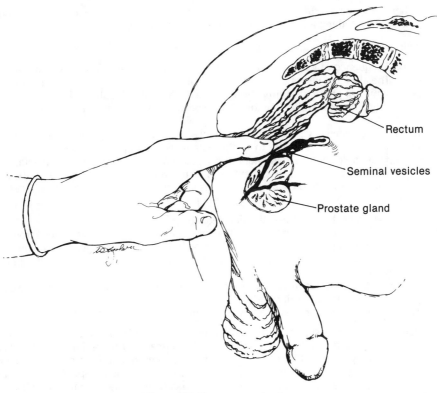

Figure 7-8. Prostate examination.

effects,* become top priorities, while cardiac auscultation may have to be deferred to a second encounter.

2. **Patient fatigue** may call for multiple brief examinations in preference to a single comprehensive one.

B. **Use of assistants.** Family members and other caregivers can be indispensable in transferring immobile patients. Sufficient help often means several people. It is much safer to examine the patient within the limits of a single body position or even in a wheelchair than to risk injury.

1. **Family members** can provide insight as well as physical assistance in positioning the patient, and often the frail patient prefers to be handled by them. However, family members are often untrained in procedures and, if unfamiliar, can be inept at them, and they may find witnessing or participating in particular procedures unacceptable (e.g., rectal examination).

2. **Nurses** are the traditional helpers with both the labor and the cognitive side of difficult examinations. Time spent developing mutual goals with the nursing staff shows respect and is richly rewarded.

3. **Patient.** Enlisting the patient's maximum capability to assist in transfers and repositioning is an essential component, which can:
   a. **Enhance functional assessment.** For example, a paraplegic who raises his trunk by pulling on a "traction triangle" demonstrates great upper-limb strength.
   b. **Improve self-esteem.** The examiner's initial impulse to help must be tempered by recognition of the patient's desire to do for him- or herself. Commanding one's own body as much as is possible sustains a besieged self-image.

---

*Ataxia and nystagmus are common with excess doses of some agents. Clouding of consciousness can occur with anticonvulsant excess. Lymph node enlargement, gingival hyperplasia, and splenomegaly are side effects of phenytoin, a major anticonvulsant. The importance of finding these things lies in the need to consider modifications of therapy, such as dose alteration or the provision of measures to minimize any of these side effects.

4. Others. Potential recruits include interns, orderlies, ward clerks, personal care attendants, or whomever is willing and is not objectionable to the patient.

C. Variations in examination technique

1. A fixed sequence of examination is indispensable for the clinician to be complete and efficient. The clinician needs to learn flexibility about content, sequence, extent, and practical performance of physical examination, especially for difficult patients.

    a. Investigation of specific symptoms and expected sources of difficulty always deserves early attention.

    b. The patient may have questions or concerns (medically well founded or otherwise) that call for a response, which helps to set the agenda. For example, inspection of the lower back and intergluteal fold is mandatory with a young man bed-bound by paraplegia, to look for early bedsores. If the same patient says, "I am worried about my prostate. My father was just diagnosed with prostate cancer," it is important to take the time to palpate this man's gland and reassure him if findings are normal.

2. Modification of the usual examination sequence

    a. Several parts of the examination of the right side of the patient may be done from the usual position, standing at the right side of the bed; the corresponding examinations of the left side may then be done from the left, rather than grouping components by sitting *versus* standing.

    b. Some parts of the facial, anterior thoracic, and abdominal examinations can be completed satisfactorily from the right side.

    c. Ophthalmoscopy and otoscopy will require that the examiner relocate.

3. Body transfers are a significant issue. Any resequencing that minimizes them saves time and energy for all parties and will almost certainly be noticed and appreciated by patient and staff.

    a. Positioning is critical for examiner and patient comfort, and for more accurate examination. The clinician can do an examination more easily and completely in a hospital bed than on an examining table, because the bed can be electrically raised and lowered, and often the upper body can be selectively and passively moved as well.

    b. Challenging settings

        (1) An **examining table** usually allows manual elevation or lowering of the upper torso and so is better for conducting examinations than a home bed.

        (2) Examination in the wheelchair is a test of the examiner's flexibility and ingenuity.

            (a) Assessment of head and neck, breasts, arms, heart, shins, and feet are all straightforward.

            (b) The back, lungs, abdomen, genitalia, rectum, and posterior thighs offer greater challenges and are at times impossible. Transfer to a bed or table is sometimes the only solution. Note that the neck must be carefully supported if the patient is quadriplegic.

    c. Side-to-side turning often permits assessment of hidden zones. For example, even a severely debilitated and bed-bound patient can often turn (or be helped to turn) to right lateral decubitus and left lateral decubitus positions; employing these two, the examiner gains access to all the structures of the occiput, posterior thorax, back, buttocks, and posterior legs. This maneuver is safe in a hospital bed and often in a home bed, less safe on an examining table (there may be no barriers to the patient's falling off), and difficult or impossible in a reclining wheelchair.

D. Alterations in physical findings may reflect artifacts of position or hypomobility, certain pathologic complications of these states, or independent pathology. The examples that follow represent common particulars and prototypes rather than an exhaustive listing.

1. Compression of lung. The clinician must be wary of overinterpretation.

    a. Compression of lung parenchyma tends to produce dullness and crackles in some dependent portions of lung in the patient lying on his or her side.

    b. Any condition that immobilizes the patient or keeps him or her bed-bound may produce some true underinflation of the lungs, suboptimal clearance of secretions, and high frequencies of pneumonia and atelectasis, which are two sources of true-positive findings.

2. Mechanical ventilators. The patient on a mechanical ventilator cannot voluntarily deep-breathe for the examiner and often has such a noisy chest-ventilator system that assessment of lung sounds is impossible.

a. **Percussion and fremitus** are not hampered by the ventilator so the clinician can use them extensively.
b. **Auscultation** of specific symmetric points on the left and right hemithoraces may uncover subtle differences easily missed against the background welter and may be directed by zones of abnormal results of the other modalities.

3. **Neurologic examination** can be troublesome.
a. **Deviation from baseline neurologic status** is the most helpful finding in a significantly impaired host. New findings, even subtle ones, carry more significance in assessment of progression and current status than do old stable deficits.
b. **Reflex sympathetic dystrophy** and other disuse and denervation changes can augment atrophy, produce hyperesthesia, and result in skin changes that mimic ischemia (e.g., dependent rubor).

4. **Stasis-related changes** in the lower limbs can mimic venous disease. This can include edema from constant gravitational pull on feet that are always dependent with an ineffective muscular pump. Misinterpretation of this edema as heart failure is not uncommon and underscores the importance of looking at the whole patient when deciding the meaning of a particular physical sign.

E. **Reliable and unreliable components of examination**

1. **Funduscopic examination** is difficult to perform on the supine patient and often in the wheelchair-bound patient. It is desirable, therefore, to consider pharmacologic pupillodilation under supervision or consultation, from preceptors or an ophthalmologist, when confronted with a negative or nondiagnostic examination in a patient whose management requires clear answers in this difficult realm.

2. **Cardiovascular assessment** by special maneuvers is sometimes feasible.
a. **Valsalva or squat** can only be accomplished by a patient who understands, wishes to help, and has reasonable motor skills and breathing reserve. The same applies to leaning forward and holding the breath in end-expiration.
b. **Sustained isometric handgrip** is less taxing on the breathing but requires equal language skill (the response to nonverbal demonstration is never satisfactory) and is contraindicated in acute coronary insufficiency.
c. **Passive straight leg-raising** is possible unless the patient objects to the manipulation, has significant arthritis of the hip, or is orthopneic.
d. **Inflating sphygmomanometers on both arms** to increase afterload is feasible in most patients.
e. **Hepatic pressure** to increase return to the right heart is feasible and so is the **use of short-acting vasoactive drugs,** such as amyl nitrite.

3. **Swallowing maneuvers** are difficult or impossible in the bedridden patient, since they may cause pulmonary aspiration.
a. **Thyroidal examination** must proceed with less use of this modality.
b. **Timing of esophageal transit** by measuring the interval from deglutition to gastric rumble is likewise limited.

4. **Rectal examination** can be done in almost all physically impaired persons.
a. **The optimal position is left lateral decubitus** with the left hip and knee fully extended, the right hip and knee fully flexed, and the trunk turned slightly prone (front side down toward the bed). The examiner then explains to the patient what is about to happen, separates the buttocks manually, and gently inserts a gloved finger.
b. Resistant or combative patients are another story, and for them, gentle and repeated explanation, "training sessions" concerning the examination, and sharing of locus of control can help.

5. **Pelvic examination** is often dismissed as impossible.
a. Difficulty may arise upon attempted transfer onto an examining table or upon seeking abduction and external rotation of the hips to a degree that in the setting of arthritis is quite painful or even impossible. The sense of vulnerability and invasion of privacy experienced with the wide exposure of the genitalia in this manner also contribute to difficulty with it.
b. The effort and time required to conduct a **bimanual examination at the bedside** are far less than for a complete examination, and the success rate in terms of gaining information is high, even in the frailest and most arthritic and immobile individuals.

(1) The technique consists of having the patient abduct the hips, with external rotation if possible, while lying supine in bed (and with full upper body support if needed for prevention of orthopnea).

(2) The examiner then inspects the perineum and genitalia and palpates the genitals and the abdominal organs per vaginam just as in any other examination.

(3) The components that are lost are speculum examination of the vagina and cervix, and Pap smear of these sites.

(4) If there is need for **speculum examination** in the patient who ought not to be moved from bed, the buttocks may be elevated with an inverted bedpan, and the speculum inserted upside down (i.e., with the handle pointing upward rather than down).

F. Other individuals with special needs

1. The effects of **braces** may include difficulty in exposing the subjacent skin and muscles and skin irritation. The patient is the best person to remove any orthosis that is hindering physical examination. Examination of function both with and without the brace can be worthwhile; however, no maneuver should be attempted that may cause a fall.

2. **Mentally retarded** patients or those with Down's syndrome usually permit a thorough and effective examination to be done. Depending on the interplay of level of intelligence and personal histories concerning socialization and abuse, there may be surprisingly complete ease about rectal and genital evaluations, or great reluctance.

3. Patients with **auditory loss** need appropriate cues, whether these be achieved through sign language, lip-reading, or other means. Medical interpreting for the deaf is not a simple matter of note-writing in most cases, nor should relatives automatically serve as interpreters in either the history or the examination.

4. The patient with **visual loss** usually presents no special difficulties. This individual has a particular need to be told what will happen next, since he or she cannot see to anticipate the examiner's intent.

5. **Neurologically impaired patients,** including hemiplegic individuals, have difficulty with positions and transfers. They may also be hyperalgesic or anesthetic in affected areas.

6. **Aphasic patients** may be able to cooperate fully if the aphasia is purely expressive and not receptive. However, hemiparesis commonly accompanies even Wernicke's aphasia, partial receptive deficits frequently coexist, and emotional difficulty is common and makes evaluation more difficult. The person with a receptive aphasia can be respectfully manipulated but is not usually able to cooperate with commands.

7. **Non–English-speaking patients** can be instructed in their own language. Medical interpreters are extremely helpful, despite the well-known difficulties they entail, such as the interposition of their own thoughts and interpretations between examiner and patient.

8. **Psychotic patients** are often physically able to have a full and proper examination but may be uncooperative or outright hostile. In this setting, consultation with the primary mental health providers may lead to behavioral or pharmacologic assistance to let the examiner do the job. Quite often, the psychotic patient is very interested in and friendly toward "physical" medicine even if antagonistic toward psychiatrists.

9. **Drug addicts** may be perfectly cooperative and even obsequious or may show a variety of unpleasantnesses up to and including outright sociopathy.

10. **Alcoholic patients** may challenge the clinician's right to take a history or perform an examination. The clinician needs to regard alcoholics as having a disease whose nature includes interpersonal deficits that are often repugnant. One useful response to an explicit or implicit challenge to the clinician's role is a gentle but forceful statement that the clinician is trying to contribute to the welfare of the patient at hand. If the alcoholic patient assents to examination on these terms, all well and good. If not, it is unproductive to argue or cajole. This may be the time to report the difficulty to a superior and leave the care of the patient to a more experienced provider.

11. **A seductive or sexualizing patient** must be taken very seriously as a significant potential threat to the clinician and ultimately a detriment to his or her own medical care.
   a. Wearing **gloves** for genital examinations minimizes inappropriate sexualization of the clinical encounter.

   b. The routine use of **chaperons** (of the same sex as the patient) for genital and rectal examinations can be helpful; the nurse–chaperon provides technical assistance and comfort to the patient as much as the traditional show of propriety.

IV. EXAMINATION OF THE MENTALLY RETARDED PATIENT

A. Techniques to maximize the examination yield

   1. Attention should be paid to the comfort and privacy of the patients. Patients are often anxious and reluctant to be examined, but allowing a known caregiver or family member to remain during the examination increases their cooperation.

   2. The examination should be evenly paced and deliberate. Multiple visits may be required to build trust and cooperation.

   3. Selective observation regarding the patient's overall level of development, cooperation, social responsiveness, and awareness of the environment can yield data about multiple organ system function.

   4. Patients in wheelchairs should be moved with assistance to an examining table to allow a comprehensive examination. Examinations in a sitting patient yield inadequate cardiac and abdominal examinations and preclude pelvic and rectal examinations.

B. Principles of the examination in mentally retarded children

   1. Developmental assessment is the fundamental task of the examination.

   2. Identifying associated abnormalities, usually congenital, should be the focus of the examination. These include concurrent neurologic, chromosomal, or cardiac disorders.

   3. Components of the examination to which particular attention should be given include:
   a. General body proportions
   b. Head circumference and shape
   c. Hair texture, skin lesions, and rashes
   d. Visual and hearing acuity
   e. Palate integrity and tongue size
   f. Heart murmurs
   g. Bone and joint deformities
   h. Gross and fine motor function and other soft neurologic findings

C. Principles of the examination in mentally retarded adults

   1. Functional assessment. Comparable to a developmental assessment in children, the focus of the examination in mentally retarded adults is to determine functional capability.
   a. Activities of daily living. Mental retardation and associated disorders can greatly influence the patient's dependence or independence in eating, toileting, and personal hygiene.
   b. Language skills, including receptive comprehension and expressive speech, need to be evaluated comprehensively. This often requires referral to audiologists and speech pathologists.
   c. Patients may range from being completely immobile to fully ambulatory. Mobility has been shown to be the single most important factor determining mortality in mentally retarded patients.

   2. Disorders associated with mental retardation may be either congenitally acquired or secondary to medication use. These include:
   a. Neurologic disease, such as seizure disorders, hemi- or quadriplegia, hearing loss, visual defects, extrapyramidal signs, Alzheimer-type dementia (especially in Down's syndrome patients), gait disorders, and tardive dyskinesia
   b. Psychiatric disorders, such as behavioral problems, depression, schizophrenia, ritualistic behavior, and autism
   c. Other disorders, such as atlantoaxial instability (especially in Down's syndrome), obesity, thyroid disease, fungal and atopic diseases of the skin, heart disease, and periodontal and dental diseases

   3. Routine well-adult care. Mentally retarded patients are as likely as any adult to acquire most medical problems. Regular breast examinations, pelvic examinations, Pap smears, rectal examinations, and stool testing for occult blood should be periodically scheduled.

D. Components of the examination requiring special attention

1. **General appearance.** Gait, stance, fine and gross motor coordination, cerebellar function, and muscle strength may be untestable and are best evaluated by **observation**.

2. **Skin integrity** is often compromised by position, contractures and incontinence, necessitating thorough examination for decubitus ulcers and desquamated areas. Fungal infections and eczema occur with greater frequency in mentally retarded patients.

3. **Eye examination** is particularly challenging. Acuity is assessed by the patient's interaction with objects and other visual stimuli. Visual evoked potentials may be helpful. Sedation may be required for the funduscopic examination.

4. **Hearing** is best assessed by an audiologist. Auditory evoked potentials may be necessary.

5. **Mouth examination** should focus on dental caries, gingival disease (e.g., hyperplasia, gingivitis), and congenital abnormalities (e.g., cleft palate).

6. **Cardiac examination** should focus on heart sounds (e.g., fixed split S_2, increased P_2) and on murmurs.

7. **Musculoskeletal examination** should emphasize **muscle tone** and passive and active **joint range of motion**. Joint deformities should be evaluated with reference to functional limitation; for example:
   a. Hand and wrist flexion contractures are common and result in the inability to hold eating utensils.
   b. Contractures at the knee, causing less than 90° extension, makes sitting in a wheelchair difficult.

8. **Neurologic examination** is essential; it should be as complete as possible despite poor cooperation. In addition to the usual questions asked in a full mental status examination, specialized assessment tools exist to evaluate cognitive and psychiatric status.
   a. Observation and history regarding **swallowing, chewing, sucking,** and **drooling** give important data on **cranial nerves V, VII, IX, X, and XII.** Cranial nerve XI is indirectly assessed by the position of the head and muscle symmetry.
   b. **Deep tendon reflexes** are difficult to obtain unless the patient is distracted or sedated.
   c. **Muscle strength, cerebellar function, and the sensory system** can usually be only grossly tested.
   d. **Abnormal reflexes** (e.g., Babinski, Hoffmann) **and frontal release signs** should be sought by testing.

V. MENTAL STATUS EXAMINATION

A. **Individuals who need to be tested.** Some clinicians believe that a full mental status examination should be done on every individual, but practical time limits suggest otherwise. A brief global assessment is always vital, but more detailed evaluation can be reserved for those most likely to be helped by the data generated.

1. **The healthy aged** ought to have mental status examinations, which can uncover early dementia that is not apparent in the history, nor in everyday life.
   a. **Altered mental status** is the commonest nonspecific presentation of physical disease in the aged.
   b. **A recorded baseline** will prove infinitely helpful in assessing deterioration and return to baseline.

2. **Individuals with medical or psychiatric problems.** A **baseline examination** is helpful at a time of stability or inactivity of a variety of medical and psychiatric problems. For example, an individual with acquired immune deficiency syndrome (AIDS) is at risk for both human immunodeficiency virus–related dementia and major psychiatric morbidity. Knowing this individual's initial mental status is useful to assess change (or lack of change) over time.

3. **Impaired individuals,** whether chronically demented, acutely delirious, psychotic, or depressed, should have a mental status examination as a part of the data base. Impairments can remit as well as worsen, so the direction of change is not predictable. Mental status examinations may uncover suicidal tendencies or other problems that pose a threat to the patient or to others.

B. Examiner conduct is important to success in this part of the examination.

    1. The clinician should make the patient physically comfortable and (if possible) mentally at ease. Otherwise, the information obtained may reflect artifacts of the interaction, rather than the true mental state of the patient.

    2. One introduction that is especially useful for the cognitive aspect of the examination is, "I have listened to your lungs and heart. To study how your brain is working, I have a series of questions that I ask of every patient." For all but the most paranoid patients, this approach obviates any fear that the individual has been singled out for the test because something is amiss.

    3. The clinician should avoid saying, "Some of these questions are very easy," because if an individual cannot answer them, he or she may feel truly inadequate.

C. Components of the mental status examination

    1. Orientation to time, place, and person constitutes only one small component of mental status testing. The common extent of observation that is recorded in a chart is that a person is "A & O × 3" [alert and oriented times three components (time, place, and person)], which is an inadequate screen. It is important to note that major psychiatric, neurologic, and functional impairments can coexist with the preservation of this level of consciousness and appropriate response to direct questioning.

    2. General appearance and behavior
        a. The degree of **socially appropriate behavior, motor activity level,** and an **estimation of the acuity of illness** are the components of this assessment. These observations are generally made in the course of the history.
        b. Stream of speech refers to **fluidity, tempo, modulation, focus,** and any suggestion of **aphasia, dysphonia,** or **psychological barriers** to communication.
        c. Mood and affect. Anger, depression, anxiety, and other recognizable deviations from equanimity are common. An unvarnished description is best (e.g., "markedly depressed woman with associated psychomotor retardation who wept when discussing her husband's death 20 years ago; labile and, at times, inappropriate with three episodes of laughter about the lack of sexual activity since her husband's death").
        d. Thought content includes all the diverse issues implicit in the name. Asking open-ended questions, such as, "What's on your mind?" help the clinician to learn the patient's thought content.
           (1) Obsessions and the more benign **formes frustes,** such as bowel fixation or fat fetishes, should be noted.
           (2) Major concerns (e.g., personal, medical, social, political, occupational, or financial) should be determined as well as their appropriateness to the patient's situation.
        e. Intellectual capacity is covered by the Folstein test described in V D. Clinicians assess intellectual function everyday, although not so reliably as by formal interview and formal mental status testing.
        f. Sensorium. This is covered by the Folstein test described in V D and includes such areas as consciousness, memory, insight, attention, and orientation.

D. Folstein mini-mental status examination has been widely used. It is effective even with the diminished attention span of individuals with impaired cognition. Its eleven questions take only 5–10 minutes. Neither its administration nor interpretation requires extensive training.

    1. The content is a series of questions and commands that test **attention, registration, memory,** and **praxis** (Figure 7-9). It concentrates only on the **cognitive aspects** of mental function and excludes questions concerning mood, abnormal mental experiences, and the form of thinking.

    2. Administering the test consists of giving the directions in the manner indicated in the detailed guidelines in Folstein's original paper.

    3. Serial repetition of this examination can be particularly helpful in assessing **recovery** from an acute confusional state or **progress** of a dementing illness. If the patient had a Folstein score of 24 last year and now has a 19, the clinician has a semiquantitative handle on progressive cognitive deterioration. A Folstein score cannot be used in isolation, just as an IQ score cannot be used in isolation. Any absence of concomitant data on ADLs and other functional measures renders the number sterile and prone to misuse.

Mini-Mental Status Examination (MMSE)

Add points for each correct response.

			Score	Points

Orientation

1. What is the:	Year		_____	1
	Season		_____	1
	Date		_____	1
	Day		_____	1
	Month		_____	1
2. Where are we?	State		_____	1
	County		_____	1
	Town or city		_____	1
	Hospital		_____	1
	Floor		_____	1

Registration

3. Name three objects, taking one second to say each. Then ask the patient to repeat all three after you have said them.   _____   3
Give one point for each correct answer. Repeat the answers until patient learns all three.

Attention and calculation

4. Serial sevens. Give one point for each correct answer. Stop after five answers.   _____   5
Alternate: Spell WORLD backwards.

Recall

5. Ask for names of three objects learned in question 3. Give one point for each   _____   3
correct answer.

Language

6. Point to a pencil and a watch. Have the patient name them as you point.   _____   2
7. Have the patient repeat "No ifs, ands, or buts."   _____   1
8. Have the patient follow a three-stage command: "Take a paper in your right   _____   3
hand. Fold the paper in half. Put the paper on the floor."
9. Have the patient read and obey the following: "CLOSE YOUR EYES." (Write it   _____   1
in large letters.)
10. Have the patient write a sentence of his or her choice. (The sentence should   _____   1
contain a subject and an object and should make sense. Ignore spelling errors
when scoring.)
11. Have the patient copy the design. (Give one point if all sides and angles are   _____   <u>1</u>
preserved and if the intersecting sides form a quadrangle.)

_____   Total 30

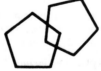

In validation studies using a cut-off score of 23 or below, the MMSE has a sensitivity of 87%, a specificity of 82%, a false-positive ratio of 39.4%, and a false-negative ratio of 4.7%. These ratios refer to the MMSE's capacity to distinguish accurately patients with clinically diagnosed dementia or delirium from patients without these syndromes.

Figure 7-9. Folstein mini-mental status examination. (Reprinted with permission from Marshall Folstein, M.D.)

4. Interpretation is generally straightforward. Scores of 23 or less commonly represent symptomatic dysfunction, and in the original report, scores below 20 were found only in psychosis and dementia (including psychotic depression with secondary cognitive impairment) and not in normal elders who maintained scores similar to those of young individuals. The mean score of individuals with dementia, which may be defined as a global intellectual deterioration without a disturbance of consciousness, is about 12.

    a. False-positive tests, some of which can be predicted, can be avoided or interpreted with greater caution.

        (1) Inattention can result from distracting pain or psychological concerns.

        (2) Depression and other psychiatric disease may cause the patient to be uninvolved, distracted, and inattentive.

        (3) Sensory loss is another obvious detractor. If the questions are heard indistinctly, performance will not represent the central processing capacity of the brain.

        (4) Motor impairment may prevent the writing of a sentence or copying of figures.

        (5) Linguistic difficulty. Individuals for whom English is not the first language are among those prone to falsely abnormal results.

        (6) Low educational level can lead to errors that do not represent attenuated cognitive function. For example, there are many adults of normal intelligence who are not literate.

    b. False-negative tests are equally important.

        (1) Inherent insensitivity of the test (i.e., a high threshold) was built in to reduce false-positives.

        (2) High educational level tends to disguise deficits for a long period. For example, an English professor may not lose the ability to spell "world" until dementia has become very advanced.

    c. Interpretation of a true-positive test is not quite as simple as implied above: There is not a one-word positive or negative outcome, and accurate diagnosis is never to be made with this instrument alone. It is a single powerful modality that must be interpreted in the context of a larger and more multidimensional data base. It is also critical to understand that abnormal cognition does not occur exclusively with permanent loss (i.e., **dementia**) but also is commonly seen in acute confusional states (i.e., **delirium**).

E. Neurologic problems versus psychopathology. Overlap is frequent, troublesome, and clinically significant. Clinicians do not want to give chlorpromazine for an unrecognized brain tumor, nor perform myelography or craniotomy for falsely localizing psychiatric symptoms. When the primary interviewer and examiner cannot tell which class of condition is present, it is reasonable and appropriate to consult representatives of either subspecialty or both.

1. Internal consistency of the diagnostic interview, the general physical examination (including neurologic), and the mental status examination helps to overcome this difficulty. A patient who is "talking crazy" but also has an acute hemiparesis is likely to be correctly identified as having a neurologic cause for the speech problem rather than a psychiatric one.

2. Guidelines for distinguishing neurologic from psychiatric processes are lengthy and imperfect. The presence of one does not exclude coexistence of the other. Indeed, they often coexist.

    a. It is characteristic of some psychiatric disorders (e.g., catalepsy) to include motor signs.

    b. Many neurologic conditions produce psychologic and interpersonal difficulties (e.g., mood disturbances in multiple sclerosis).

    c. Manifest anxiety and depression of psychologic origin frequently complicate neurologic disease and may dominate the clinical picture, obscuring the underlying neurologic disease.

REFERENCES

Crocker AC: Medical care for adults with developmental disabilities. *JAMA* 260:1455, 1988

Dahlquist LM, Gil KM, Kalfus GR, et al: Enhancing an autistic girl's cooperation with gynecological examinations. *Clin Pediatr* 23:203, 1984

DeGowin RL: *DeGowin and DeGowin's Bedside Diagnostic Examination,* 5th ed. New York, Macmillan, 1987

Del Guercio LRM: *Multi-lingual Manual for Medical History-taking.* Boston, Little, Brown, 1972

DeMyer W: The patient's mental status and higher cerebral functions. In *Technique of the Neurologic Examination: A Programmed Text,* 3rd ed. New York, McGraw-Hill, pp 329–358, 1980

Eyman RK, et al: The life expectancy of profoundly handicapped people with mental retardation. *N Engl J Med* 323:584–589, 1990

Eyman RK, Cheney RH, Givens CA, et al: Medical conditions underlying increasing mortality of institutionalized persons with mental retardation. *Ment Retard* 24:301–306, 1986

Folstein MF, Folstein SE, McHugh PR: "Mini-mental state": a practical method of grading the cognitive state of patients for the clinician. *J Psychiatr Res* 12:189–198, 1975

Havens LL: Taking a history from the difficult patient. *Lancet* 1:138–140, 1978

Kosan AS: Dental treatment of the handicapped patient. *NY State Dent J* 51:351–353, 1985

Launer J: Taking medical histories through interpreters: practice in a Nigerian outpatient department. *Brit Med J* 2:934–935, 1978

Lembo NJ, Dell'Italia LJ, Crawford MH, et al: Diagnosis of left-sided regurgitant murmurs by transient arterial occlusion: a new maneuver using blood pressure cuffs. *Ann Intern Med* 105:368–370, 1986

MacDonald EP: Medical needs of severely developmentally disabled persons residing in the community. *Am J Ment Defic* 90:171–176, 1985

Merker EL, Wernsing DH: Medical care of the deinstitutionalized mentally retarded. *Am Fam Physician* 29:228–233, 1984

Peters L: Women's health care: approaches in delivery to physically disabled women. *Nurse Pract* 7:34, 36–37, 48, 1982

Pueschel SM, et al: Atlantoaxial instability in Down syndrome: roentgenographic, neurologic, and somatosensory evoked potential studies. *J Pediatr* 110:515–521, 1987

Reisman G, Scanlan J, Kemp K: Medical interpreting for hearing-impaired patients. *JAMA* 237:2397–2398, 1977

Rohde P: The withdrawn patient. *Practitioner* 220:223–227, 1978

Rubin IL, Crocker AC (eds): *Developmental Disabilities: Delivery of Medical Care for Children and Adults.* Philadelphia, Lea & Febiger, 1988

Strub RL, Black FW: *The Mental Status Examination in Neurology,* 2nd ed. Philadelphia, FA Davis, 1985

Ziring PR, Kostner T, Friedman D, et al: Provision of health services for persons with developmental disabilities living in the community: the Morristown model. *JAMA* 160:1439–1444, 1988

STUDY QUESTIONS

Directions: Each of the numbered items or incomplete statements in this section is followed by answers or by completions of the statement. Select the **one** lettered answer or completion that is **best** in each case.

1. A 47-year-old woman comes in because her 42-year-old sister has just been diagnosed as having breast cancer. The clinician's first maneuver should be to

(A) have the patient prepare for breast examination

(B) reassure the patient that she has nothing to worry about

(C) obtain a full risk-factor history

(D) get a family history of all cancer

(E) order a mammogram

2. A 21-year-old male college student presents with the following CC: "I feel something funny in the right side of my scrotum." As the clinician begins the examination, the patient's penis becomes tumescent. The clinician should then

(A) proceed with the examination

(B) stop the examination and leave the room

(C) ask the patient to dress immediately

(D) acknowledge the involuntary erection and proceed with the examination

(E) reassure the patient that this is not an unusual phenomenon and ask whether he would like to proceed or discontinue the examination

3. A new patient, a 35-year-old woman, has on physical examination a unilateral inverted nipple. The clinician should now

(A) ask her if anyone in her family has cancer of the breast

(B) ask her if she has ever noticed that her right nipple looks different from her left

(C) continue with palpation without comment

(D) order a mammogram

(E) refer the patient to a surgeon

4. Patient satisfaction studies have shown that increasing numbers of women are requesting all of the following modifications of the pelvic examination procedure EXCEPT

(A) elevation of the head of the examining table to a 45° angle

(B) reduced or modified draping to allow patient–examiner eye contact during the examination

(C) the use of a plastic rather than a metal speculum

(D) speculum warmed to body temperature

(E) use of a mirror to allow the patient to observe the examination

5. A 25-year-old newly married woman becomes tense and agitated upon insertion of the vaginal speculum. To facilitate the completion of the examination, the clinician should do all of the following EXCEPT

(A) check the lubrication and temperature of the speculum

(B) stop the examination and talk with the patient about her reaction

(C) check the width of the speculum blade relative to the introitus

(D) tell the patient to breathe deeply and relax, then proceed immediately with the examination

(E) place the index finger at the introitus and exert gentle downward pressure against the perineal muscles

6. The male genital examination is best done under which of the following conditions?

(A) Patient supine with legs flat and spread

(B) Patient supine with knees flexed and spread

(C) Patient standing with examiner seated facing him

(D) Patient in left lateral decubitus position

(E) Patient and examiner both standing

7. What is the body position in which the buttocks and rectum can be most effectively examined in the bed-bound patient?

(A) Right lateral decubitus, left hip and knee flexed
(B) Right lateral decubitus, both hips and knees flexed
(C) Supine
(D) Prone
(E) Lithotomy

8. Which of the following tests is most likely to be of use in characterizing a cardiac murmur in a profoundly retarded adult?

(A) Passive straight leg-raising
(B) Sustained handgrip
(C) Valsalva maneuver
(D) Squatting on command to alter hemodynamics
(E) Posterior auscultation

9. All of the following problems are likely to interfere with a complete pelvic examination EXCEPT

(A) osteoarthritis of the hips
(B) dementia
(C) congestive heart failure, decompensated
(D) history of sexual abuse
(E) physician-phobia

10. Thorough examination of the narcotics addict offers several difficulties to the examiner. All of the following factors must be kept in mind in approaching this population EXCEPT

(A) examinations are frequently terminated by inappropriate behavior of the patient, regardless of the examiner's skill and patience
(B) security or other staff should be at hand in case of attempted violence
(C) there is an increased incidence of infection with HIV
(D) there is an increased incidence of infection with hepatitis B virus
(E) pre-medication is necessary if the addict is to be tractable enough to be examined

11. In evaluating a 20-month-old infant with an apparent developmental delay, all of the following tests or examinations would be likely to yield important diagnostic information EXCEPT

(A) audiologic testing
(B) a complete developmental assessment
(C) a complete cardiac examination
(D) karyotyping for chromosomal abnormalities
(E) fasting serum glucose

12. All of the following components of a periodic health evaluation of an asymptomatic, previously healthy 45-year-old mentally retarded woman should be performed EXCEPT

(A) pelvic bimanual examination
(B) Pap smear
(C) chest x-ray
(D) breast examination
(E) mammogram

13. In examining a 6-year-old nonverbal child with mental retardation, which of the following components of the physical examination are likely to be most useful?

(A) Thorough mental status examination
(B) Complete abdominal examination
(C) Careful period of observation
(D) Thorough lung examination
(E) Complete eye examination

14. The clinician's observations on mood and affect are best recorded in the

(A) history: informant, reliability
(B) history: HPI
(C) history: psychiatric part of ROS
(D) physical: general appearance
(E) physical: mental status examination

15. A Folstein score of 13 out of 30 points is most characteristic of

(A) dementia
(B) blindness (inability to read some test items)
(C) deafness (inability to hear some oral test items)
(D) normal cognitive function
(E) depression

16. A patient with a chronic psychiatric disease has all of the signs listed below. Which sign most strongly suggests that a neurologic disorder is present as well?

(A) Delusions and hallucinations
(B) Reflex asymmetry (2+ left knee, 3+ right knee)
(C) Pupillary diameters of 3 mm on the left and 3.5 mm on the right
(D) Nonreactivity on plantar stimulation
(E) Complete amnesia for recent events

ANSWERS AND EXPLANATIONS

1. The answer is C. [*II A 1 a*] History always comes before physical examination under circumstances such as this. It has been demonstrated that the decisions regarding follow-up of a patient with a family history of breast cancer, especially with other risk factors, requires a special approach. Before examining the patient, all the historic information necessary regarding breast cancer risk factors should be gathered, such as parity, nursing, hormonal use, and other family history of breast cancer.

2. The answer is E. [*II C 1*] The event of a penile erection during the genital examination is a fearsome (to the patient even more than the examiner) event. Tumescense of the corpora cavernosa is a subtentorial and involuntary event, is apt to occur on any stimulation, and is something that the patient cannot control. Because the examiner should be aware of the incidental nature of the erection, he or she must be prepared to take the lead in responding and acknowledging what is happening. To discontinue the examination without consultation with the patient is to send a message of disgust or insensitivity. If the examiner lets the patient join in the negotiations about the next step, the probability of accomplishing the mutual goal of ascertaining the cause of the scrotal symptom is greatly increased.

3. The answer is B. [*II A 1 a*] The history should always be taken before proceeding with the examination. If an abnormality is noted on the examination, it should be determined how long it has been present. Inversion of a nipple may be a long-standing phenomenon and of little consequence. Failure to acknowledge the difference in the two nipples may lead to confusion, which might be cleared by simple inquiry. Referral for mammogram or for surgical consultation before getting an adequate history may lead to unnecessary expense and anxiety for the patient.

4. The answer is C. [*II B 2 d*] Elevating the patient's head and shoulders and using a draping technique that allows the patient and clinician to maintain eye contact can make the patient more comfortable and make her feel more like a participant in the examination, than an inanimate "object." A warm speculum is not only more comfortable but minimizes involuntary perineal muscle spasm stimulated by touching with a very cold instrument. Many women have expressed an interest in their own anatomy; a mirror enables these women to observe the examination. The plastic and metal specula are equally acceptable to patients and should be the choice of the examiner.

5. The answer is D. [*II B 3 b*] A speculum that is too large, very cold, too hot, or inadequately lubricated may induce involuntary muscle contractions. Patients may be startled or even have pubic hair caught in the speculum blades. The patient should be asked what happened that caused her muscles to tense. Perhaps she has had a bad prior experience and needs simple reassurance at this point. After assessing the above possibilities and correcting them accordingly, downward pressure should be applied against the posterior introitus, toward the anus, with a fingertip. This motion serves to relax the perineal muscles. To proceed with the examination without checking possible correctable problems is to ask for a less than optimal examination and a disturbed patient.

6. The answer is C. [*II C 1 b, c*] The best access to the scrotal structures and the inguinal ring is with the patient standing and the examiner seated at eye level with the parts to be examined. The patient in a supine or decubitus position does not allow for the gravity advantage for the best examination. Also, the examiner must take into consideration the control issues of the patient being in the superior position during this sensitive examination. If both the examiner and patient are standing, the examiner cannot readily inspect and palpate the dependent genital organs.

7. The answer is A. [*III C 3 a–c, E 4 a*] By convention, the ideal body position for rectal examination is the left lateral decubitus. However, there is no reason why the patient cannot lie on whichever side is more comfortable. In any case, the dependent leg—that is, the leg on the bed—is kept straight, the upper leg is flexed at the waist and knee, and the trunk is twisted toward the bed. The effect of these maneuvers is to present the slightly spread buttocks toward the examiner, facilitating both inspection of the perianal skin and digital rectal palpation; none of the other positions accomplishes this as effectively.

8. The answer is A. [*III E 2*] Profoundly retarded individuals, while typically highly cooperative and eager to please, are often unable to comprehend and assist with maneuvers that require active participation. The advantage of straight leg-raising is that it can be accomplished readily in this setting (unless the subject resists, which is extremely unusual); it is also an excellent choice in the patient who is physically feeble, since the work of the maneuver is done by the examiner. The other choices (i.e., sustained handgrip, Valsalva maneuver, or squatting on command) either require the patient's participation or, in the case of posterior auscultation, are seldom helpful.

9. The answer is B. [*III E 5, F 8*] Arthritic hips cause pain on attempted wide external rotation, the position required for the usual speculum examination. Some demented persons are extremely modest, others show disinhibition, but most are amenable to pelvic examination if the examiner (and chaperon) display the same skills needed to soothe any other patient. The supine position produces breathlessness in heart failure. Patients who find encounters with clinicians unusually highly charged or who have been subjected to sexual abuse need particularly gentle examiners and are even more liable than other patients to find the pelvic examination distasteful and frightening.

10. The answer is E. [*III E 9*] Addicts often relate poorly to health care workers, and unsatisfactory encounters are commonest. Some addicts can be violent, but most will not exhibit more than verbal outbursts in the health care setting; nonetheless, it is important to be sure that colleagues are within earshot until the individual has demonstrated appropriate behavior or has been separated from implements of harm. It is unwarranted and medically counterproductive to medicate patients before they have been evaluated, and this applies to addicts as well as to all others. Although health care workers fear the HIV more than hepatitis B virus (HBV), HBV actually represents the greater threat of contagion.

11. The answer is E. [*IV B 1–3*] The most important aspect of the examination of a 20-month-old infant is a complete developmental assessment. Cardiac and chromosomal abnormalities often accompany developmental disabilities. Poor hearing alone may be a cause for developmental delay and needs to be evaluated thoroughly. There is no routine recommendation for fasting serum glucose, since diabetes has no association with developmental delay.

12. The answer is C. [*IV C 3*] The evaluation of a mentally retarded patient should be identical to that of a patient without mental retardation. Recommendations for healthy 45-year-old women include regular pelvic examinations, Pap smears, breast examinations, and mammograms for all patients over the age of 40. Chest x-ray is not recommended for any age-group at any time as a routine procedure.

13. The answer is C. [*IV D 1–8*] The most information can be obtained by careful observation and inspection, especially in a nonverbal patient. A thorough mental status examination would not be possible in a nonverbal patient. Complete eye examination would also be extremely difficult in a young child. It is unlikely that an abdominal examination or a lung examination would yield useful diagnostic information.

14. The answer is E. [*V C 2 c*] Mood and affect bear on all the components named in the question. If they are strikingly abnormal, they are likely to be mentioned briefly at the outset. Affect is often discussed in the HPI, but it is the affect in the past, not at the present moment. The history should not include the examiner's observations made during the interview. Current affect is fully characterized in detail in the mental status examination.

15. The answer is A. [*V D 4*] Normal individuals usually score 26 or above out of 30 on the Folstein test. Individuals with sensory deficits lose only a few points. Depressed individuals typically show scores in the 20s. A score lower than 20 strongly suggests dementia, delirium, or very poor cooperation with the testing procedure.

16. The answer is B. [*V E*] Reflex asymmetry should not result from psychiatric disturbance, does not occur in normal persons, and is difficult to fake. Delusions and hallucinations can occur in neurologic disease but are commoner in psychiatric disorders. Minor anisocoria is present in many normal hosts, as is nonreactivity on plantar stimulation. Psychiatric causes of amnesia are commoner than neurologic etiologies.

8
Pediatric Clinical Encounter

Paula S. Algranati

I. PEDIATRIC HISTORY

A. Overview

1. **Parents** are the usual source of the pediatric history, the exception being adolescents who usually provide their own histories.
   a. **Accuracy of reporting** is dependent on the parents' innate abilities as observers. Parental interpretation of their observations also influences the reporting.
      (1) The **parent's perspective** is influenced by proximity to the patient (e.g., the perspective of the working parent vs. the perspective of the parent at home).
      (2) The **parent's perceptions** of a child's vulnerability to illness may magnify minor problems into major concerns.
      (3) **Hidden agendas.** Listening to "how" a parent reports the history in addition to "what" the parent says, may reveal the "real" concerns of the parent.
   b. **Clarification of the history.** Exploring how the problem has affected the child's day-to-day functioning (e.g., playing, sleeping, drinking) can help parents to see the problem from the child's vantage point.

2. **Children.** The potential for the child to contribute to the history is often overlooked. Techniques for obtaining a history directly from the child include the following:
   a. **Posing questions at a developmentally appropriate level** will maximize the child's ability to respond (e.g., the 5-year-old is able to "point to the ear that hurts" but is unable to respond to the question, "Why did you misbehave?").
   b. **Using humor cautiously** (e.g., joking but not teasing, friendliness without intrusiveness) may help to put the child at ease.
   c. **Uncovering hidden agendas** and addressing them when feasible may improve compliance (e.g., children who are concerned about receiving immunizations may be reluctant to admit that they do not feel well).
   d. **Clarifying what will transpire,** using developmentally appropriate language, enhances cooperation. The child hears everything, both tone and content, that transpires between the parent and the clinician.

3. **Adolescent**
   a. **Confidentiality.** Prior to obtaining the history, the clinician should explain to the patient, and the parent if present, that under usual circumstances the content of the encounter between the patient and the clinician is confidential. This reinforces the clinician's role as the adolescent's advocate.
   b. **Sensitive issues,** such as sexuality or puberty, are approached in an open and matter-of-fact manner. Preparation for discussion of sensitive issues requires that the clinician:
      (1) Acquires a working knowledge of expected patterns and normal variations of adolescent growth and development and of common age-related problems
      (2) Examines his or her internal values and prejudices, thereby reducing the likelihood of making judgmental statements and fostering the ability for making objective recommendations

B. Comprehensive pediatric history.
A complete history is obtained in the outpatient setting whenever a new patient is seen for either a well-child or a problem visit (except that which is trivial in nature) and whenever a child is admitted to the hospital. An outline of the comprehensive history follows. Details are provided below only in areas that differ significantly from the standard adult history (see Chapter 3). Specific age-related content is discussed in I C.

1. **Chief complaint (CC).** The reason for the visit is recorded as a direct quote from a parent or the patient.

2. **History of present illness (HPI).** Narrative description of the evolution of the CC is given in the HPI, including relevant past medical history and relevant review of systems.

3. **Past medical history (PMH)**
   a. **Prenatal, natal, and neonatal history**
      (1) **Prenatal**
         (a) **Maternal**
            (i)   Age
            (ii) G (gravida status)
            (iii) P (para status)
            (iv) Ab (abortus status)
            (v)   EDC (due date)
         (b) **Pregnancy**
            (i)   Prenatal care
            (ii) Complications
            (iii) Medications
            (iv) Substance abuse
      (2) **Natal**
         (a) Onset of labor: spontaneous or induced, including indications for induction
         (b) Duration of labor
         (c) Duration of rupture of membranes prior to delivery
         (d) Meconium staining of amniotic fluid
         (e) Medications during labor and delivery
         (f) Presentation (vertex vs. breech)
         (g) Vaginal or cesarean section, including indications for cesarean section
         (h) Maternal response to the experience of labor and delivery
      (3) **Neonatal**
         (a) Birth date, birth weight, and gestational age of newborn
         (b) Apgar scores and condition of infant at delivery
         (c) Resuscitation required
         (d) Problems in nursery (e.g., jaundice) and therapy administered
         (e) Discharge from hospital of both mother and infant, including reasons for prolongation of hospitalization, if applicable
   b. **Childhood illnesses and recent exposures**
   c. **Immunizations and reactions**
   d. **Medications**
   e. **Allergies** (i.e., medication, others)
   f. **Injuries**
   g. **Hospitalizations, surgery, and transfusions**
   h. **Prior screening results** (e.g., hearing, vision, newborn screens), including the date, results, and recommendations
   i. **Nutrition**
      (1) Infant feeding history (e.g., breast, formula, solids), including timing, problems, and satisfaction level
      (2) Childhood eating history, including likes, dislikes, and actual diet
   j. **Growth and development**
      (1) **Developmental milestones.** Ages at attainment of major developmental milestones should be listed, such as lifts head off bed, rolls over, sits alone, pulls to stand, walks alone, holds cup or spoon, smiles, babbles, says first meaningful word, says two-word phrases, talks in sentences, dresses alone, ties shoelaces, and skips.
      (2) **Growth and motor development** should be noted, such as infant and child growth patterns as well as parental concerns about growth rate, motor development, and progress of puberty. Prior measurements should be recorded when available.

4. **Review of systems (ROS).** A few general questions are posed within each major system. Further detail is pursued, depending on the response to general inquiry, CC, and age of patient. Only topics that are uniquely pediatric are listed below. Standard topics of inquiry are listed in Chapter 3. Age-specific content for the pediatric ROS may be found in I C.

    a. General. Activity level, days of missed school, poor or excessive growth

    b. Skin. Birthmarks

    c. Head, ears, eyes, nose, throat (HEENT), and neck. Abnormal size or shape of head, crossed eyes

    d. Lymphatics

    e. Breasts. Premature or delayed puberty

    f. Cardiovascular and respiratory systems

    g. Gastrointestinal system. Colic, soiling

    h. Genitourinary system. Bedwetting, premature or delayed puberty

    i. Musculoskeletal system. Congenital deformities, scoliosis

    j. Neurodevelopment and psychiatric. Delayed development, school progress

5. Psychosocial history. Questions explore the child's life-style; environment; and behavioral, emotional, and cognitive functioning. Choice and phrasing of questions are tailored to the specific patient.

    a. Affective development. Inquiry focuses on the child's mood, behavior, relationship with peers, siblings, and other family members. Topics include temperament, adjustment to rules and discipline, peer interactions, ability to adapt to new situations, favorite activities, strengths, and weaknesses.

    b. Cognitive development. Inquiry focuses on prior and present intellectual functioning and may include a discussion of language development, speech problems, school readiness, school progress, and functioning.

    c. Habits and day-to-day functioning

        (1) Sleep. Usual patterns, past or present night waking, nightmares, night terrors

        (2) Toileting. Age of attainment of bowel and bladder control, enuresis, encopresis

        (3) Habits. Thumb-sucking, body and head-rocking, nail-biting, tics

        (4) Sexuality. Sex awareness and experiences

        (5) Substance abuse. Problems with alcohol, cigarettes, and other drugs

        (6) Other parental concerns

    d. Household and family (as in the adult)

    e. Child's self-image. The child is asked to discuss his or her own perceptions of personal strengths and weaknesses, likes and dislikes, and concerns. The adolescent is asked if concrete plans have been formulated for future employment or education.

6. Family history (FH). This is obtained in the same manner as in the adult (see Chapter 3 I F) with the addition of **congenital anomalies** and **deaths in infancy** or **childhood (causes)**.

C. Interval history and age-related topics. The interval history is a global update of the patient's health and psychosocial status. The interval history is obtained at every **well-child visit.** Pertinent components of the interval history are also explored during **problem visits** to gain further insight into the patient's problem or effect of the problem on the patient's day-to-day functioning. Questions are geared to the **age** and **developmental stage** of the child.

1. Infants (ages 2 weeks to 12 months)

    a. General care. Inquiry focuses on:

        (1) Daily functioning, such as feeding (e.g., method, scheduling, problems), sleep (e.g., schedules, night waking), and bowel and bladder functioning

        (2) Parental care, such as injury prevention (e.g., use of car seat, child-proofing), provision of appropriate toys, and tooth care

    b. Growth and development. Inquiry focuses on:

        (1) Affective development as evidenced by:

            (a) Infant's effect on the environment (**synchrony**)

            (b) Parents' perceptions of the infant's behavioral style (**temperament**)

            (c) The older infant's demonstration of preferential response to caretakers as demonstrated by separation and stranger anxiety, beginning at 6–9 months (**attachment**)

        (2) Cognitive development. The infant (9–12 months) shows an interest in:

            (a) Searching for objects hidden while he watches (**object permanence**)

            (b) "Windup" toys (**causality**)

        (3) Physical development as evidenced by:

            (a) Sleep–wake cycle patterns (**state organization**)

            (b) Parental perceptions of the infant's growth and strength

            (c) Reports of motor accomplishments

    c. Developmental milestones are assessed by a combination of the history and physical examination. Expected findings for age are found under the neurodevelopment examination (see III B 9). Milestones in the following areas are sought:

      (1) Hearing, vision, and language

      (2) Gross motor abilities

      (3) Fine motor abilities

      (4) Personal and social interaction abilities

    d. General health (interval update of ROS and PMH). Inquiry focuses on:

      (1) Symptoms (e.g., teething) the infant may have had

      (2) Medicine exposure, including over-the-counter medications (e.g., vitamins, acetaminophen)

      (3) Immunization reactions or contraindications

      (4) Perceptions of the infant's vision and hearing

      (5) Self-soothing (e.g., thumb-sucking) or self-stimulating (e.g., head-banging) behaviors

      (6) Results of prior screening procedures

    e. FH (interval update of family health and psychosocial histories). Inquiry focuses on:

      (1) Adjustment of family members to the new infant

      (2) Return to work or school, including child care arrangements

      (3) Smokers in the household

2. Toddlers (ages 15 months to 4 years). Part of the history (especially in the areas of daily life) can be obtained directly from the older toddler.

    a. General care. Inquiry focuses on:

      (1) Daily functioning, such as diet (e.g., content, utensil use, weaning, mealtime behavior, concerns about decreased appetite), sleep (e.g., schedules, struggles), and bowel and bladder control (e.g., toilet training)

      (2) Parental care, such as injury prevention (e.g., use of a car seat, child-proofing, stranger awareness) and tooth care (e.g., avoidance of bottle in bed, first dental examination at 3 years of age)

    b. Growth and development. Inquiry focuses on:

      (1) Affective development as evidenced by:

        (a) "Negative" behaviors (autonomy–independence struggles)

        (b) Lack of impulse control

        (c) Heightened stranger anxiety (15–18 months)

        (d) Separation difficulties (**attachment**)

        (e) Discipline style

        (f) Temperament

        (g) Play behavior (e.g., "lovey" toy, pretend, parallel play)

        (h) Peer interactions

        (i) Adjustment to day care or nursery school

        (j) Dressing up in clothes of the opposite sex (gender identity is not yet fixed)

      (2) Cognitive development as evidenced by:

        (a) Emergence of the toddler's understanding of things or individuals not actually present (**representation,** 18 months)

        (b) Emergence of "what's this" questions (2 years)

        (c) Parent's perceptions of school readiness (4–5 years)

        (d) Progress in language, the most important cognitive issue for ages 2–5

          (i) The 2-year-old child makes his or her desires known verbally, uses several words regularly, and responds by pointing when asked to locate a common object.

          (ii) The 3-year-old child speaks in short sentences, uses "me" or "you" correctly, and responds to simple directions.

          (iii) The 4-year-old child can tell someone his name, discuss simple aspects of daily life, and uses some plurals and past tenses.

      (3) Physical development as evidenced by:

        (a) The degree to which the toddler is "always moving" and enjoys "rough" play

        (b) Parental responses to toddler behaviors

        (c) Parental concerns regarding delays in walking, appearance of extremities, and deceleration of growth rate

    c. Developmental milestones are assessed by the combination of the history and physical examination. Expected findings for age are found under the neurodevelopment examination (see III C 9). Milestones in the following areas are sought:

        (1) Language acquisition
        (2) Gross motor abilities
        (3) Fine motor abilities
        (4) Personal and social interaction

    d. General health (interval update of ROS and PMH). Inquiry focuses on:

        (1) Symptoms the toddler may have had
        (2) Medicine exposures
        (3) Immunization reactions or contraindications
        (4) Parent's perceptions of the toddler's vision and hearing (and readiness for formal screening)
        (5) Habits (e.g., thumb-sucking, pica, masturbation)
        (6) Results of prior screening procedures (e.g., lead, tuberculosis)
        (7) Speech intelligibility (75% by age 3, almost 100% by age 4)
        (8) Disfluency (stuttering), letter substitutions, hesitancies

    e. FH (interval update of family health and psychosocial histories). Inquiry focuses on:

        (1) Toddler's effect on the household, including sibling rivalry
        (2) "Goodness of fit" between the toddler's behaviors and abilities vs. expectations of parents
        (3) Major changes in household structure (e.g., marital status, employment, new infant)

3. School-age child (ages 5–10 years). The clinician involves the school-age child as an active participant while obtaining a history. The adolescent visit may be previewed by asking the parent to return to the waiting room after major concerns are elicited.

    a. General care. Inquiry focuses on daily functioning, such as:

        (1) Diet (e.g., content, scheduling, attempts at weight change)
        (2) Sleep (e.g., schedules, struggles, night waking)
        (3) Elimination (e.g., independent functioning, soiling, bedwetting)
        (4) Dental care
        (5) Exercise (e.g., participation, organized sports)
        (6) Play (e.g., preferences, peer involvement)
        (7) Safety (e.g., use of seat belts, water and fire safety)
        (8) Risk-taking behavior (e.g., fire setting, substance abuse)

    b. Growth and development. Inquiry focuses on:

        (1) Affective development as evidenced by:

            (a) Peer interactions ("best" friend)
            (b) Gender identity (fixed at age 5)
            (c) Conflicts with rules and authority figures
            (d) Decreasing reliance on parents (autonomy–independence issues)
            (e) Responsibilities at home
            (f) Child–parent communication
            (g) Mood
            (h) Temperament

        (2) Cognitive development as evidenced by:

            (a) School adjustment, school functioning (e.g., actual grades, preferences, problems and remediations, recent changes in performance, absenteeism)
            (b) Ability to focus on multiple aspects of a problem, establish hierarchies, use logic, and acknowledge other points of view (**concrete operations,** 8 years)

        (3) Physical development. The clinician should determine if there is an awareness of upcoming puberty or evidence that puberty has begun. The pre- or early pubertal child requires "privacy" when discussing this subject.

    c. Developmental milestones are assessed by a combination of the history and physical examination. **School** and **athletic progress** supply important information about major areas of development. Expected findings for age are found under the neurodevelopment examination (see III D 6). Milestones in the following areas are sought:

        (1) Language abilities
        (2) Gross motor abilities
        (3) Fine motor abilities
        (4) Personal and social interaction

    d. General health (interval update of ROS and PMH). Inquiry focuses on:
      (1) Somatic complaints (e.g., limb pains, headaches, recurrent abdominal pain)
      (2) Illnesses the child may have experienced
      (3) Immunization reactions or contraindications
      (4) Habits (e.g., thumb-sucking, nail-biting, tics)
      (5) Vision, hearing, and speech abilities (and results of prior screens)
      (6) Puberty-related concerns
    e. FH (interval update of family health and psychosocial histories). Inquiry focuses on:
      (1) The effect of the child's school entry on the family
      (2) Major changes in household structure
      (3) Whether the preadolescent's "declaration of independence" is a source of family stress

4. Adolescent (ages 12–16 years). The adolescent is the **primary historian.** If necessary, time is allotted for parents' special concerns. Optimally, parents are not present when the adolescent is interviewed. Confidentiality is discussed at the beginning of the encounter. Sensitive issues (e.g., substance abuse, sexuality, and self-perceptions) are best discussed after rapport has been established.
    a. General care. Inquiring about a "typical day" is a nonthreatening way to begin an adolescent history. Inquiry focuses on aspects of daily life, such as:
      (1) Diet (e.g., content scheduling, attempts at weight change)
      (2) Sleep (e.g., patterns, difficulties)
      (3) Dental care
      (4) Exercise (e.g., participation, team sports, injuries)
      (5) Leisure activities (e.g., preferences, peer involvement, reading, television)
      (6) Injury prevention (e.g., seat belts, driving habits of self and peers)
    b. Growth and development. Inquiry focuses on:
      (1) Affective development as evidenced by:
        (a) Relationships with adults. Rules, privileges, and responsibilities at home are discussed as well as the adolescent's ability to confide in his or her parents and activities shared with adults. The clinician should not assume that the adolescent lives with both parents.
        (b) Relationships with peers. "Best" friend or confidant, dating experience, similarities and differences in values, and interests of peers are discussed. Asking the adolescent if friends experiment with substances of abuse (e.g., smoking, drinking, drugs) or other risk-taking behaviors is a nonthreatening way to introduce these topics. This may be followed by the question, "Do you ever . . . too?" Further information about the extent of the involvement or the desire to stop is explored if necessary.
        (c) Self-assessment of overall well-being. Using a scale of 1–10 or asking for a "weather report" of "how life has gone so far" provides evidence of the adolescent's overall sense of happiness. Other topics to discuss include strengths, weaknesses, concerns, and wishes.
      (2) Cognitive development as evidenced by:
        (a) School performance (e.g., actual grades, preferences, problems, remediations, recent changes in performance, absenteeism)
        (b) Ability to reason hypothetically and think abstractly (e.g., stage of **formal operations,** age 12)
        (c) Concrete plans for future employment or education (older adolescent)
      (3) Physical development as evidenced by knowledge and concerns about puberty, pubertal changes, development, growth, strength, and sexual identity. The clinician should acknowledge the difficulty in discussing sexuality while emphasizing its necessity because of the impact on the patient's health. Asking the adolescent if friends are involved in sexual relationships is a nonthreatening way to introduce this topic. This may be followed by the question, "Have you ever been involved in a sexual relationship?" Assumptions about consent, heterosexuality, and homosexuality should be avoided.
    c. Developmental milestones are assessed by monitoring:
      (1) School performance
      (2) Athletic and extracurricular activities
      (3) Tanner staging (Tables 8-3, 8-4, and 8-5)

    d. General health (interval update of ROS and PMH). Inquiry focuses on:

       (1) Somatic complaints (particularly skin, musculoskeletal, genitourinary systems)

       (2) Illnesses the patient may have experienced

       (3) Habits, (e.g., nail-biting, tics, compulsions)

       (4) Self-assessment of vision, hearing, speech, and results of recent screens (e.g., scoliosis)

       (5) Complaints related to puberty and sexuality, which should be pursued further if prior discussion is incomplete. Specifically, the clinician offers the opportunity to discuss the following subjects:

          (a) Male patients. Experience with, or concerns about, erections, wet dreams, birth control, pregnancy, sexually transmitted diseases, and testicular self-examination

          (b) Female patients. Experience with, or concerns about, menarche, birth control, pregnancy, sexually transmitted diseases, and breast self-examination

    e. FH (interval update of family health and psychosocial histories). Relationships with family have been explored earlier. The clinician summarizes prior discussion and clarifies concerns raised earlier.

D. Focused history. The focused history is obtained whenever the clinician is investigating a patient's problem. The history is focused on the HPI and relevant ROS. Additional information from the **age-appropriate interval history** may also be required to gain insight into the patient's problem or effect on the patient's day-to-day functioning (e.g., quality of eating, drinking, sleeping).

II. PEDIATRIC PHYSICAL EXAMINATION

A. Overview

    1. Resistance to examination. Patient age, behavior during the history portion of the encounter, and chart review may indicate which patients will resist. Contributing factors include:

      a. Developmentally related fears, such as stranger and separation anxiety, which begin during the latter half of the first year, and exaggerated fears of bodily harm, which are common in 5- or 6-year-old children

      b. Failure to understand what's happening during the encounter (related to level of cognitive development)

      c. Innate temperament or personality. Chart review revealing statements, such as "slow to warm up" or "gregarious and outgoing," may predict whether or not the patient is likely to cooperate for an examination.

      d. Prior frightening or painful medical experiences (e.g., the 3-year-old with multiple visits for otitis media may be wary of the ear examination)

      e. Lack of appropriate limit-setting by parents

      f. Fussiness and irritability. Observation of the child's overall state of health, alertness, and mood helps to predict which patients will resist.

    2. Countering resistance. Techniques to maximize compliance (by adjusting the manner of approach and examination sequencing) include:

      a. Entering the room gradually, avoiding direct eye contact (initially), speaking in a soft friendly voice, and sitting away from the patient if the child has stranger anxiety

      b. Examining the child in the parent's lap (or with the parent close by) if the child has separation anxiety

      c. Using the child's physical and cognitive abilities to distract, entertain, and familiarize him or her with the examination

        (1) The child may be allowed to manipulate or practice with instruments (e.g., the stethoscope is transformed into a telephone).

        (2) Noises and conversation can be helpful (e.g., "guessing" what the toddler ate for lunch softens the abdomen during palpation).

      d. Pacing the encounter to fit the child's innate temperamental style. The shy, "slow to warm up" child requires more time before actually being touched. The child who adapts poorly to change requires advance notice of upcoming maneuvers.

      e. Altering the examination sequencing by beginning with the least intrusive aspects of the examination (e.g., observe motor skills and inspect skin) and proceeding from the periphery of the body inward rather than head-to-toe sequencing (e.g., count fingers or toes first)

f. Engaging the parent as an ally to distract or soothe the child (e.g., give a hungry baby a bottle)

g. Asking the parent to set appropriate limits to release the clinician from the "bad guy" role

h. Taking advantage of opportunities as they arise (e.g., the cardiac auscultation may be performed in a sleeping child without protest; a hungry infant sucking on a bottle may allow funduscopic examination)

3. Observation to obtain data. The relative importance of this technique as part of the physical examination is maximal in pediatrics. Observation will supply data related to:

a. Parent–child relationship. Clinicians must observe and listen to the content and manner of parent–child interactions.

b. Child's affect and temperament. The child's behavior out of and within the examination room is observed.

c. Developmental milestones
   (1) Gross motor skills are observed as the child moves around the room or on the examining table.
   (2) Fine motor skills are observed as the child plays with crayons or blocks.
   (3) Speech content and clarity is displayed when the child converses with parent or sibling.

d. Other physical findings
   (1) General impressions about growth and body proportions (e.g., Does the head size seem too large for the body?)
   (2) Obvious congenital anomalies (e.g., asymmetry of facial features, cleft lip, low-set ears, pidgeon breast)
   (3) Gait patterns
   (4) Skin lesions

4. Measurements and vital signs in children. Because of the evolving nature of physical findings in children, it is particularly important to assess pediatric measurements and vital signs correctly.

a. Length or height. Supine length is measured in infants and children up to age 2 or 3; beyond that age, erect height is measured. Length or height is assessed at every well-child visit and whenever there are concerns about growth or development. This measurement is also necessary for calculations of surface area (or meter square) in administering intravenous fluid therapy.
   (1) Supine length is measured on a flat, hard surface; two adults may be required for restraint. The recumbent length is the distance between the vertex and the soles of the feet. This is an imprecise measurement, especially in the newborn who has normal flexion contractures at the hips and knees.
   (2) Standing height is measured with the child in bare or stocking feet, which is the same technique used with adults.
   (3) Length or height is recorded on the appropriate age and sex chart at the patient's exact age.
      (a) Length or height measurements in children between the ages of 2 and 3 years may be recorded on either the "Birth to 36 Months" chart (supine length only) or the "2–18 Years" chart (erect height only).
      (b) The toddler's length or height must be recorded on the chart that reflects the norms appropriate to the method used.

b. Weight. The child is weighed wearing a diaper or underwear and a hospital gown.
   (1) Weight is recorded on the appropriate age and sex growth chart at the patient's exact age.
   (2) Weight is measured at every well-child visit, at most illness-related visits, and whenever calculations for medication of fluid therapy are required.

c. Head circumference. A tape measure surrounds the head to obtain the **maximal occipital–frontal circumference** (Figure 8-1).
   (1) Head circumference is recorded on the appropriate age and sex chart at the patient's exact age.
   (2) Head circumference is measured at every well-child visit during the first year (the period of maximal brain growth) and whenever there are concerns about growth, development, or neurologically related systems.

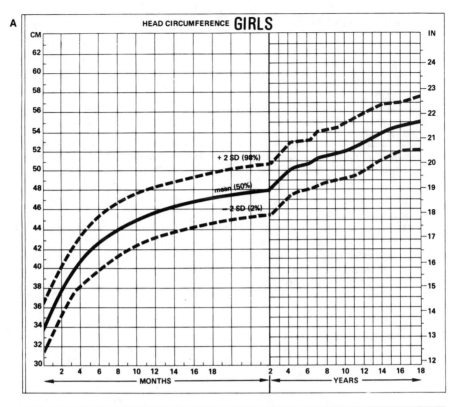

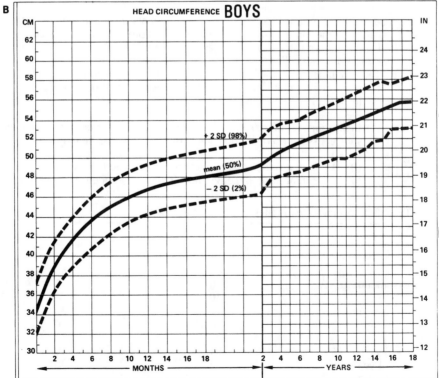

Figure 8-1. Head circumference. *A,* Girls; *B,* boys. (Reprinted with permission from Nellhaus G: Composite international and interracial graphs. *Pediatrics* 41:107–108, 1968.)

Table 8-1. Normal Respiratory Rates in Children

Age	Respirations/min
Newborn	30–75
6–12 months	22–31
1–2 years	17–23
2–4 years	16–25
4–10 years	13–23
10–14 years	13–19

Reprinted with permission from Cloutier MM: Pulmonary diseases. In *Pediatrics*. Edited by Dworkin PH. Baltimore, Williams & Wilkins, 1987, p 266.

   d. Respiratory rate. If feasible, respiratory rate is determined when the child is at rest and is not crying. It is most accurate when the child is sleeping.
     (1) Respiratory rate is determined by observing the rise and fall of the chest or by chest auscultation, as long as the child is not consciously "breathing in and out" to cooperate with the examiner
     (2) Normal respiratory rates decrease with advancing age throughout childhood, increase with physical activity, and are lowest in the sleeping child.
     (3) Respiratory rates are measured in the newborn, in the hospitalized child, and in ill children, particularly those with respiratory, cardiac, or neurologic concerns (Table 8-1).
   e. Heart rate. Heart rate is determined by palpation of a peripheral pulse, by cardiac auscultation, or by observation of pulsations through an open fontanelle.
     (1) Normal heart rates decrease with advancing age throughout childhood. Heart rates increase with physical activity, fever, and anxiety.
     (2) Heart rates are measured in the newborn and in the hospitalized child. Heart rates are also measured in ill children, particularly those with concerns about cardiac, respiratory, or hydration status (Table 8-2).
   f. Blood pressure. Routine blood pressure measurements are determined using the right brachial artery in the same manner as in adults. Blood pressure is determined at every well-child visit beginning at 3 years of age and whenever there are concerns about cardiac or renal status or serious illness.
     (1) The **cuff** (inner inflatable bladder not the outer cloth covering) should completely encircle the circumference of the child's arm (with or without overlap).
       (a) It should be wide enough to cover approximately three quarters of the length of the upper arm.
       (b) Inappropriate cuff size selection accounts for most errors in pediatric blood pressure assessment. When choosing between two sizes, the larger cuff should be selected.
         (i) A cuff that is too small will overestimate blood pressure.
         (ii) A cuff that is too large will not significantly underestimate blood pressure.

Table 8-2. Average Heart Rates in Children at Rest

Age	Average Rate	Two Standard Deviations
Birth	140	50
First month	130	45
1–6 months	130	45
6–12 months	115	40
1–2 years	110	40
2–4 years	105	35
6–10 years	95	30
10–14 years	85	30
14–18 years	82	25

Reprinted with permission from Lowrey GH: *Growth and Development of Children*, 8th ed. Chicago, Year Book, 1986, p 246.

(2) **Normal blood pressure** increases with advancing age throughout childhood. Systolic blood pressure rises with anxiety (Figure 8-2).
- **(a)** Lower extremity systolic blood pressure, using the popliteal artery, is normally 10–30 mm higher than **upper extremity systolic blood pressure**.
- **(b)** The **fourth Korotkoff sound** (K4) [muffling] is used in the standards for **diastolic pressure in children** up to the age of 12.
- **(c)** The **fifth Korotkoff sound** (K5) [disappearance] is used in the standards for **diastolic pressure in adolescents** 13–18 years of age.

g. Temperature. Rectal temperature is determined in children too young to cooperate for the **oral** method. Some offices and hospitals use an **ear probe** instead of an oral or rectal thermometer. Temperature is determined in the newborn, the hospitalized child, and in the outpatient who is ill.
- **(1)** The normal Farenheit temperature range is approximately: 97.5° F–100.4° F rectally. Rectal temperature is approximately 1° higher than oral temperature.
  - **(a)** Normal temperature increases with physical activity, hot ambient temperature, and heavy clothing.
  - **(b)** Normal temperature decreases (by a total of approximately 1°) with advancing age from newborn to adolescent.
- **(2)** There is a normal diurnal variation in body temperature. Temperature rises to its highest point by early evening and falls to its lowest point at midnight. The diurnal variation may encompass as much as 2°.
- **(3)** Forehead strips do not measure core temperature accurately.

B. Comprehensive pediatric physical examination. The complete physical examination is performed in the outpatient setting whenever a patient is seen for **well-child care** or a **problem visit** involving generalized or vague complaints (minor problems merit a more focused examination). All **ill infants** (e.g., under 4–6 months) require a comprehensive physical examination, regardless of the problem. In addition, the **child admitted to the hospital,** regardless of the CC, requires a comprehensive examination. An outline of the comprehensive examination follows to be used once techniques have been mastered. Details are added only in areas that differ significantly from the standard adult physical examination (see Chapter 6). Examination sequencing and age-related procedures (and techniques) are discussed in III.

1. Identifying information. Demographic data should include objective statements of the patient's name, age, and sex.

2. Measurements (age-dependent and CC-dependent)
- **a.** Length or height
- **b.** Weight
- **c.** Head circumference
- **d.** Respiratory rate
- **e.** Heart rate
- **f.** Blood pressure
- **g.** Temperature

3. Observations and findings
- **a. General appearance.** The importance of these observations in the pediatric population cannot be overstated. Clues to underlying serious infection or other covert pathologic processes may be found by observing the general appearance. This is particularly true in the preverbal age-group. Observations of various global characteristics, such as well or sick, state of nutrition (e.g., well-nourished, obese, thin), and hygiene. General impression of physical development, obvious dysmorphic features, degree of alertness, irritability (and consolability), and cooperation. Age-related examination emphasis is provided in III.
- **b. Skin, hair, and nails.** Note any birthmarks (see III A 3 d).
- **c. HEENT.** Fontanelle size; suture approximation; corneal light reflex; alternate cover test; tympanic membrane examination, including pneumatic otoscopy; inspection for bifid uvula; palpation of soft palate for submucous cleft; speech clarity (e.g., letter substitutions) and content; teeth are counted.
- **d. Neck.** Webbing
- **e. Chest, lungs, and heart.** Femoral pulses vs. right radial pulse
- **f. Breasts.** Tanner stage
- **g. Abdomen**
- **h. Genitalia, anus, and rectum.** Anal patency; Tanner stage

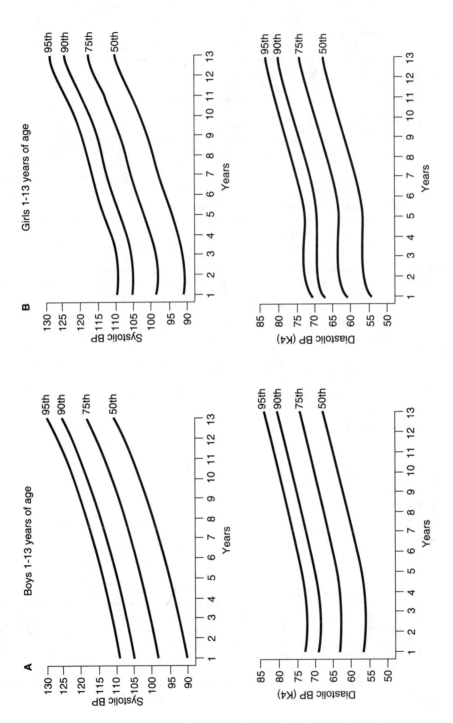

Figure 8-2. Age-specific percentiles of blood pressure measurements. (Reprinted with permission from the Task Force on Blood Pressure Control in Children: Report of the second task force on blood pressure control in children—1987. *Pediatrics* 79:6–7, 1987.)

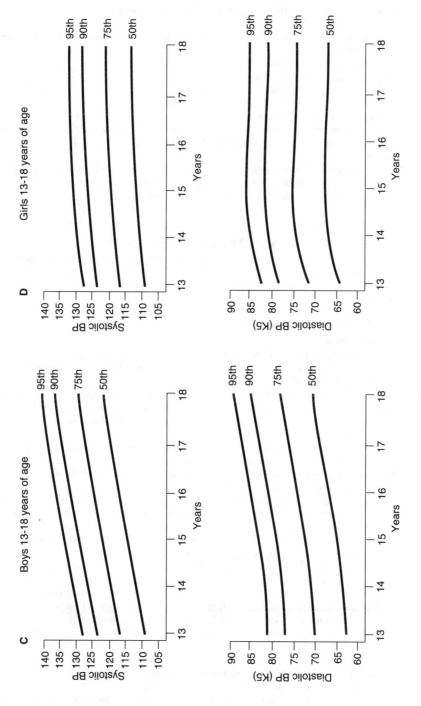

Figure 8-2. Continued.

     i. Back
     j. Upper and lower extremities. Check for Gower's sign (see III C 9 b).
     k. Neurologic and developmental examination
         (1) Gestational age
         (2) General appearance and mental status
         (3) Cranial nerves (I–XII). Assess as completely as possible.
         (4) Gross motor skills
         (5) Fine motor skills. Assess age-related task ability (e.g., pincer grasp, transferring, copying figure)
         (6) Coordination. Age-related
         (7) Station and gait. Age-related
         (8) Unwanted movements
         (9) Sensory. Cortical sensation in older children
        (10) Reflexes. Primitive reflexes
        (11) **Cognition.** Informal assessment by inquiring about school performance. If significant concerns are identified, formal testing may be required (e.g., WISC-R or Stanford Binet)
        (12) **Developmental milestones** are assessed by an objective list of age-appropriate tasks or screening instrument (e.g., collection of age-appropriate tasks or Denver Developmental Screening Test). If significant delays are identified, formal testing may be required.

III. AGE-RELATED PHYSICAL EXAMINATIONS. Most clinical situations (e.g., well-child visit, hospital admission, problem visit for complex or vague complaints) require a comprehensive examination. The examination is tailored to fit the patient's age, developmental stage, and complaints. This section reviews expected age- and stage-related normal findings, common variations of normal, and areas of special emphasis.

    A. Physical examination of the newborn
      1. General principles
        a. The parent–infant interaction is observed for the presence or absence of bonding. Does the parent seem interested and concerned about the infant? Does the parent look at, touch, or speak to the infant?
        b. A complete physical examination is performed with special attention to screening for congenital anomalies, birth trauma, neonatal medical problems, and assessment of gestational age. A **head-to-toe sequence** is feasible with the following exceptions:
          (1) Chest auscultation is performed at the onset if the infant is calm and quiet.
          (2) Screening for congenital hip dysplasia should be deferred until the end of the examination as this is uncomfortable and will evoke a cry.
        c. Gestational age is most accurate when assessed by examination rather than by maternal history. Gestational age assessment is based on the fact that a variety of neurologic and physical findings evolve in an orderly and predictable manner as gestation progresses. Premature and postmature infants are at increased risk for various perinatal and neonatal problems.
          (1) **Categories.** Infants are categorized by gestational age into three groups.
            (a) **Premature** (37 weeks of gestation or less)
            (b) **Full term** (38–42 weeks of gestation)
            (c) **Postmature** (greater than 42 weeks of gestation)
          (2) **Scoring systems** (e.g., Dubowitz) assign weighted numerical values to specific physical and neurologic findings to determine gestational age. These scores are summed, and the totals are correlated with specific weeks of gestation. Some clinicians use physical findings alone, some use neurologic findings alone, and some use a combination of both.
         (3) **Prematurity**
           (a) **Physical findings that suggest prematurity** include:
             (i) Thin smooth skin that is red or dark pink
             (ii) Absence of palpable breast tissue or breast tissue that is less than 1 cm in diameter
             (iii) Ear pinnae that are soft without definite cartilage and are easily folded into various positions without ready recoil

(iv) Thick layer of vernix (cheesy white material) covering the skin

(v) Abundant lanugo (soft downy hair) on the back

(vi) Absence of creases on the soles of the feet or creases on the anterior third only

(vii) Immature genitalia (testes in the canal in boys and prominent clitoris and labia minora in girls)

(viii) Skull bones that are soft

(b) Neurologic findings that suggest prematurity. Neurologic findings are assessed when the infant is quiet and calm. The premature infant has an overall "floppy" tone; the range of passive motion of the extremities far exceeds that of the term and older infant. Findings include:

(i) Little or no flexion of the extremities with posture at rest. The full-term newborn has a fully flexed posture.

(ii) Poor overall tone

(iii) Scarf sign. This sign is elicited in a supine infant when the hand is drawn across the neck toward the opposite shoulder. In the premature infant, the elbow reaches beyond the midline or to the opposite anterior axillary lines. The elbow does not reach the middle of the thorax in the full-term infant (Figure 8-3).

(iv) The heel approaches or reaches the head when the foot is moved toward the head while the pelvis is held flat (**heel-to-ear maneuver**). The heel does not reach the head in a full-term infant (Figure 8-4).

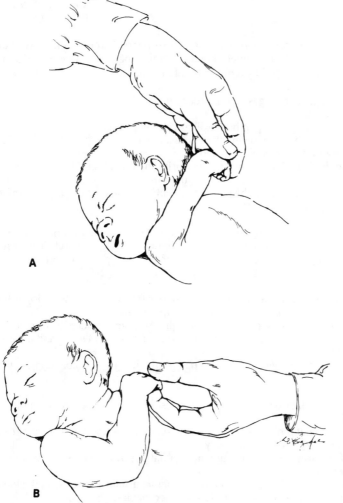

A

B

Figure 8-3. Scarf sign. *A,* Premature newborn. The elbow reaches the opposite anterior axillary line. *B,* Full-term newborn. The elbow does not reach the midline of the thorax. (Adapted with permission from Klaus MH, Fanaroff AA: *Care of the High Risk Neonate,* 3rd ed. Philadelphia, WB Saunders, 1986, p 82.)

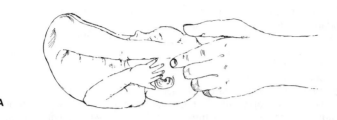

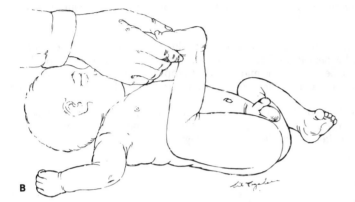

Figure 8-4. Heel-to-ear maneuver. *A,* Premature newborn. The heel reaches the head. *B,* Full-term newborn. The heel does not reach the head. (Adapted with permission from Klaus MH, Fanaroff AA: *Care of the High Risk Newborn.* Philadelphia, WB Saunders, 1973, p 44.

      (v) A semicircular posture when the infant is suspended prone in the air with the chest resting on the examiner's hand (**ventral suspension**). A more horizontal posture is maintained by a full-term infant (Figure 8-5).

    (4) Postmaturity

      (a) Physical findings that suggest postmaturity include:

        (i) Long fingernails

        (ii) Skin that is thick and parchment-like with deep cracks

        (iii) Deep sole creases, involving the entire surface

        (iv) Skull bones that are well calcified

      (b) Neurologic findings that suggest postmaturity include all of the mature neurologic criteria of the term infant (e.g., mature posture or scarf sign) plus fully developed primitive reflexes of the term infant with fewer exceptions than a term infant might display (see III A 10 b)

2. General appearance. Observations are made with the infant at rest for overall impression (e.g., maturity, color, activity, gross abnormalities in body size or configuration) and signs of respiratory distress, which may be audible (e.g., grunting) or visible (e.g., nasal flaring).

3. Skin

  a. Normal **acrocyanosis,** involving the perioral skin or skin of the extremities, is distinguished from true **cyanosis,** involving nail beds and mucous membranes.

  b. The presence of **jaundice** is assessed in natural sunlight. Assessment includes the extent of head-to-toe involvement, which roughly correlates to actual bilirubin level, and determination of scleral icterus.

  c. **Normal fair skin tone** is distinguished from true **pallor** (involving pale bulbar conjunctival vessels).

  d. **Common birthmarks**

    (1) Salmon patch or stork bite is a flat pink to red lesion over the eyelids, nasal bridge, and nape of the neck.

    (2) Port wine stain is a flat pink to red lesion most commonly found on the face or neck but may be found anywhere on the body.

    (3) Forerunner of the strawberry hemangioma is a flat hypovascularized area with telangiectasia within.

    (4) Mongolian spot is a ''black and blue'' colored macule, usually located over the lower spine and buttocks. It is commoner in dark skinned babies.

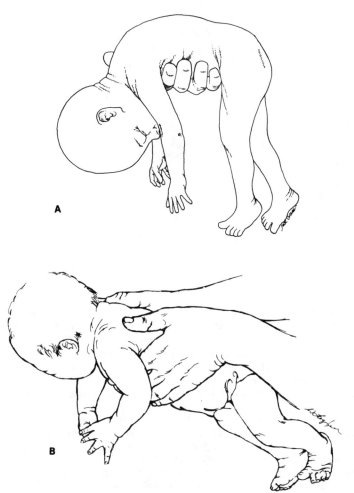

Figure 8-5. Ventral suspension. *A,* Premature newborn. *B,* Full-term newborn. (Adapted with permission from Klaus MH, Fanaroff AA: *Care of the High Risk Newborn.* Philadelphia, WB Saunders, 1973, p 44.

e. **Benign newborn rashes**
   (1) **Erythema toxicum** has a "flea bite" appearance of scattered erythematous macules, some of which may contain papulopustular centers; the distribution of this rash characteristically changes from hour to hour.
   (2) **Milia** consist of small yellowish white papules most commonly found on the bridge of the nose, chin, or cheeks.
   (3) **Miliaria rubra** consists of tiny papules or vesicles that may have a surrounding red halo base and is found on the face and neck.
   (4) **Transient neonatal pustular melanosis** consists of vesiculopustular lesions found all over the body. The lesions rupture within a few days and leave pigmented macules with a surrounding fine scale. It is commoner in dark skinned infants.

4. **Head and neck**
   a. **Head circumference** is measured.
   b. **Shape and symmetry of skull and face** are noted. Pressure on the head during labor and delivery may produce:
      (1) Molding of the head into an elongated or asymmetric shape
      (2) Caput, ill-defined area of firm, pitting scalp edema, which crosses suture lines
      (3) **Cephalohematoma,** a circumscribed area of swelling, which usually does not cross suture lines and has a "mushy" or tense center
   c. **Cranial sutures** are not fused at birth (Figure 8-6).
      (1) Suture lines are palpated for **ridging** or **overriding,** which may result from pressure during labor and delivery or for unusually **wide separation** (i.e., more than a fingertip), which may result from increased intracranial pressure.

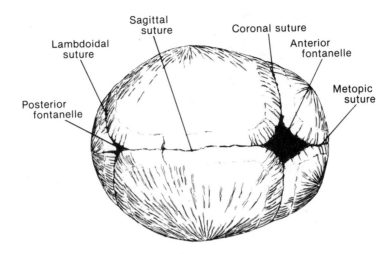

Figure 8-6. Cranial sutures and fontanelles.

    (2) Fontanelle borders are outlined with the fingertip for estimation of size: The anterior fontanelle is diamond shaped (average size is 2 × 2 cm up to 3 × 4 cm); the posterior fontanelle is approximately a fingertip in diameter. When the infant is held upright, the anterior fontanelle is flat (neither sunken or bulging) [see Figure 8-6].

  d. Eyes may "cross" intermittently up to 3 months of age. This is normal as long as there is no paralysis of the extraocular muscles.

    (1) A **red reflex** (observed through the ophthalmoscope) excludes lens opacities (e.g., cataracts) and retinoblastoma.

    (2) Scleral hemorrhage is a consequence of the birth process and resolves spontaneously.

    (3) Eyelids may be swollen during the first 48 hours if silver nitrate was instilled at birth.

  e. Ears are examined for placement and configuration. Normal placement means that the top of the external ear does not appear posteriorly rotated and that the ear is not "low set" (i.e., when an imaginary horizontal line is drawn through the medial canthi of the eyes, more than 1/10–1/5 of the total height of the external ear should fall above that line).

    (1) Ear canals are filled with vernix caseosa.

    (2) Tympanic membranes are examined only in ill newborns or if a congenital anomaly is suspected.

  f. Nose

    (1) Most newborns are obligate nose breathers.

    (2) Sneezing in moderation is the newborn's normal mechanism for clearing the nasal passages of amniotic fluid and debris.

  g. Lips, mouth, and palate are observed for symmetry with the newborn at rest and during crying.

    (1) Benign white papules may be observed at the junction of the hard and soft palate (**Epstein's pearls**) or on the gum lines (**epithelial pearls**).

    (2) The hard palate is inspected for an abnormally high arch, which may accompany other craniofacial anomalies.

    (3) The soft palate is palpated to rule out a submucous cleft.

    (4) The uvula is inspected for absence of a bifid appearance, which may accompany other craniofacial anomalies.

  h. The neck is assessed for **webbing** (seen in Turner's syndrome), masses (head should be extended during inspection and palpation to rule out masses or swellings, such as goiter or thyroglossal duct cyst), and mobility.

5. Chest

  a. Clavicles are palpated for crepitance, an indication of a fracture, which is usually the result of a difficult delivery.

  b. Breast engorgement and secretion of a milky substance ("witches milk"), resulting from the withdrawal of maternal hormones, are noted several days after birth.

    c. Rate and rhythm of respirations are noted. Short pauses in respirations are normal as long as the pauses do not exceed 20 seconds and are not associated with limpness, pallor, cyanosis, or bradycardia.

    d. Murmurs

       (1) A soft blowing **systolic ejection murmur,** usually heard at the upper left sternal border, may be present transiently during the first few days of life secondary to changing cardiovascular dynamics.

       (2) The benign **midsystolic murmur of peripheral pulmonic stenosis** is heard along the distribution of the peripheral pulmonary arteries; therefore, it is as loud in the right chest as in the left. This murmur disappears by 3 months of age.

6. Abdomen. Palpation is best accomplished while the infant is sucking.

    a. Inspection of the "brand new" moist **umbilicus** reveals the presence of two thick-walled arteries and one thin-walled vein. The absence of an umbilical artery is associated with many other congenital anomalies.

    b. The **liver edge** of the newborn is normally palpated 1–2 cm down from the costal margin in the midclavicular line. A **spleen tip** may be palpable in the normal newborn.

    c. Kidneys are palpated for approximate size (2×4 cm) and masses.

       (1) The right kidney is lower and, therefore, easier to feel. Experienced examiners may not always be able to locate both kidneys.

       (2) The kidneys are palpated using either one hand (thumb over the abdomen and fingers under the back) or two hands (one hand under the back and one hand on the abdomen).

    d. Femoral pulses are palpated and compared to the right brachial pulse for delay or diminishment to rule out the likelihood of a coarctation of the aorta. The pedal pulses are substituted if difficulty palpating the femoral pulses is encountered.

7. Genitalia and anus. Careful inspection for congenital anomalies is especially important. Inspection for anal patency and palpation for inguinal masses is performed in boys and girls. Swelling and ecchymoses of external genitalia may be noted for several days after breech presentations.

    a. Boys

       (1) The penis is inspected for approximate length (3–4 cm stretched length), ventral bend (chordae), and location of the urethral meatus.

       (2) Retractile testes, which are located in the inguinal canal but may be "milked down" into the scrotum, must be differentiated from true undescended testes, which are either not palpable or impossible to "milk down."

    b. Girls. The clitoris, urethra, and vagina are visualized to rule out anomalies and ambiguous genitalia.

       (1) In the full-term infant, the normal-sized clitoris is covered by the labia when the legs are in the adducted position.

       (2) The vagina is inspected for imperforate hymen and for posterior labial fusion, which obscures the separation of the vaginal introitus from the urethral meatus.

       (3) Vaginal discharge or bleeding and labial swelling, resulting from the withdrawal of maternal hormones, are noted several days after birth.

8. Extremities. Extremities are inspected at rest for asymmetries of shape, angulation, and bulk. They are also observed for symmetry during movement to rule out a fracture or nerve injury.

    a. Flexion contractures (mild) of the elbows, knees, and hips are present during the first weeks of life in term newborns.

    b. Congenital hip dysplasia. Examination to rule out this condition begins by evaluating symmetry of medial thigh creases, gluteal folds, approximate leg lengths, and degrees of hip and knee flexion (Figure 8-7).

       (1) This is followed by the **Ortolani maneuver,** which determines if a posteriorly dislocated hip can be relocated into the acetabulum, and the **Barlow maneuver,** which determines if a hip can be posteriorly dislocated out of the acetabulum. These maneuvers may be performed on one hip at a time while the opposite side of the pelvis is stabilized with the examiner's free hand or both hips simultaneously.

         (a) The examiner stands at the feet of a supine infant.

         (b) The hip is placed in 90° of flexion, and the knee is fully flexed. The examining hand grasps the upper thigh so that the second and third fingers lie on the posterolateral thigh over the greater trochanter, and the thumb lies on the anteromedial thigh just distal to the inguinal fold; the flexed leg rests against the examiner's palm.

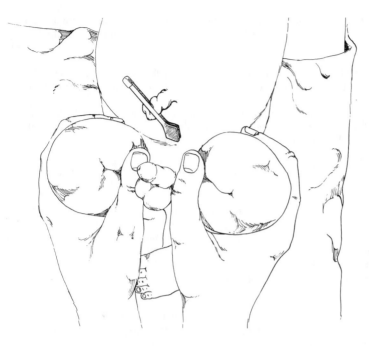

Figure 8-7. Bimanual examination of the hips for congenital dislocation. (Adapted from the Standing Medical Advisory Committee and the Standing Nursing and Midwifery Advisory Committee for the Secretaries of State for Social Services and for Wales: *Screening for the Detection of Congenital Dislocation of the Hip.* London, England, Department of Health and Social Security, 1986, p A4.)

    (c) As the hip is gently abducted, the examiner applies gentle upward (towards the ceiling) pressure on the posterolateral thigh to relocate a posteriorly displaced hip back into the acetabulum (Ortolani maneuver). If a dislocated hip has been relocated back into the acetabulum, the clinician may feel or hear a "clunk."

    (d) With the hips in the adducted position, downward (towards the floor) pressure is applied by the thumb onto the anteromedial thigh to dislocate an unstable hip posteriorly (Barlow maneuver). If a hip has been dislocated by this maneuver, the clinician may feel or hear a "clunk."

  (2) Cartilagenous "clicks," which usually emanate from the knees, must be distinguished from true "clunks." This distinction is difficult and requires considerable experience performing these maneuvers.

 c. Tibial bowing laterally at the midsection (mild) is a common consequence of intrauterine positioning.

 d. Angulation and flexibility of the feet. When the heel is held between the examiner's thumb and forefinger, the forefoot is frequently curved towards the midline (**metatarsus adductus**) as a consequence of intrauterine positioning (Figure 8-8). Mild degrees of this problem are common and self-resolving. If the forefoot rigidly resists straightening, orthopedic correction will be necessary.

9. Back. The spine should appear straight and intact. It is palpated along its full length.

 a. A **dimple** over the lower spine is common and is not usually clinically significant as long as it is not the lead point for a sinus tract or skin defect.

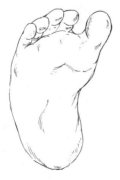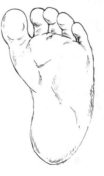

Figure 8-8. Metatarsus adductus.

b. Mass lesions (e.g., hemangiomas or other soft tissue masses) or hairy tufts that lie directly on the spine must raise the suspicion of an underlying abnormality of neural tube development.

10. Neurologic examination

a. General neurologic impressions include:

(1) **State** (e.g., sleeping, awake) **and degree of alertness**

(2) **Fluidity and spontaneity of movements**

(a) The term newborn may display a few beats (but not sustained) clonus of the extremities.

(b) The term newborn may display an occasional Moro reflex with normal handling.

(c) The term newborn should not feel "floppy" when handled.

(3) **Quality of cry.** The healthy term newborn has a loud and lusty cry.

b. Reflexes

(1) **Primitive reflexes** supply the examiner with information about the overall integrity of the neurologic system. They are evaluated for presence and symmetry. Primitive reflexes are not fully developed in the premature infant. They include the following:

(a) **Moro reflex** consists of the symmetric abduction of the upper extremities with extension of the fingers and a lesser abduction of the lower extremities, followed by a return to the normal flexed posture. This reflex is elicited by cradling the head and upper body of a supine infant in the examiner's hands and abruptly (gently) lowering the hands back towards the surface on which the infant is lying (Figure 8-9).

(b) **Sucking reflex.** The infant spontaneously and firmly sucks on a nipple or finger placed in the mouth.

(c) **Rooting reflex.** The infant turns the head (and begins to suck) when the skin of the face just lateral to the outer corner of the mouth is stroked.

(d) **Placing and stepping.** While the infant is held upright (under the axillae), the top of the foot is scraped along the lip of a table or bassinet, the infant will flex the foot and "place" it onto the table surface. When the sole of the foot touches the table

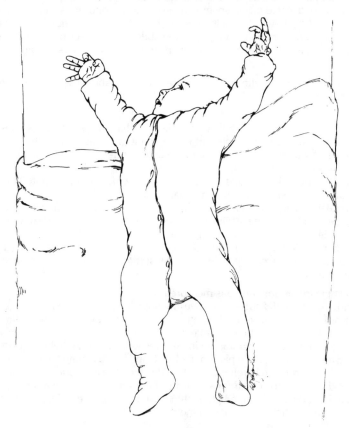

Figure 8-9. Moro reflex.

surface, the infant will bring the other foot forward and begin to take several ''steps.''

   (e) **Reflex grasp.** The infant will spontaneously close the fist when an object is placed within the palm.

(2) **Plantar reflex** may result in flexion or extension in the normal newborn.

c. **Vision** is assessed by observing:

   (1) Pupillary reflexes
   (2) The infant blinking in response to bright light
   (3) The infant, while quiet and alert, fixing on and following the examiner's face as the examiner moves slowly from side to side

d. **Hearing** is assessed by the introduction of a novel sound (e.g., a bell) and watching the infant ''alert'' by quieting movements and opening eyes.

11. **Development** is assessed by the determination of gestational age, the response to sensory stimuli, and by the neurologic examination.

B. Physical examination of the infant (ages 2 weeks to 12 months)

1. **General principles**

   a. **Observation of the parent–infant interaction** includes watching how the parent holds, feeds, and comforts the infant.

   b. **A complete physical examination** is performed with special attention to growth and early motor development. During the first few months, renewed attention is focused on screening for congenital anomalies. **A head-to-toe sequence** for most of the examination is feasible during the first 4–6 months because of the compliant nature of the young infant.

      (1) **Chest auscultation** is performed at the onset if the infant is quiet and calm.

      (2) Following auscultation, the examiner returns to the head and proceeds downward, **deferring the tympanic membrane, pharynx,** and **hip examinations** until the end as these intrusions are likely to evoke protest even in very young infants.

      (3) Once the infant acquires a **fear of strangers** and **separation anxiety,** a head-to-toe sequence becomes less feasible. Compliance is maximized by beginning with the least intrusive maneuvers (e.g., observations of skin, body proportions, muscles of facial expression) and by beginning palpation peripherally prior to moving centrally (e.g., count fingers and toes before palpating the abdomen). Noises or toys can be used to distract the infant. If necessary, the entire examination may be performed with the infant in the parent's lap.

2. **General appearance** is noted with attention to facial appearance, overall mood, motor activity, and body proportions.

3. **Skin**

   a. Newborn **rashes** (e.g., erythema toxicum, miliaria, milia) and the scales of transient neonatal pustular melanosis may be present in the infant under age 1 month.

   b. **Infantile acne** may be found on the face of the infant under 3 months. The appearance of this rash is the same as in the adolescent.

   c. **Seborrhea** is a yellow-tinged, greasy, scaly eruption, which is concentrated on the scalp (called cradle cap), eyebrows, behind the ears, and skin folds.

   d. **Atopic dermatitis** (eczema) is a red, dry eruption, which during infancy involves the face (especially the cheeks) and the extensor surfaces of the extremities. There may be overlying crusts or vesicles, and there is frequently marked excoriation.

   e. **Strawberry hemangioma** grows rapidly during the first year of life and appears as a raised, bumpy (like a strawberry) red to purple lesion. Most strawberry hemangiomas regress completely during middle childhood.

4. **Head and neck.** Head circumference is measured.

   a. Palpable ridging of **cranial sutures** resolves by approximately 6 months of age.

   b. The **posterior fontanelle** closes by 2 months of age, and the **anterior fontanelle** closes between 6 and 18 months (up to age 2 may be normal).

   c. **Vision** is assessed grossly by noting the infant's response to bright light, by observing the infant following a light or boldly patterned object, and by observing the older infant reach out for a toy. The corneal light reflex and alternate cover test are performed in infants (over 3–6 mos) and toddlers to screen for strabismus (abnormal ocular alignment).

      (1) **Corneal light reflex.** When a light is shined on the eyes, the reflection of light on the corneas (corneal light reflex) is symmetric.

     (2) **Alternate cover test.** With the infant fixing on an object, the examiner alternately occludes the line of sight of one eye, then the other (back and forth) without allowing an intervening period of binocular vision (and without touching the eyes). Any movement of the eye, which has just been uncovered, raises a suspicion of strabismus.

  d. **The ear canal** of the infant is directed upwards. Pulling the pinna down and posteriorly facilitates visualization of the tympanic membrane. **Pneumatic otoscopy** (i.e., the otoscope with an attached rubber or plastic tube and bulb) enables the clinician to assess mobility of the tympanic membrane.

     (1) Pneumatic otoscopy requires a firm seal between speculum and ear canal. Therefore, the largest sized speculum that fits easily into the canal (at this age, size 2.5–3 is appropriate) is used.

     (2) The ear examination may be performed with the infant supine on the examining table or while sitting in the parent's lap. To avoid injury to the ear canal, the infant must be firmly restrained (Figure 8-10).

  e. *Candida albicans* infection (**thrush**) presents as a white coating on the tongue or buccal mucosa, which resists scraping.

  f. The infant is observed for evidence of a **lateral head tilt** or **chin rotation** (e.g., congenital muscular torticollis).

5. Chest

  a. Auscultation of the nose followed by chest auscultation assists the examiner in distinguishing sounds emanating from the upper airway from those emanating from the lungs.

  b. During crying, the inspiratory phase of breathing is easily appreciated. Expiratory sounds are best appreciated during quiet breathing.

  c. **Innocent systolic ejection murmurs** may be appreciated during the first year of life. An innocent murmur is present without underlying cardiac pathology and has the following characteristics:

     (1) It is generally soft (not louder than a grade 2 or 3).

     (2) It occupies the ejection portion of systole (i.e., begins after the first heart sound) except for the continuous murmur of the venous hum.

     (3) It does not radiate widely from the point of origin.

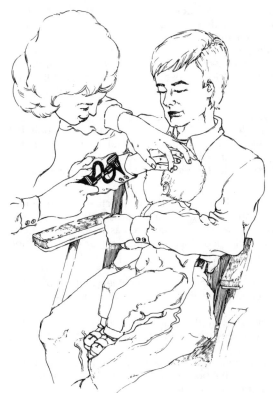

Figure 8-10. Ear examination with infant in parent's lap.

(4) It may change in intensity with repositioning the patient (supine to prone).
(5) It is never accompanied by other adventitious sounds.
(6) The innocent murmur of peripheral pulmonic stenosis may be heard up to age 3 months. Disappearance by this age confirms the diagnosis retrospectively.

6. Abdomen
   a. After the umbilical cord falls off, an **umbilical hernia** may be noted as an outpouching around the umbilicus.
   b. A separation of the medial rectus sheath known as a **diastasis recti** is commonly found in the infant.

7. Genitalia
   a. **Labial adhesions** may form after birth and occlude the vaginal orifice. These may separate over time from the minor trauma associated with diaper changes or during early adolescence under the influence of estrogen hormone.
   b. **Diaper rashes** are common and predictable during infancy.
      (1) Generic or **ammonia diaper rash** appears as an area of red, dry confluent inflammation; the groin creases are usually spared.
      (2) *Candida* **diaper rash** appears as a bright red area of confluent inflammation in the groin with accompanying tiny red "satellite" papules just beyond the margins of the rash. This rash may involve the groin creases.
   c. **Phimosis,** tightness of the foreskin so that it cannot be drawn back from over the glans penis, is physiologic in infant boys.

8. Extremities
   a. Examination for **congenital hip dislocation** continues throughout infancy. Movement of a dislocated or dislocatable hip (Ortolani and Barlow maneuvers) into or out of the acetabulum becomes impossible after early infancy. Thereafter, the most significant evaluation of the hips consists of noting the normally symmetric and full (almost 90°) abduction of the hips when they are held in flexion with the infant in the supine position.
   b. During initial attempts at ambulation, the infant has a **wide-based gait,** which functions to improve stability. The legs and feet gradually come together as the infant grows and gains confidence and agility.
   c. Once the legs come together, the parents may note **intoeing.** Forces at the hip joint (excess femoral anteversion) along the shaft of the tibia (internal tibial torsion) or at the feet (metatarsus adductus) may be responsible for intoeing.
      (1) To assess the degree of **hip rotation,** the infant is placed in the prone position with the hips in extension (flat on the table) and knees flexed to 90° (Figure 8-11). During infancy and young childhood, external rotation exceeds internal rotation, but they are approximately equal in older children. In the presence of **excess femoral anteversion,** the degree of internal rotation is greater than normal (e.g., greater than 60°).
      (2) To examine for **internal tibial torsion,** the child is placed in the sitting position on the end of the examining table with the legs dangling over the side and knees pointing straight ahead. In the presence of internal tibial torsion, the lateral malleolus is rotated so that it is placed more anteriorly than the medial malleolus.
      (3) The feet are evaluated for **metatarsus adductus,** which may have been overlooked in the newborn period (see Figure 8-8).

9. Neurologic and developmental examination. Observing the infant "practice" new developmental achievements offers the clinician the opportunity to evaluate gross and fine motor muscle strength and coordination; cranial nerve evaluation is enhanced as well. The examiner mentally reviews the standard components of the neurologic examination during observation of milestones and adds remaining maneuvers as necessary.
   a. Age-specific neurodevelopment
      (1) The **2–4-week-old** infant regards the human face, follows an object as it is moved 90° to either side from the midline, reacts to sound, lifts head slightly when prone, and has a reflex grasp.
      (2) The **2-month-old** infant smiles responsively, follows an object as it is moved from side-to-side past the midline, turns head and eyes to sound, raises head 45° when prone, and babbles and coos.
      (3) The **4-month-old** infant shows excitement with familiar people, follows an object as it is moved through 180°, laughs, raises the body on arms when prone, rolls front to back, sits with support, and has a brief purposeful grasp.

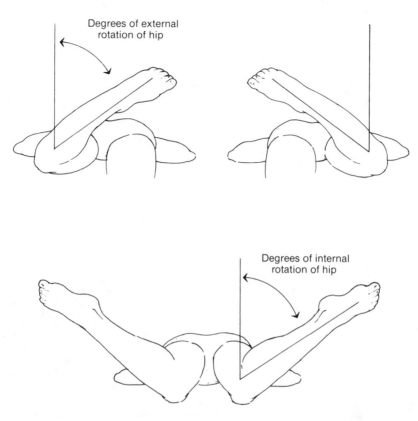

Figure 8-11. Assessment of external and internal rotation at the hip. (Reprinted with permission from Staheli LT: Torsional deformity. *Pediatr Clin North Am* 24:803, 1977.)

        (4) The **6-month-old infant** squeals, may sit alone, bears some weight when held erect, rolls back to front, reaches, transfers small objects from one hand to the other, and turns body to sound.

        (5) The **9-month-old infant** babbles mama or dada nonspecifically, sits alone, pulls to stand, transfers well, and plays peekaboo.

        (6) The **12-month-old infant** says mama or dada with meaning (and possibly other meaningful words), cruises, has a pincer grasp (i.e., picks up small objects with thumb and forefinger), plays social games (e.g., pat-a-cake and waves bye-bye), and looks for objects hidden in his presence.

    b. Primitive reflexes, which appear at birth (e.g., Moro reflex) or during the first month of life (e.g., tonic neck reflex), may be normally elicited up to 4–6 months of age (Figure 8-12). Delayed disappearance of these may reflect a problem with neuromaturation.

    c. Delayed appearance of other primitive reflexes, which normally emerge later, may also reflect a problem with neuromaturation. For example, a parachute reflex is elicited in an infant beginning at approximately 6–9 months of age. This reflex is elicited by holding the infant in ventral suspension and then abruptly tilting the head toward the floor. Both arms should extend symmetrically as if protecting oneself from falling.

    d. Head lag when pulled by the hands from a supine to sitting position should no longer be present in a 6-month-old infant.

C. Physical examination of the toddler (ages 15 months to 4 years)

  1. General principles

    a. Observation of the parent–child interaction includes listening to and observing limit-setting and ease of separation. The younger toddler may be expected to cling to the parent and resist examination. The lap examination continues to be helpful. The clinician may allow the child to explore the room during history taking, while observing the activity level, motor abilities, language development, and gait.

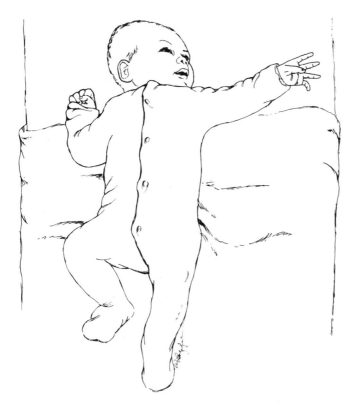

Figure 8-12. Tonic neck reflex. A tonic neck reflex is elicited in a supine infant whose shoulders are held level by rotating the head to one side. The extremities on the side that the head faces will extend, and the extremities on the opposite side will flex. The reflex should appear symmetric when the head is turned to either side.

    b. A complete physical examination is performed with special attention to vision, hearing, dentition, language development, tympanic membranes, and gait.

        (1) Often, the 3- or 4-year old child will cooperate by sitting on the examination table independently and allow a **head-to-toe examination** while conversing about familiar aspects of daily life (e.g., television, nursery school).

        (2) Praise for "acting like a big boy or big girl," allowing choices (e.g., "which ear shall be looked at first"), and reviewing simple aspects of the medical history directly with the child not only enhance cooperation but initiate the patient in an independent physician-patient relationship.

2. General appearance is noted with attention to facial appearance, overall mood, and motor and verbal abilities. **Blood pressure** is obtained at well-child visits beginning at age 3.

3. Skin (atopic dermatitis). The dry skin and excoriations may involve any area of the skin, but during the toddler and middle childhood years, the antecubital and popliteal fossae are predominantly involved.

4. Head and neck

    a. Eyes. By age 4, many children can cooperate for formal **visual screening.** This may be accomplished by using a wall chart (e.g., a Snellen test), which uses "tumbling E's" or pictures of common objects. The corneal light reflex and alternate cover test are performed to screen for strabismus. Children before their 5th birthday should read at least the 20/40 line. Failure to accomplish this or a two-line difference in acuity between the eyes, even in the passing range, warrants ophthalmologic referral.

    b. Ears. By age 4, many children can cooperate for formal **audiologic screening.** This is accomplished with the use of a pure tone audiometer. Failure of hearing screen is defined as an inability to respond to sounds of 1000 Hz or 2000 Hz at 20 dB or 4000 Hz at 25 dB in either ear when cooperation has been judged adequate. Failure to pass a hearing screen merits an otoscopic examination and may require formal audiologic testing. The high incidence of middle ear disease in the toddler age-group requires careful examination of the tympanic membranes for color, landmarks, and mobility.

    c. Oral hygiene is evaluated. Teeth should be counted and inspected for stains and decay. By age 24–36 months, most toddlers will have a full complement of 20 primary teeth.

d. **Speech and language.** Listening to the content and clarity of the patient's speech confirms the history obtained from the parent about language development and speech disfluencies. Letter substitutions, such as "w" for "r" in "rabbit" or "d" for "th" in "that" are common and developmentally appropriate during the toddler years.

e. **Large tonsils and shoddy cervical lymphadenopathy** are common findings in the toddler and often reflect the high frequency of upper respiratory infections in this age-group.

5. **Chest**

   a. **Auscultation of the lungs** includes careful evaluation of both inspiratory and expiratory phases. Lung sounds during end expiration may be difficult to hear but may be more easily appreciated if the examiner applies gentle inward pressure on the thorax (during expiration).

   b. **Innocent murmurs** are often first heard during the toddler years. The following are three innocent murmurs:

      (1) **Still's murmur** is a soft, vibratory systolic ejection murmur. It is heard loudest halfway between the lower left sternal border and the apex. It decreases in intensity when the patient sits up and increases in intensity with fever, exercise, and anxiety.

      (2) **Venous hum** is a continuous murmur (heard in both systole and diastole). This is the only innocent murmur that is heard during diastole. It is heard best in the right infraclavicular area. It may be softened or extinguished by turning the patient's head away from the site of the murmur or by compression of the ipsilateral internal jugular vein. It disappears when the patient lies down.

      (3) **Carotid bruit** is a systolic ejection murmur that is heard over the carotids. It diminishes as auscultation proceeds towards the aortic or pulmonic areas.

6. **Abdomen**

   a. The toddler's abdomen retains an infantile **protuberant shape,** which is accentuated by a normal lower lumbar lordosis.

   b. Toddlers are often ticklish and resist abdominal palpation.

      (1) Conversing during the examination (e.g., telling the child that the examiner is going to "guess" what was eaten for breakfast) is a useful distractor.

      (2) Placing the patient's fingers under or over the examiner's and asking the patient to "press down for me" enhances deep palpation.

      (3) Fecal material is commonly palpated as small, round, hard, mobile "balls" in the left lower quadrant; occasionally, a sausage-shaped stool mass may outline the descending colon.

7. **Genitalia**

   a. Itchy **vaginal discharge** is usually a benign and nonspecific problem. However, the possibility of sexual abuse must always be excluded. The presence of perineal or anal warts (or bruises or lacerations) makes this diagnosis especially likely.

   b. By age three, 90% of boys will have a fully retractable **foreskin.**

8. **Extremities**

   a. The young toddler's **feet appear flat** because fat pads obscure the longitudinal arch of the feet.

   b. Increased **femoral anteversion** is the commonest cause for intoeing. Examination to confirm this diagnosis and rule out metatarsus adductus and internal tibial torsion is required when intoeing is observed.

   c. **Toe walking** may be a transient phenomenon seen in the newly ambulating child. Careful neuromuscular examination is required as the child with spastic diplegia or muscular dystrophy may also demonstrate toe walking.

9. **Neurologic and developmental examination**

   a. **Age-specific neurodevelopment**

      (1) The **15-month-old child** walks alone, has a pincer grasp, bangs two blocks together, scribbles spontaneously, indicates wants by some method other than crying, and says mama or dada specifically.

      (2) The **18-month-old child** descends stairs unaided (may slide on belly), may throw a ball overhand, turns pages of a book, uses a spoon, piles a block on top of another, identifies body parts, and says three words other than mama.

      (3) The **2-year-old child** climbs stairs alone, kicks a ball, makes a pile of four blocks, holds a cup securely, and uses pronouns, such as mine, me, you, or I.

(4) The **3-year-old child** pedals a tricycle, can copy a vertical line or draw a circle, begins to share toys and play interactive games with peers, and answers the question, "What is he doing?" when shown a picture book.

(5) The **4-year-old child** can point to many body parts, heel walk, begin to perform rapid opposing movements of thumb and forefinger, supply two out of three correct answers when asked for name, age, and address, repeat four numbers with one error, and crudely copy a drawing of two circles atop each other.

b. **General neurologic examination** includes observing for a **Gower's sign,** which is seen in children with muscle weakness in the lower back or pelvic girdle (e.g., Duchenne muscular dystrophy). The child with a Gower's sign will get up off the floor from a prone position in the following manner:

(1) Buttocks are lifted up in the air.

(2) The rest of the back comes off the floor.

(3) The hands are "walked" up along the lower extremities (for bracing) until the upright position is reached.

D. Physical examination of the school-age child (ages 5 years to 10 years)

1. General principles

a. **Observation of the parent–child interaction** includes listening to "how" the parent talks "about" the child and "to" the child. Statements exemplifying parental support and acceptance or excessive criticism and rigidity are noted.

b. **A complete physical examination** is performed with special attention to growth, dentition, scoliosis screening, breasts, and genitalia.

(1) The older school-age child is supplied with a gown to wear over underwear. In addition, a drape is used during the examination in the same manner as in the adult examination.

(2) When the interview is concluded, if the parent is absent, the clinician inquires as to whether or not the child would like the parent to be present during the examination. Female patients to be examined by male clinicians always require a chaperon (e.g., parent, nurse) during the physical examination.

(3) Children between 5 and 8 years of age may have some **special concerns** about "getting a shot" or other painful procedures. By openly addressing this concern with reassurance if feasible, the patient is given two messages:

(a) The clinician respects the patient's concerns.

(b) The clinician is being truthful.

(4) The school-age child does not usually display major resistance to the general examination. If he or she does, the examiner should reflect on the possible explanations.

(a) The child is still experiencing some difficulties with separation (not rare in 5-year-old children).

(b) The child has a "slow to warm up" or "shy" temperament. This child may manifest similar difficulties at school.

(c) The child may have poor limit-setting at home.

(d) The child may have been physically abused.

(e) The child may be very ill or in severe pain.

2. Head and neck

a. **Vision.** Children 5 years of age or older should read a majority of the 20/30 line. Failure to do that or a two-line difference in visual acuity (even in the passing range) between eyes requires ophthalmologic evaluation.

b. Teeth

(1) Shedding of primary teeth begins around 6 years of age usually with the loss of the lower central incisors. Eruption of permanent dentition begins within 1–2 years.

(2) The top teeth should overlap the bottom teeth all the way around the mouth. The clinician should also observe that the child bites down on the back teeth.

3. Chest

a. **Sternal bowing** (inward pectus excavatum, outward pectus carinatum) and chest wall asymmetries become more noticeable in this age-group as the thoracic cage elongates and the "pot belly" thins out.

b. Breasts of both sexes are inspected. Tanner stage is noted in girls (Table 8-3).

(1) In girls, breast budding (the onset of puberty) may begin as early as 8 years of age or as late as 13 years of age.

Table 8-3. Tanner Stages of Female Breast Development

Stage I	Preadolescent: The juvenile breast has an elevated papilla (nipple-shaped projection) and small flat areola.
Stage II	The breast bud forms under the influence of hormonal stimulation. The papilla and areola elevate as a small mound, and the areolar diameter increases.
Stage III	Continued enlargement of the breast bud further elevates the papilla. The areola continues to enlarge; no separation of breast contours is noted.
Stage IV	The areola and papilla separate from the contour of the breast to form a secondary mound.
Stage V	Mature: The areolar mound recedes into the general contour of the breast. The papilla continues to project.

Reprinted with permission from Hofmann AD, Greydanus DE: *Adolescent Medicine*, ed 2. Norwalk, Connecticut, Appleton & Lange, 1989, p 31. Adapted from Tanner JM: *Growth at Adolescence.* Oxford, Blackwell, 1962.

      (2) Initial development may be asymmetric.
   c. Pulmonary flow murmur is an innocent murmur, which is often first appreciated in the school-age child.
      (1) This is a systolic ejection murmur, which is loudest in the recumbent patient at the upper left sternal border; it may disappear in the upright position.
      (2) The heart sounds are normal. This includes normal S2 splitting.
  4. Genitalia. The genitalia of both sexes is inspected. Tanner stage of male genital development and of male and female pubic hair development is noted (Tables 8-4 and 8-5).
   a. Girls
      (1) The premenarchal girl may have a normal watery, nonpurulent, non–foul-smelling vaginal discharge.
      (2) Pubic hair development in girls begins approximately 6 months after the onset of breast budding. The opposite sequence may occur in normal girls but is much less common.

Table 8-4. Tanner Stages of Pubic Hair Development

	Male	Female
Stage I	Preadolescent: No pubic hair is present; a fine vellus hair covers the genital area.	Preadolescent: No pubic hair is present; a fine vellus hair covers the genital area.
Stage II	A sparse distribution of long, slightly pigmented hair appears at the base of the penis.	A sparse distribution of long, slightly pigmented straight hair appears bilaterally along the medial border of the labia majora.
Stage III	The pubic hair pigmentation increases; it begins to curl and spread laterally in a scanty distribution.	The pubic hair pigmentation increases; it begins to curl and spread sparsely over the mons pubis.
Stage IV	The pubic hair continues to curl and becomes coarse in texture. An adult type of distribution is attained, but the number of hairs remains fewer.	The pubic hair continues to curl and becomes coarse in texture. The number of hairs continues to increase.
Stage V	Mature: The pubic hair attains an adult distribution with spread to the surface of the medial thigh. Pubic hair grows along the linea alba in 80% of males.	Mature: The pubic hair attains an adult feminine triangular pattern with spread to the surface of the medial thigh.

Reprinted with permission from Hofmann AD, Greydanus DE: *Adolescent Medicine*, ed 2. Norwalk, Connecticut, Appleton & Lange, 1989, p 29. Adapted from Tanner JM: *Growth at Adolescence.* Oxford, Blackwell, 1962.

Table 8-5. Tanner Stages of Male Genital Development

Stage I	Preadolescent: The testes, scrotum, and penis are the same as in childhood.
Stage II	As a result of canalization of seminiferous tubules, the testes enlarge. The scrotum enlarges, developing a reddish hue and altering in skin texture. The penis enlarges slightly.
Stage III	The testes and scrotum continue to grow. The length of the penis increases.
Stage IV	The testes and scrotum continue to grow; the scrotal skin darkens. The penis grows in width, and the glans penis develops.
Stage V	Mature: The testes, scrotum, and penis are adult in size and shape.

Reprinted with permission from Hofmann AD, Greydanus DE: *Adolescent Medicine*, ed 2. Norwalk, Connecticut, Appleton & Lange, 1989, p 30. Adapted from Tanner JM: *Growth at Adolescence*. Oxford, Blackwell, 1962.

    b. Boys
        (1) The first sign of puberty in boys is testicular enlargement and scrotal skin thinning and reddening. This occurs between the ages of 9½ and 13½.
        (2) Unless there are special concerns about pubertal development, testicular size is ordinarily assessed by estimated length. (An orchiometer is used for exact measurement.)
        (3) The prepubertal testicle measures approximately 1½–2 cm in length.
        (4) Pubic hair development in boys begins between the ages of 10 and 15 years of age.

5. Back
    a. The **scoliosis examination** is especially important in the school-age child and adolescent as progression of a curve is common during the period of rapid growth.
        (1) The spine and paraspinal structures are inspected and palpated with upper body clothing removed.
        (2) The back is inspected with the patient erect and during forward bending from the waist. The examiner stands first behind and then to the side of the patient and observes for lateral curvatures of the spine and symmetry of shoulders, scapulae, posterior ribs, and iliac crests.
    b. The school-age child or adolescent may have a mild **kyphosis** (bowing out) of the upper back or a mild **lordosis** (bowing in) of the lower lumbar area, which disappears on forward bending from the waist.

6. Neurologic and developmental examination. Most aspects of the general neurologic examination may be performed in a manner similar to that of the adult. The child's school functioning, athletic achievements, and behavior are important components of the overall neurodevelopmental assessment.
    a. Age-specific neurodevelopment. Some examples of tasks to observe (or additional history items) in the examination setting include:
        (1) The **5-year-old child** can walk on tiptoes, dress and undress without supervision, tell a simple story, define many simple words, cut and paste, and has a beginning comprehension of right and wrong.
        (2) The **6-year-old child** can skip, tie shoelaces, repeat four numbers, and has an increased facility with coloring and drawing.
        (3) The **8-year-old child** can hop twice on one foot then smoothly alternate to hop twice on the opposite foot, can perform rapid alternating movements of thumb to each finger of the same hand in rapid succession, and can accurately repeat five numbers.
        (4) The **10-year-old child** can stand heel to toe in a straight line with eyes closed for 15 seconds and can crumple up paper into a ball without using a table surface (5 seconds with the dominant hand and 7 seconds with the nondominant hand).
    b. "Soft" neurologic signs may be noted during the neurodevelopment examination. These

findings are considered normal in a younger child but when still present in an older child suggest neuromaturational delay. Examples of soft signs in the school-age child include:
  (1) Dystonic posturing of arms or hands when walking on heels.
  (2) Mirror movements of the opposite hand while performing rapid alternating movements with thumb and fingers.
  (3) Substantial movements of tongue or mouth while writing.

E. Physical examination of the adolescent (ages 12–16 years)

  1. General principles
  a. The clinician inquires about preference for a chaperon prior to the physical examination. For medical–legal reasons, the female patient who is examined by a male clinician requires a chaperon.
  b. The adolescent's intense **preoccupation with body image** is magnified during the physical examination.
    (1) Providing thorough explanations as the examination proceeds diffuses anxiety.
    (2) Offering reassurances about normal findings diffuses anxiety.
    (3) Insuring privacy and respecting modesty (e.g., gown, drape, curtain drawn, door securely closed) diffuses anxiety.
  c. **A complete physical examination** is performed with special attention to growth, skin, dentition, scoliosis, sports screening, breasts, and genitalia.

  2. Skin
  a. Careful inspection of all skin surfaces is very important in this age-group as many adolescents experience at least one **skin rash** (i.e., acne, eczema, superficial fungal infection, or psoriasis).
  b. Most adolescents experience **acne.** The face, neck, back, and upper chest may be involved in this condition.
    (1) The first manifestation of acne is the comedo. A closed comedo (whitehead) is a small, flesh-colored papule. An open comedo is a blackhead.
    (2) The later manifestations of acne are pustules, nodules, and cysts.
  c. **Atopic dermatitis** (eczema) in this age-group concentrates on the face and neck but may also involve other body surfaces and skin creases.

  3. Head and neck
  a. **Vision** is screened at least once during this period, even if prior screening has been normal. This is a high-risk period for the development of myopia.
  b. **Sinus transillumination** may be performed in the adolescent if indicated; it is unreliable prior to adolescence.
  c. **Hearing** is screened at least once during this period (more often if prior screening has been abnormal).
  d. **Teeth** are inspected for caries, adequacy of occlusion, and eruption of molars.
    (1) Second molars erupt during early adolescence (ages 12–13).
    (2) Third molars ("wisdom teeth") erupt during late adolescence (ages 17–21).
  e. **Thyroid examination** is especially important as thyroid problems are common in teenagers (particularly in girls). Examination of the gland is performed in the same manner as in adults. The size of the lateral lobes is compared to the patient's terminal thumb phalanx. Thyromegaly is suspected if the size of either lobe exceeds this measurement.

  4. Chest
  a. **Breasts** of both sexes are inspected.
    (1) **Female breast** examination includes determination of Tanner stage (see Table 8-3) and inspection and palpation in the manner of the adult examination.
    (2) **Gynecomastia** is relatively common in pubertal boys; it may last up to several years. Gynecomastia may involve one or both breasts.
  b. **Cardiac auscultation** may reveal occasional **premature beats,** which are of no concern if occurrence is limited to no more than 6 or 7 a minute, if they are abolished by exercise, and if they are isolated findings (i.e., there are no signs or symptoms of cardiac disease). The **pulmonary flow murmur** is the commonest innocent murmur heard in this age-group. It is especially easy to hear in the anxious patient.

5. **Genitalia**
   a. **Girls.** The external genitalia are examined with attention to monitoring pubertal development (Tanner staging of pubic hair; see Table 8-4) and ruling out vulvar lesions and vaginal discharge.
      (1) The vaginal mucosa in the pubertal girl is dull pink as compared to the thicker red mucosa in the prepubertal girl.
      (2) The hymen is inspected to rule out total occlusion of the vaginal orifice.
      (3) Physiologic leukorrhea is a whitish vaginal discharge that is not associated with pruritus or inflammation.
      (4) Pelvic examination is performed if the patient is sexually active or desires to become sexually active. Other indications include significant dysmenorrhea or abnormal periods, abnormal pubertal development, vulvar lesions or vaginal discharge, lower abdominal or pelvic pain, or a history of diethylstilbestrol (DES) exposure in utero.
   b. **Boys.** The genitalia are examined with attention to monitoring pubertal development (Tanner staging of genitalia and pubic hair; see Tables 8-4 and 8-5), ruling out penile and scrotal lesions, penile discharge, testicular masses, hernia, hydrocele, and varicocele.

6. **Back.** Examination for scoliosis is important throughout this age period as curves may progress significantly in the absence of symptoms.

7. **Extremities**
   a. A thorough extremity examination is performed as adolescents frequently manifest problems (particularly in the knees and hips).
   b. The adolescent athlete commonly requires **orthopedic screening** before participating in sports. The clinician may perform the traditional physical examination for this purpose. Alternatively, the clinician may perform the orthopedic screening examination with further examination when abnormalities are noted (Table 8-6).

8. **Closure.** At the conclusion of the adolescent examination, it is particularly important to review findings with an emphasis on normalcy (when appropriate).

F. **Focused physical examination.** The focused physical examination is performed whenever the clinician is investigating a particular clinical problem.

   1. Physical examination is **limited to the regions and systems** most likely to be involved in the patient's problem.

   2. In pediatrics, the focused physical examination is most commonly performed in children with **illnesses of a minor nature** (e.g., minor skin rashes or upper respiratory illnesses).

Table 8-6. Orthopedic Screening Examination

Athletic Activity (Instructions)	Observation
Stand facing examiner	Acromioclavicular joints; general habitus
Look at ceiling, floor, over both shoulders; touch ears to shoulders	Cervical spine motion
Shrug shoulders 90° (examiner resists)	Trapezius strength
Abduct shoulders 90° (examiner resists at 90°)	Deltoid strength
Full external rotation of arms	Shoulder motion
Flex and extend elbows	Elbow motion
Arms at sides, elbows 90° flexed; pronate and supinate wrists	Elbow and wrist motion
Spread fingers; make fist	Hand or finger motion and deformities
Tighten (contract) quadriceps; relax quadriceps	Symmetry and knee effusion; ankle effusion
"Duck walk" four steps (away from examiner with buttocks on heels)	Hip, knee, and ankle motion
Back to examiner	Shoulder symmetry; scoliosis
Knees straight, touch toes	Scoliosis, hip motion, hamstring tightness
Raise up on toes, raise heels	Calf symmetry, leg strength

Reprinted with permission from American Academy of Pediatrics Committee on Sports Medicine: *Sports Medicine: Health Care for Young Athletes.* Elk Grove Village, Illinois, American Academy of Pediatrics, 1983, p 87.

3. The focused physical examination is **inappropriate when the CC is a general one** (e.g., fatigue). In these cases, a comprehensive examination is required.

4. The focused physical examination is **inappropriate when the patient is an ill infant** (under 4–6 months), regardless of the problem.

REFERENCES

American Academy of Pediatrics Committee on Psychosocial Aspects of Child and Family Health: *Guidelines for Health Supervision,* ed. 2. Elk Grove Village, Illinois, American Academy of Pediatrics, 1988

Amiel-Tison C: Neurologic evaluation of the maturity of newborn infants. *Arch J Dis Child* 43:89, 1968

Athreya BH, Silverman BK: *Pediatric Physical Diagnosis.* Norwalk, Connecticut, Appleton-Century-Crofts, 1985

Barness LA: *Manual of Pediatric Physical Diagnosis,* ed 5. Chicago, Year Book, 1981

Boyle WE Jr, Hoekelman RA: The pediatric history. In *Primary Pediatric Care.* Edited by Hoekelman RA. St. Louis, CV Mosby, 1987, pp 52–63

Dworkin PH, Wible KL, Sutherland MC, et al: *Manual of Pediatric Anticipatory Guidance.* Morgantown, West Virginia, Department of Pediatrics, West Virginia University Medical Center, 1986

Dubowitz L, Dubowitz V, Goldberg C: Clinical assessment of gestational age in the newborn infant. *J Pediatr* 77:4, 1970

Goldenring JM, Cohen E: Getting into adolescent heads. *Contemp Pediatr* July:75–90, 1988

Gundy JH: The pediatric physical examination. In *Primary Pediatric Care.* Edited by Hoekelman RA. St. Louis, CV Mosby, 1987, pp 63–110

Hoekelman RA: The physical examination of infants and children. In *A Guide to Physical Examination and History Taking,* ed. 4. Edited by Bates B. Philadelphia, JB Lippincott, 1987, pp 525–529

Hofmann AD, Greydanus DE: *Adolescent Medicine,* ed 2. Norwalk, Connecticut, Appleton & Lange,1989

Rudolph AM (ed): *Pediatrics,* ed 17. Norwalk, Connecticut, Appleton-Century-Crofts, 1982

Solomon R: *Pediatric Experiences in Year II Clinical Sciences.* East Lansing, Michigan, Department of Pediatrics and Human Development, College of Human Medicine, Michigan State University, 1986

Sweet AY: Classification of the low-birth-weight infant. In *Care of the High Risk Neonate.* Edited by Klaus MH, Fanaroff AA. Philadelphia, WB Saunders, 1973, pp 36–57

Telzrow RW: Anticipatory guidance in pediatric practice. *J Cont Educ Pediatr* 20:14–27, 1978

Vaughan VC, McKay RJ, Behrman RE (eds): *Nelson Textbook of Pediatrics,* ed 11. Philadelphia, WB Saunders, 1979

STUDY QUESTIONS

Directions: Each of the numbered items or incomplete statements in this section is followed by answers or by completions of the statement. Select the **one** lettered answer or completion that is **best** in each case.

1. When queried, the parents of a 1-month-old infant comment that their infant's nap times are very irregular. At times, she sleeps for a few minutes, and at other times, she sleeps for many hours. Their concern revolves around the developmental issue known as

(A) synchrony
(B) attachment
(C) autonomy/independence
(D) state organization
(E) causality

2. A 6-year-old girl is brought to the clinician by her mother who states that her daughter awoke with an earache. The patient resists attempts to engage her in conversation. All of the following issues are likely to be responsible for her reluctance to cooperate EXCEPT

(A) fear of strangers
(B) fear of a painful procedure
(C) shy temperament
(D) no prior limit-setting by parents
(E) fear of separation

3. True statements about pediatric blood pressure measurement include all of the following EXCEPT

(A) routine blood pressure measurement begins at 3 years of age
(B) the cuff should completely encircle the circumference of the arm
(C) normal blood pressure increases with advancing age
(D) lower extremity blood pressure is normally 10–30 mm lower than upper extremity blood pressure
(E) the fifth Korotkoff sound (disappearance) is used in the standards for diastolic blood pressure in adolescents

4. In the newborn examination, physical findings that suggest prematurity include all of the following EXCEPT

(A) thick layer of vernix
(B) abundant lanugo
(C) absent sole creases
(D) prominent labia majora
(E) ear pinnae without ready recoil

5. Characteristics of innocent murmurs include all of the following EXCEPT

(A) changes in intensity with repositioning the patient
(B) does not radiate widely from point of origin
(C) sound is low in intensity
(D) sound begins after S1
(E) sound is accompanied by clicks or rubs

6. The mother of a 13-year-old girl is concerned because she does not think that her child has entered puberty. After the patient is examined, the clinician happily confirms that the child has definite signs of early puberty. The commonest manifestation of initial pubertal development in girls is

(A) axillary hair
(B) breast buds
(C) physiologic leukorrhea
(D) pubic hair
(E) red vaginal mucosa

Directions: Each item below contains four suggested answers of which **one or more** is correct. Choose the answer

A   if **1, 2, and 3** are correct
B   if **1 and 3** are correct
C   if **2 and 4** are correct
D   if **4** is correct
E   if **1, 2, 3, and 4** are correct

7. Accurate methods of determining body temperature include

(1) oral thermometer
(2) ear thermometer
(3) rectal thermometer
(4) forehead thermometer

Questions 8–12

A 2-year-old boy is scheduled for a routine well-child visit.

8. Routine measurements to obtain at this child's visit include

(1) height or length
(2) head circumference
(3) weight
(4) blood pressure

9. The mother of this toddler states that her child is doing well. Routine interval history may include questions about

(1) appetite
(2) lack of impulse control
(3) letter substitutions
(4) best friends

10. Prior to beginning the physical examination, the clinician should attempt to "make friends" with the patient, using which of the following techniques?

(1) Demonstrating that the hammer can be used to bang on the table top
(2) Bouncing the child on the examiner's knee
(3) Making clicking noises with the examiner's beeper
(4) Explaining that there will be "no shots" today

11. The clinician should listen while the child converses with his mother. The 2-year-old with normal language development

(1) uses plurals
(2) discusses simple aspects of daily life
(3) uses "me" or "you" correctly
(4) uses several words regularly

12. The clinician is ready to perform a physical examination on the toddler. Areas to emphasize include

(1) inspection of teeth for numbers and staining
(2) observation of gait for intoeing
(3) observation of corneal light reflex
(4) inspection of tympanic membrane during pneumatic otoscopy

(end of group question)

Directions: The group of items in this section consists of lettered options followed by a set of numbered items. For each item, select the **one** lettered option that is most closely associated with it. Each lettered option may be selected once, more than once, or not at all.

Questions 13–15

For each aspect of the interval history, select the age-group in which this issue is most important.

(A) Newborn
(B) Infancy (2 weeks to 12 months)
(C) Toddler (15 months to 4 years)
(D) School-age child (5–10 years)
(E) Adolescent (12–16 years)

13. Progress in toilet training

14. Emergence of stranger anxiety

15. Emergence of somatic complaints

ANSWERS AND EXPLANATIONS

1. The answer is D. [*I C 1 b (3) (a)*] Interval history during early infancy includes questions about the infant's physical and affective development. Many behaviors during early infancy are "predictably unpredictable." An example of this phenomenon is the infant's sleep–wake cycles (state organization). As the infant matures, predictability and individuality emerge. Synchrony (the infant's effect on the environment), attachment (the infant's preferential response to caretakers), and autonomy–independence (e.g., negative behaviors) refer to areas of affective development during infancy and the toddler years. Causality is a milestone of cognitive development (e.g., interest in windup toys), which emerges during the latter part of the first year.

2. The answer is A. [*II A 1 a; III D 1 (4) (a)–(c)*] The pediatrician may encounter a school-age child who is reluctant to converse or cooperate for examination. Reasons for reluctance include the child with an innately shy temperament, lack of discipline at home, prior frightening experiences in the medical setting, and developmentally related fears. The fear of painful procedures is a common fear of young school-age children. The fear of strangers and of separation from ones' parents usually begin during the latter half of the first year of life. Stranger anxiety would be distinctly uncommon in the 6-year-old child. Its presence ought to stimulate the clinician to inquire further about the child's behavior and temperament and about previous frightening experiences.

3. The answer is D. [*II A 4 f*] Routine pediatric blood pressure measurement begins at 3 years of age. The cuff should completely encircle the circumference of the extremity. The fifth Korotkoff sound is used in the standards for diastolic blood pressure in children ages 13–18, and the fourth Korotkoff sound is used in the standards for diastolic pressure in children up to the age of 12. Lower extremity blood pressure should be slightly higher (10–30 mm) than upper extremity blood pressure. When upper extremity blood pressure exceeds that of the lower extremities, a coarctation of the aorta should be suspected.

4. The answer is D. [*III A 1 c (3) (a) (iii)–(vii)*] Observation of various external characteristics of the newborn is helpful in estimating gestational age. Findings that suggest prematurity include a thick layer of vernix (a cheesy white material) covering the skin, abundant lanugo (fine downy hair) most noticeable on the back and shoulders, absence or paucity of creases on the soles of the feet, ear pinnae that are soft and easily folded into bizarre positions, soft skull bones, absent breast buds, and a hypotonic extended resting posture. Premature genitalia is suggested by prominent labia minora in girls or testes in the inguinal canal in boys.

5. The answer is E. [*III B 5 c*] An innocent murmur by definition is a murmur without underlying heart disease. As such, it is never accompanied by other signs (e.g., clicks, rubs, or cyanosis) or symptoms of heart disease. Except for the venous hum, which is a continuous murmur heard throughout the cardiac cycle, all innocent murmurs begin after the first sound and occur within systole. Innocent murmurs are generally soft, do not radiate widely, and may change in intensity with repositioning of the patient.

6. The answer is B. [*III D 3 b (1), 4 a (2)*] The sign that heralds the beginning of puberty for most girls is breast budding. This is followed approximately 6 months later by the beginning of pubic hair growth. The opposite sequence may occur, but it is far less common (only found in approximately 15% of normals). Axillary hair growth occurs approximately 2 years after the appearance of pubic hair.

7. The answer is A (1, 2, 3). [*II A 4 g*] Rectal temperature has traditionally been used to determine body temperature in children too young to cooperate for oral temperature. Recently, some pediatricians have begun using a device that is inserted into the ear canal. This device measures infrared energy emitted from the eardrum. It is noninvasive and works quickly. Its accuracy in children is presently under investigation. Forehead strips do not accurately reflect core temperature.

8. The answer is B (1, 3). [*II A 4 a–c, f*] Standing height or supine length and weight are measured at all well-child visits. Head circumference is measured in all well children for the first 6–12 months. If there are special concerns about neurologic, developmental, or growth status, head circumference is measured in an older child as well. Blood pressure is measured at well visits beginning at age 3 or whenever there are special concerns about cardiac or renal status, or serious illness.

9. The answer is A (1, 2, 3). [*I C 2*] The interval history for the toddler focuses on behavioral issues and language development. Growth rate (compared to early infancy) has diminished considerably by this age. The "typical" 2-year-old child is enmeshed in autonomy–independence struggles and displays "out of control" behavior. Any and all spheres of daily life are potential battlegrounds for the toddler to exert autonomy (e.g., mealtimes: poor appetite and lack of table manners; nighttime: bedtime struggles and night awakening). Letter substitutions (e.g., "w" for "r" in rabbit) are common during the early years of language development and do not mean that the toddler has a speech problem. Young toddlers engage in parallel play. The formation of special alliances (e.g., "best friend") does not routinely occur until school age.

10. The answer is B (1, 3). [*II A 2*] Techniques to maximize compliance should maximize what is known about the patient's age and developmental stage. The 2-year-old is likely to be wary of strangers and of being separated from his mother. As long as the clinician does not approach the child directly, the child may feel comfortable enough to play with the examiner's instruments (or be interested in the actions of a beeper). Bouncing the child on the examiner's knee in the early stages of the encounter is too intrusive and will frighten the patient. The toddler does not have the ability to think rationally and, therefore, will not benefit from a discussion about "no shots" today.

11. The answer is D (4). [*I C 2 b (2) (d) (i)*] Mastery of language is the major cognitive issue during the preoperational period of development. The 2-year-old uses several words regularly, makes his or her desires known verbally, and when asked for the location of common objects, will correctly respond by pointing. Children who manifest significant delays in language development require further evaluation. This evaluation may consist of a complete physical examination, audiologic testing, and referral to a speech and language expert.

12. The answer is E (all). [*III B 4 c, d, C 4 a–c, 8 b*] During the toddler years, a complete physical examination is performed with special attention to vision, hearing, dentition, language development, tympanic membranes, and gait. Teeth are counted and inspected for stains and decay. By age 2–2½, most toddlers will have a full complement of 20 primary teeth. Intoeing at this age most commonly results from internal tibial torsion or femoral anteversion; both are self-resolving when mild. Sadly, strabismus may occasionally go undetected until age 2, in which case the corneal light reflex may be asymmetric. The high incidence of middle ear disease during infancy and toddler years requires careful inspection of the eardrum and observation of mobility during pneumatic otoscopy.

13–15. The answers are: 13-C, 14-B, 15-D. [*I C 1 b (1) (c), 2 a (1), 3 d (1)*] Interval history is a global update of the patient's health and psychosocial status. Questions about bowel and bladder functioning are pursued at all well-child visits. Questions specifically related to toilet training do not assume importance until the child is developmentally ready for training; this usually occurs no earlier than 18 months. According to Brazelton, the child is not ready for training until he or she is able to walk and sit well, wants to please his or her parents, and desires to develop control over these bodily functions.

Stranger anxiety is a manifestation of attachment and emerges between 6–9 months. The earliest manifestation of attachment is demonstrated by the young infant's preferential response to a parent's voice. This is followed by the infant's demonstrating visual recognition of caretakers and a response of pleasure or excitement towards them. Stranger and separation anxiety emerge after these developments.

Prior to the school years, chronic "aches and pains" are unusual. During school age, recurrent abdominal pain, headaches, and limb pains are common enough to merit routine discussion during interval history. In this age-group, most recurrent "aches and pains" do not have a definite identifiable organic etiology. Their occurrence is usually attributed to a combination of factors, including the environment, individual physiology, and personality.

Geriatric History and Physical Examination

Henry Schneiderman
Anthony J. Ardolino

I. GERIATRIC MEDICAL HISTORY

A. Communication faculties

1. **Hearing impairment** is a common disorder in the geriatric population; thus, examiners should do the following:
   a. Situate themselves as close as comfortably possible and at ear level with the patient
   b. Minimize both audible and visual distractions at the interview site
   c. Speak in a slow, modulated, moderately loud voice
   d. Confirm that they are being understood, repeating phrases if necessary

2. **Visual impairment** may contribute to miscommunication. Hand gestures and other nonverbal cues must be avoided.

3. **Language.** Examiners must use terminology that is easily understood, not technical words or jargon.

B. Content issues

1. **Presenting symptoms.** The chief complaint (CC) is often a multisystem complex in elderly patients. The symptoms are often vague and nonspecific due to a greater likelihood of chronic illness and multisystem involvement.

2. **History of present illness (HPI)**
   a. **Classic presentations.** Acute illness may not present in a textbook manner in the elderly patient since classic presentations are usually derived from a young cohort of patients. For example, acute appendicitis in elderly patients sometimes presents as back pain, not right lower quadrant pain.
   b. **Chronic illnesses.** Patients over 65 years of age are more likely to have one or more chronic diseases, the symptoms of which can modify the HPI.
   c. **Caregivers.** It is often necessary to obtain a corroborating history from a spouse or caregiver.
      (1) Many patients have a history of a memory deficit or dementia or an acute illness that causes a change in mental status (e.g., stroke or meningitis).
      (2) Data from other sources can be misleading, but such data are important and occasionally essential. However, these data should not be used to invalidate the patient's own history.
      (3) Symptoms supplied by demented patients are always important and should be pursued.
   d. **Multiple medication use** is common; however, the reliability of a medication history decreases as the number of drugs increases.

3. **Patient profile (PP)**
   a. **Comprehensive assessment of the patient's independence or dependence** in the activities of daily living (ADLs) should be explored, including getting in and out of bed, preparing meals, eating, toileting, ambulation, as well as higher functions, such as shopping for food or driving a car. Information about these activities is crucial in determining how the patient functions in the environment.
   b. **Household members** should be listed.
   c. **Physical environment.** It is important to determine how the patient lives.

        (1) What type of housing does the patient own or rent?

        (2) Are there stairs or elevators?

        (3) Are there unsafe factors present, such as throw rugs or inadequate heating?

  d. Support systems must be fully determined, including family, friends, and professional services, such as visiting nurses and home health aides.

  e. Financial information, including insurance, is essential at all levels of patient care. Even the type of medication prescribed may be predicated by the source of payment.

  f. Diet in elderly patients is often poorly balanced. Economic factors and taste modifications (i.e., medication side effects or decreased taste buds) may lead to a bland and largely carbohydrate diet.

  g. Alcohol and drug use remain problems for all age-groups.

        (1) Alcoholism is present in 10%–20% in the elderly population with major health effects.

        (2) Abuse of prescription medications, such as tranquilizers and narcotic analgesics, exceeds that of illegal street drugs.

4. Past medical history (PMH)

  a. Chronic medical conditions increase in likelihood and number over age 65. Each condition must be explored in detail in the elderly patient.

  b. Immunization history should be obtained, especially for influenza, pneumococcal, and hepatitis B vaccines and for tetanus toxoid.

  c. Surgical and obstetric histories are often critical to the HPI. Exact dates are difficult to obtain; therefore, the emphasis should be on the type and number of procedures.

  d. Trauma history, including falling, may be pertinent to the HPI and associated disorders (e.g., alcohol use or osteoporosis).

  e. Medication history should be obtained. Pill bottles should be brought in by the patient so that existing prescriptions can be compared with the patient's reported usage.

5. Family history. The interview should focus on siblings, children, and grandchildren, rather than on parents and grandparents.

6. Review of systems (ROS) in elderly patients should emphasize symptom complexes that occur with frequency, such as:

  a. Visual impairment

  b. Hearing impairment

  c. Urinary incontinence

  d. Sexual dysfunction

  e. Gait abnormalities and arthritic complaints

  f. Altered cognition

  g. Depression

7. Special clinical situations

  a. Cognitively impaired patients present a particular challenge to clinicians who take the medical history.

        (1) Memory deficits and decreased intellectual functioning influence the reliability of factual information, especially the past medical history and medication use.

        (2) Symptoms are often vague and subtle but nonetheless crucial to the diagnosis of genuine medical illness. For example, treatable phobic disorders and depression occur with greater frequency in demented patients than normal individuals. Symptoms of these disorders often present as changes in overall functioning (e.g., decreased social interaction or psychomotor retardation) and are not well articulated by patients.

        (3) New symptoms of gait instability, falls, urinary or fecal incontinence, or a rapid change in cognitive function should alert the examiner to a likelihood of organic disease. These may be the only clues to an acute, reversible condition.

        (4) Corroborating data are useful to substantiate a medical history.

  b. Depression is commonly encountered among elderly patients.

        (1) As with many diseases, the presentation of depression is not classic. Symptoms that suggest psychomotor retardation, such as decreased energy, listlessness, decreased appetite, or cognitive impairment, are often clues.

        (2) Depression often accompanies other diseases, such as Alzheimer-type dementia, alcohol abuse, or cancer.

        (3) Prescription medications alone or in combination often produce side effects that mimic endogenous depression in elderly patients.

        (4) Depression can significantly alter or mask symptoms of other acute or chronic illness.

II. GERIATRIC PHYSICAL EXAMINATION

A. Overview. Although disability is disproportionately represented among the aged, many elderly individuals are hearty, ambulatory, and fully functional.

1. **Initial evaluation.** Sufficient time must be allowed to carry out a thorough physical examination, remembering the following:
   a. Many aged individuals have long problem lists, making it necessary for clinicians to develop priorities for problems in order of their potential for causing harm.
   b. The frail, elderly patient may easily become exhausted by a comprehensive, full-length assessment attempted at one visit.
   c. A good examination is often requested, required, noted, and remembered appreciatively.
   d. Laboratory results can be misleading. For example, many elderly women have asymptomatic bacteriuria; thus, a urinalysis and culture may lead a clinician to conclude erroneously that the source of a fever has been discovered and fail to consider pneumonia, myocardial infarction, or adverse drug reactions.

2. **Family members and caregivers.** The protectiveness of a caregiver may prevent the examiner from fully assessing the patient's capability. The clinician must, therefore, direct the caregiver to allow the patient to proceed unassisted when feasible.

3. **Chronicity and acuity** are important determinants of the sequence of obtaining a data base. For example, a prominent cardiac murmur that has been present for 20 years may not need immediate attention, but a fever should be worked up on the first visit.

4. **Disrobing,** while indispensable to an adequate examination, is embarrassing for old and young patients alike.
   a. Getting into a hospital gown may present a major barrier to individuals impaired by age or disease, such as arthritis.
   b. A warm room and sufficient covering must be provided so that elderly patients do not get chilled.
   c. As with all patients, modesty must be preserved by keeping certain body areas, such as breasts, abdomen, genitalia, and thighs, covered when they are not being examined.

B. Interpretation. It is essential to recognize common abnormalities associated with true pathology and to distinguish them from the normal changes associated with the aging process.

1. **Vital signs and statistics**
   a. **Body temperature**
      (1) Hypometabolic states, such as hypothyroidism or accidental (environmental) hypothermia, must be considered with temperatures below 36° C or 35.5° C.
      (2) Normal body temperatures in elderly individuals must be viewed with circumspection because infection does not always produce fever in these individuals, even when they are bacteremic.
   b. **Blood pressure**
      (1) Blood pressure rises slightly in normal aging, but 140/90 still defines the baseline for **hypertension**.
      (2) Treatment of hypertension in elderly patients lowers cardiovascular mortality.
   c. **Orthostatic changes.** Shifts in pulse and blood pressure with changes in body position must be interpreted in context.
      (1) To be meaningful, pulse and blood pressure must be assessed in one position and then again after assuming a more gravity-dependent position for 3 minutes. The best sequence is moving from a supine to a sitting position; however, it is also valid to move from a sitting to a standing position.
         (a) The pulse should normally rise by less than 10 beats a minute on becoming upright.
         (b) The systolic pressure should fall no more than 10 mm Hg, and the diastolic pressure should *rise* slightly.
         (c) If there is a fall in the diastolic pressure, with or without an excessive fall in the systolic pressure and with an increase in the pulse rate, there is significant orthostatic hypotension, the cause of which may be hypovolemia.
         (d) If the pressures fall and there is no compensatory pulse rise, then autonomic neural dysfunction is present. Diabetic neuropathy, pharmacologic therapy (beta-blockade), or other processes may be responsible.

(2) Since the assessment of orthostatic pulse and blood pressure changes can precipitate illness if performed thoughtlessly, several warnings should be heeded.

   (a) If patients develop lightheadedness, chest pain or tightness, weakness, wooziness, or dyspnea, the test should be stopped at once, and they should be returned immediately to the supine position.

   (b) In patients suspected of intravascular volume depletion (dehydration), pulse and blood pressure are taken in the supine position.

   (i) If symptoms are present or if significant baseline tachycardia or hypotension is present, no orthostatic measurements are made.

   (ii) Otherwise, the clinician can raise the patient to a sitting position; if no symptoms develop, measurements can be made.

   (iii) If pulse and blood pressure are unchanged, measurements can be repeated with the patient standing, if indicated.

   (c) It is never appropriate to proceed to a standing position if orthostatic symptoms, hypotension, or tachycardia develops in the seated position.

d. Weight should not change with age. Obesity is common and, in some populations, so is malnutrition. Accurately measured weight is correctly called a vital statistic and is an essential part of the geriatric physical examination.

e. Respiratory rate. Studies confirm that the respiratory rate is the vital sign most likely to change in elderly individuals early in an acute illness. For example, in patients with a respiratory tract infection, the respiratory rate sometimes rises several days before the source of the acute process can be localized.

2. Mental status examination is covered in Chapter 7 V.

3. Breast and genital examinations are important in the evaluation of symptoms and in detecting presymptomatic remediable disorders.

a. Breast examinations are sometimes omitted because patients and clinicians alike mistakenly believe that breast cancer incidence declines in old age or that the biology of the disease is less lethal in the elderly. Both of these myths have been thoroughly disproven.

b. A common abnormality on genital examination in older women is **atrophic vulvovaginourethritis**. Symptoms tend to be underreported, and complications can include pruritus, tenderness, dyspareunia, urinary incontinence, and psychological stress. Treatment is simple and effective.

c. In elderly men, **prostatic palpation** via rectal examination may reveal a hard nodule suggestive of cancer. The benefits of an early diagnosis are significant.

   (1) The clinician need not be concerned about the timing of blood work in relation to prostatic palpation because it is now known that this examination does not cause a false elevation of serum acid phosphatase, a laboratory marker of metastatic prostate cancer.

   (2) Although a large prostate on palpation suggests the cause when urethral obstruction is present, the converse inference cannot be safely made. A prostate that feels small from the character of the accessible posterior lobe may have an enlarged median bar on its anterior, inaccessible surface that disrupts urethral function.

4. Skin ages in a number of familiar ways (e.g., wrinkling). **Turgor** diminishes so that "tenting" of the skin should not be taken to imply volume depletion as it does in young individuals. Orthostatic measurements provide more reliable data for that assessment.

5. Oral examination involves the removal of dentures since they may cover irritative and infectious processes or even neoplasms in the mucosae.

a. Ill-fitting dentures are a major cause of weight loss and failure to thrive. Severe gingivitis can have a similar impact.

b. To diagnose oral cancers in high-risk elderly individuals—that is, those who drink alcohol to excess and use tobacco—the tongue must be grasped with a gauze and retracted laterally toward each side, thus adequately exposing the sides of the tongue and the floor of the mouth—common sites for malignancies.

6. Pulmonary examination may be normal or may include crackles or other abnormalities. A common error is the automatic equation of bibasilar pulmonary crackles with heart failure. For example, crackles caused by simple atelectasis associated with immobility and inactivity may clear after several deep breaths and coughs.

7. Cardiovascular examination may reveal systolic murmurs, fourth heart sounds, and diminished peripheral pulses in many vigorous old people.

    a. Murmurs. The decision to pursue a murmur must be based on the same criteria as in young individuals, such as the clinical context and the particular characteristics of the murmur; for example, diastolic murmurs deserve diagnostic attention since they are more likely to represent major valvular pathology in need of further study or therapy.

    b. Fourth heart sounds are present in many normal individuals over the age of 50. In the absence of symptoms or signs of organic heart disease, it is prudent to record and then dismiss this finding.

    c. Diminished peripheral pulses vary in significance.

        (1) Loss of **foot pulses** in patients confined to bed by a primary neurologic disorder may have little clinical consequence. Absent foot pulses in an ambulatory elder who is free of claudication and has normal, warm feet is similarly unimportant.

        (2) Diminished **carotid pulses** deserve more attention. **Gentle carotid palpation** is the rule because undue pressure on diseased carotids can cause a stroke or an arrhythmia.

        (3) The **superficial temporal arteries** should be palpated in elderly persons just anterosuperior to the tragus. If these arteries are tender, knotty, or pulseless, and if the patient has headaches, polymyalgic symptoms, or visual symptoms, the clinician should think of giant cell (temporal) arteritis, a major cause of preventable blindness.

8. Abdominal examination commonly reveals a variety of anomalies.

    a. Palpable intracolonic stools may feel like a mass. It is wise to reexamine the patient after the colon has been emptied. If the mass disappears, as it often does, the problem is solved.

    b. Vertically oriented masses suggest aortic ectasia or aneurysm, which can be distinguished by ultrasound.

    c. Lower abdominal swelling often suggests a distended urinary bladder with urethral obstruction, which may be unaccompanied by symptoms. This may be confirmed by ultrasound if physical examination proves inconclusive.

9. Musculoskeletal examination provides:

    a. Documentation of the evident, such as arthritic changes in fingers

    b. Functional information, such as how well the patient can open a jar, walk across a room, or sit down on a toilet

    c. A chance to observe stance, gait, and sitting upright unsupported

10. Neurologic examination. The range of neurologic abnormalities in the aged is enormous. In addition to the critical issue of mental status addressed in Chapter 7, several other issues can be briefly delineated.

    a. The most commonly diminished test result in the healthy elderly individual is **vibratory sensation** at the toes and the ankles; to eliminate false-positives, the function in the dorsal columns can be checked through routine assessment of position sense.

    b. Elderly individuals can have **false-positive signs** in several areas. For example, many patients with dementia but without meningitis have positive meningeal signs.

    c. Achilles reflexes (ankle jerks). These can be lacking in the absence of demonstrable, pathologic cause, although some authorities dispute this.

    d. Cogwheel rigidity is common in elderly individuals. This finding suggests parkinsonism but is not diagnostic. Note that tremor is also common in healthy, elderly individuals as well as parkinsonian patients.

    e. Special senses are critically important. No assessment is complete without including **hearing** and **vision**. Losses in both are common in the elderly (see I A 1, 2).

        (1) They may impact profoundly on daily life as well as on such specific medical issues as drawing the correct insulin dose in a syringe.

        (2) The importance of these functions for bidirectional communication is obvious, but it is striking how often written records omit any reference to these essential data.

11. Examination of the home environment. Disorder of living space, a smell of urine, and collapse of previously sociable personal grooming and hygiene are predictors of significant trouble.

REFERENCES

Davis PB, Robins LW: History-taking in the elderly with and without cognitive impairment. *J Am Geriatr Soc* 37:249–255, 1989

Gambert SR, Duthie EH, Wiltzius F: The value of the yearly medical evaluation in a nursing home. *J Chronic Dis* 35:65–68, 1982

Gordon SR, Jahnigen DW: Oral assessment of the edentulous elderly patient. *J Am Geriatr Soc* 31:797–801, 1983

Hodkinson HM: Non-specific presentation of illness. *Br Med J* 4:94–96, 1973

Impallomeni M, Flynn MD, Kenny RA, et al: The elderly and their ankle jerks. *Lancet* 1:670–672, 1984

Jackson JE, et al: Reliability of drug histories in a specialized geriatric outpatient clinic. *J Gen Intern Med* 4:39–43, 1989

Kerzner LJ, Greb L, Steel K: History-taking forms and the care of geriatric patients. *J Med Educ* 57:376–379, 1982

McFadden JP, Price RC, Eastwood HD, et al: Raised respiratory rate in elderly patients: a valuable physical sign. *Br Med J* 284:626–627, 1982

Murden RA, Cohn SL: Myocardial infarction caused by hypotension during physical examination maneuvers in the elderly. *J Am Geriatr Soc* 36:1120–1122, 1988

Puxty JAH, Fox RA, Horan MA: The frequency of physical signs usually attributed to meningeal irritation in elderly patients. *J Am Geriatr Soc* 31:590–592, 1983

Skrastins R, Merry GM, Rosenberg GM, et al: Clinical assessment of the elderly patient. *Can Med Assoc J* 127:203–206, 1982

Steel K: History-taking from elderly patients. *Hosp Prac* May:70–71, 1985

Tinetti ME: Performance-oriented assessment of mobility problems in elderly patients. *J Am Geriatr Soc* 34:119–126, 1986

Wright WB: How to examine an old person. *Lancet* 1:1145–1146, 1977

STUDY QUESTIONS

Directions: Each of the numbered items or incomplete statements in this section is followed by answers or by completions of the statement. Select the **one** lettered answer or completion that is **best** in each case.

1. All of the following techniques are useful in communicating with the hearing-impaired elderly patient EXCEPT

(A) sitting at eye level in front of the patient
(B) removing audible and visual distractions
(C) raising the voice as high as necessary to be heard
(D) repeating phrases to test comprehension
(E) writing the questions down

2. An 85-year-old previously healthy man is hospitalized with a fractured hip. All of the following factors are important to the decision to send the patient home where he lives alone in an apartment EXCEPT

(A) the apartment is on the second floor, and there is no elevator
(B) he is unable to get in and out of bed on his own
(C) he has no relatives or close friends in the area
(D) he has had two myocardial infarctions, 1 and 5 years ago
(E) his food is delivered by a nearby supermarket

3. A 90-year-old woman has a new onset of breast carcinoma. In obtaining this patient's family history (FH), on which individual should the clinician focus?

(A) Mother
(B) Father
(C) Maternal grandmother
(D) Sister
(E) Daughter

4. A 75-year-old man presents with symptoms of a new onset of mental status changes. He reports poor memory, poor attention span, and insomnia. All of the following statements provide useful diagnostic information for the clinician EXCEPT

(A) his spouse of 50 years has recently expired
(B) he drinks three to four alcoholic drinks a day with a recent increase
(C) his internist recently added two new medications to his usual four chronic medications
(D) he has a medical history of arthritis and hypertension
(E) he was previously treated for depression 5 years ago

5. Alzheimer-type dementia could be mimicked by many disorders in the elderly, including all of the following EXCEPT

(A) depression
(B) alcohol abuse
(C) cancer
(D) medication use
(E) coronary artery disease

6. A 100-year-old patient is observed to be tachypneic at 28 beats a minute. Nurses record a normal body temperature. The clinician finds localized crackles in the right upper lobe. A chest radiograph is normal. What is the most logical explanation for these findings?

(A) Renal failure with volume overload
(B) Age-related changes in respiratory tract
(C) Age-related neurologic change in respiratory center set point
(D) Atelectatic crackles with resolution
(E) Pneumonia

7. A 64-year-old woman presents with all the following symptoms. Pelvic examination may help to clarify the source of all of them EXCEPT

(A) urinary incontinence
(B) new bilateral edema of the legs
(C) anemia
(D) weight loss
(E) severe foot pain

8. Oral examination is important in all of the following patients EXCEPT

(A) a patient with congestive heart failure
(B) a patient with dentures
(C) a heavy smoker
(D) an alcoholic individual
(E) a patient with AIDS

9. A mass is felt in the left lateral abdomen of a 92-year-old woman. The most appropriate next step in characterizing the mass is

(A) a scratch test
(B) a urethral catheterization to drain the bladder and see if it changes
(C) laxatives, enemas, or time to empty the colon and see if it changes
(D) ultrasound examination
(E) reexamination in the left lateral decubitus position to see if it changes

10. An 86-year-old man has diminished vibratory sensation at the knees and toes, although his reflexes are intact, temperature sensation is normal, and he feels well apart from headaches. What is the most likely explanation?

(A) Peripheral neuropathy
(B) Normal age-related change
(C) Spinal cord lesion
(D) Small strokes
(E) Brain or brain stem tumor

Directions: The item below contains four suggested answers of which **one or more** is correct. Choose the answer

A if **1, 2, and 3** are correct
B if **1 and 3** are correct
C if **2 and 4** are correct
D if **4** is correct
E if **1, 2, 3, and 4** are correct

11. A 70-year-old man with dementia collapses and loses consciousness suddenly. His pulse is 115 and weak, respirations are 28 a minute, blood pressure is 115/65, and temperature is 37° C. Diagnoses that are likely with this man's presentation include

(1) acute myocardial infarction
(2) pulmonary embolism
(3) severe infection with septicemia
(4) drug toxicity

Directions: The group of items in this section consists of lettered options followed by a set of numbered items. For each item, select the **one** lettered option that is most closely associated with it. Each lettered option may be selected once, more than once, or not at all.

Questions 12–16

Match the pulse and pressure readings listed on the right with the most likely diagnosis.

(A) Normal host
(B) Isolated systolic hypertension
(C) Autonomic neuropathy (e.g., diabetic neuropathy)
(D) Hypovolemia (dehydration)
(E) Hypertension

	Age	Sex	Pulse, supine	Blood pressure, supine	Pulse, sitting	Blood pressure, sitting
12.	74	F	60	140/80	65	128/85
13.	59	M	62	140/80	85	135/75
14.	68	M	72	138/76	74	124/63
15.	81	F	88	154/86	92	150/88
16.	63	M	64	145/92	66	147/94

ANSWERS AND EXPLANATIONS

1. The answer is C. [*I A 1 a–d*] In communicating with the hearing-impaired patient, it is essential to minimize outside distractions. Communication is improved if the patient can also watch the examiner's face. Repeating and writing down phrases are useful adjuncts. While a moderately loud voice aids in communication, patients who are truly hearing-impaired will not benefit from an extremely loud voice.

2. The answer is D. [*I B 3 a*] The disposition of elderly patients is often dependent upon items obtained in the PP and is often less dependent upon the medical history. The fact that the patient lives in a second floor walk-up apartment, that he has no support system in the area, and that his food can be delivered all influence his ability to live alone. Obviously being unable to get in and out of bed jeopardizes his ability to live independently. The patient's cardiac history is not relevant to where he will be sent.

3. The answer is E. [*I B 5*] In obtaining a FH from an elderly patient, it is important to shift the focus from prior generations to children and grandchildren. While the presence of breast carcinoma in the mother, maternal grandmother, or sister may have influenced the surveillance for breast carcinoma in this patient, once it has been diagnosed, this information is less important. In this particular patient, the father's history is not relevant to the risk for breast cancer. It would be most important to focus on the daughters or grand-daughters to assess their risk for breast carcinoma.

4. The answer is D. [*I B 7 a, b*] The patient described in the question most likely has a new onset of depression. A past history of depression, a recent loss of a family member, and a history of alcohol use or abuse contribute to this diagnosis. An alternative explanation may be a drug interaction, as this effect is more likely with multiple medications. The history of arthritis and hypertension is irrelevant in this case, other than the fact that the medication used to treat these disorders may be contributing to the mental status changes.

5. The answer is E. [*I B 3 g, 7 b (1), (2); II B 7*] Depression often presents in the elderly with psychomotor retardation suggestive of a dementing process. Alcohol abuse, cancer, and medication use could all present in similar ways. Coronary artery disease should have no effect on mental status.

6. The answer is E. [*II B 1 e*] The absence of fever does not exclude infection, especially in very old patients. Alterations in the physical examination often precede those on the chest film, so the clinician need not invoke a process that changed between examination and radiograph to explain the apparent disparity between the two studies. Tachypnea is not expected with age, and while crackles may be heard in a very few normal individuals at any age, in the context of tachypnea, the clinician must seek another cause.

7. The answer is E. [*II B 3*] Pelvic examination may reveal a mass that is obstructing venous or lymphatic return from the legs, thus explaining new edema. A pelvic malignancy might be the source of bleeding (vaginal or internal), potentially causing anemia and also weight loss. Various findings of atrophic vaginitis, urethritis, and cystocele could explain urinary incontinence. It would be difficult or impossible to connect foot pain with findings on pelvic examination.

8. The answer is A. [*II B 5*] Oral examination adds little useful information in the patient with heart failure. By contrast, all the patients listed in the question (i.e., patients with dentures, heavy smokers, alcoholics, and patients with AIDS) are at increased risk of intraoral malignancies, serious infections, or both.

9. The answer is C. [*II B 8 a*] Most often masses in the left lateral abdomen prove to be intracolonic feces, which disappear when the patient is reexamined 1 or 2 days later, particularly after several good bowel movements. With lateralization, a bladder source is unlikely, and, in any case, the patient may be able to empty the bladder perfectly without the intrusion of a catheter. Laboratory and imaging studies are not indicated. Reexamination in another body position is futile, and the scratch test is irrelevant.

10. The answer is B. [*II B 10 a*] The selectivity of the deficit makes a supraforaminal lesion and a peripheral neuropathy impossible. We are not told if position sense is impaired: If it is, the posterior column of the spinal cord becomes a possibility, but an isolated vibratory deficit can occur as a normal aging change. The practical point is that when diminished vibratory sensation is encountered, position sense must be tested carefully to make the branch point.

11. The answer is E (all). [*II B 1*] Any of the processes listed in the question (i.e., acute myocardial infarction, pulmonary embolism, severe infection with septicemia, and drug toxicity) can cause a sudden loss of consciousness. It is often thought that drug toxicity develops less suddenly; however, while serum and tissue levels rise, there is sometimes an "iceberg effect," resulting in the sudden appearance of symptoms as a threshold is exceeded. The absence of fever does not exclude infection.

12–16. The answers are: 12-A, 13-D, 14-C, 15-B, 16-E. [*II B 1 b, c*] Normal blood pressure is 140/90 or less in adults. If only the systolic pressure is elevated, this is called isolated systolic hypertension; if the word "hypertension" is used without further qualification, it is presumed that both the systolic and the diastolic elements are high. The normal response to standing upright is a slight rise in pulse rate, a small drop in systolic pressure, and a small rise in diastolic pressure. With volume depletion, both the systolic and the diastolic pressure often drop more considerably; however, if the host has intact vascular reflexes, the pressures may be maintained, or nearly so, by a marked increase in heart rate. This is the situation depicted in the 59-year-old man, where the pressures are almost steady, but at the cost of a 23-beat rise in heart rate. If the pressures drop and there is no compensatory increase in heart rate, the autonomic response is dysfunctional, as shown in the 68-year-old man.

10
Approach to Clinical Problem-Solving
Janice L. Willms

I. INTRODUCTION. Once the student has mastered the basic data-acquisition skills—interviewing, taking the medical history, and conducting the physical examination—the next challenge becomes that of **putting the data to work**. From the medical history and physical examination, the student must develop a **problem list;** from the problem list, the student must develop a **differential diagnosis;** and from the differential diagnosis, **diagnostic** and **management plans** evolve. This chapter presents a sequential method of organization and planning for action based upon the information available.

II. PROBLEM LIST. Unlike the differential diagnosis, the problem list is not speculative. It is a tabular list of the patient's problems defined at any given time. The problem list is **primary, reduced to concrete terms,** and **dynamic**. Ongoing modification of the problem list as data are obtained and as the patient's condition changes is an efficient and accurate way of communicating to the health care team the immediate status of the patient.

A. Definition of a problem. A problem is anything that demands action (**active problem**) or requires notation because it is essential to the comprehensive care of the patient (**inactive problem**). Active problems can require action at one or more of three levels:

1. Diagnostic action. This category includes unresolved problems, including symptoms, signs, or abnormal laboratory tests, that cannot be converted into plans for management or resolution without additional data. Only when a definite cause for the problem is defined may it be converted to a diagnosis or rendered inconsequential (inactive or resolved).

a. A symptom, such as shortness of breath, the cause of which is unclear, may constitute a problem. If the cause is not absolutely known, the symptom must be listed **at the level at which it is absolute**—that is, as "shortness of breath."

b. A sign, such as sinus tachycardia, is listed as a problem if its cause is unknown or if either the patient or the clinician feels it needs further diagnostic workup.

c. A laboratory finding, such as hypokalemia or hypernatremia, may be defined as a problem.

2. Therapeutic action. If a symptom, sign, or abnormal laboratory test is either sufficiently well understood to justify treatment or is clearly threatening to the patient's well-being, it may be entered as a problem requiring therapeutic action.

a. Known diagnosis with dangerous presentation. A patient with known diabetes mellitus may present with hyperglycemia and acidosis. Since the cause of the abnormal laboratory values is presumed to be the underlying disease and since both abnormalities require immediate therapy, the problem may be entered as "diabetes mellitus with hyperglycemia and metabolic acidosis."

b. Unknown diagnosis with dangerous presentation. Occasionally, a problem requires therapeutic action for the patient's safety, even when its basis is not clearly understood. For example, a child with a history of febrile convulsions may present with a temperature of 105° F, necessitating antipyretics while the cause of the fever remains unknown. Thus, the single problem, "fever," demands both treatment *and* further diagnostic workup simultaneously.

3. Patient education
a. Preexisting problems may need to be reviewed with the patient.
b. Diagnostic or therapeutic intervention may need a patient's contractual agreement.
c. A discussion of prognosis with long-term management plans is necessary.

B. Derivation of the problem list

1. **Medical history.** After acquiring, recording, and reviewing the medical history, the clinician may begin to identify problems, most of which will fall into one of three groups:
   a. **Preexisting diagnoses**
   b. **New or unresolved symptoms or signs**
   c. **Social, health habit, or financial problems.** Known or suspected drug allergies, tobacco or alcohol abuse, and unemployment, leading to financial or social problems, may all be defined as problems that require some level of intervention or education.

2. **Physical examination.** Upon review of the physical examination, **all abnormalities** requiring some sort of action and inactive problems requiring notation, such as a surgical scar that indicates the patient no longer has an appendix, should be listed at the level at which their implications are understood.

3. **Laboratory data base.** If laboratory data have been obtained, they are scanned for abnormalities. The primary problem list is updated if these are entered as independent problems requiring action.

C. Discriminating active from inactive problems

1. **Active problems.** The active problem list should be separated from the inactive list, so that any reader can clearly discriminate between the two. Double columns with active problems on the left and inactive problems on the right facilitate the conversion of an active problem to an inactive one simply by using an arrow from one column to another (see Figure 10-1).

2. **Inactive problems.** There is no consensus among clinicians about the need to maintain an inactive problem list. However, since this chapter is concerned with the comprehensive data base, which should be available on every patient, an inactive problem list is described. The list should include all concurrent conditions, which might conceivably resurface or alter consideration of an active problem, and all past conditions, ignorance of which might affect the approach to the active problems. Examples of valid inactive problems in a patient with a broken hip include:
   a. **Positive PPD.** The knowledge of the PPD positivity is essential to full awareness of potential problems in this patient.
   b. **Organ removal** [usually designated as "S/P (status-post) cholecystectomy"]. Although this might not be important to the patient's broken hip, it may be important if the patient presents later with an acute abdomen.

D. Modifying and updating the problem list. The problem list is intended to be a comprehensive, dynamic, and up-to-date summary of the patient's status. As the patient's problems are refined and altered, so must items on the problem list be either subsumed, resolved, or inactivated.

1. **Subsumption of a problem.** As the diagnostic workup proceeds or as therapeutic interventions change the course of the illness, separate problems on the primary list may be clarified as belonging to a single diagnosis.
   a. When the health care team becomes certain that problems can be grouped, a cluster of symptoms, signs, or abnormal laboratory results may be **subsumed** under a single heading. For example, a patient presenting to the emergency room may have the following primary problem list:
      (1) **Problem 1:** Shortness of breath
      (2) **Problem 2:** High blood pressure
      (3) **Problem 3:** Peripheral cyanosis
      (4) **Problem 4:** Bilateral pulmonary rales
      (5) **Problem 5:** Low serum oxygen saturation
   b. Although members of the health care team may suspect acute pulmonary edema as the basis for all of these symptoms and signs, they may not be comfortable ascribing all of them to a single problem until a chest x-ray shows the signs of pulmonary edema and a treatment trial for pulmonary edema results in resolution of all five problems. At this point, the problem list may be altered to reflect this **refinement in definition:** Problems 1–5 are now subsumed under Problem 1, which is refined from "shortness of breath" to "pulmonary edema."

2. **Resolution of a problem**
    a. When a problem **disappears completely,** either via nature or interventions of the health care team, the problem may be designated as **resolved,** usually with the date upon which the problem disappeared with no expectation of recurrence. For example, *Mycoplasma* pneumonia in an otherwise healthy adult is placed in the resolved category when it clears completely.
    b. Caution must be exercised in designating a problem resolved if it was a symptom or sign of an underlying process, which could cause the problem to reappear; for example, acute symptoms of pulmonary edema reduced by intensive treatment are not listed as resolved until the cause of the symptom complex has also been corrected.
        (1) If the underlying pathology is a toxic exposure from which the patient can be protected, resolution may have been achieved.
        (2) If the basic pathophysiology is cardiomyopathy, the patient should be considered at risk for recurrence. Here, clinical judgment must dictate how the problem list will be modified to indicate that although the acute pulmonary edema is currently resolved, the patient remains at risk for exacerbation of the symptom complex.

3. **Inactivation of a problem.** A problem may be moved to the **inactive list** when it no longer requires intervention.
    a. A broken arm, once set and fully healed, requires no future consideration and is considered resolved.
    b. The control of pulmonary tuberculosis renders it **inactive** but not resolved; relapse is always possible.
    c. When a surgical procedure is successful, and the patient is well, resolution of the problem requiring the surgery has been achieved, but the absence or alteration of the organ involved is redesignated as inactive; for example, a gastric resection for bleeding ulcer resolves the bleeding problem, but there must be an inactive listing of the surgical procedure, such as "S/P partial gastrectomy." Absence of part of the stomach is important information for the management of any future complications related to the altered anatomy (Figure 10-1).

Figure 10-1.

Sample Case: Derivation of the Problem List

Medical history

L.P. is a 50-year-old female magazine editor who comes in with a 3-month history of fatigue.
CC: "I am so tired all the time."
HPI: Patient states that she was in her usual state of health until about 3 months ago, when she began to notice easy fatigability, intermittent low-grade fever, and rare back and lower right flank pain, sometimes radiating into the right lower quadrant. These symptoms have remained static except for the fatigue, which she feels has been getting progressively worse.

Problem 1: Fatigue

Onset was insidious about 3 months ago. The symptom is characterized as "low energy." She feels inadequately rested after a night's sleep and finds that she has increasing difficulty getting through her usual 9-hour workday, the routine of meals and housework, and her night school class. She has stopped some of her social and community service activities because of the fatigue. She denies feeling sad, anxious, or depressed. Her appetite has remained good, and she has lost no weight. She finds that a nap at midday on weekends, a new thing for her, permits her to carry out the essential functions of the day.

Problem 2: Low-grade fever

When she began feeling tired, she also became aware of feeling hot and then chilly, usually at night, but sometimes in the late afternoon. She began recording her temperature 2 months ago and found that she has a 99.6–100° F temperature in the evenings several times a week. This seems to occur in cycles: 2–3 days with fever, then 2–3 days without fever. She denies shaking chills, night sweats, rashes, or sore throat. She has not been out of the United States in over 18 months. There is no known exposure to ticks or to persons with infectious diseases. She denies cough, GI symptoms, or GU symptoms over this period of time.

Problem 3: Back and flank pain

The patient has had two episodes of severe right flank and right lower quadrant pain in the past 3 months. Each lasted less than 6 hours and resolved spontaneously. She sought no medical attention on either occasion and tends to minimize these symptoms. For the past month, she has been aware of vague low-back pain, which is not incapacitating. For the past week, the low-back pain has been persistent, low-grade, and has seemed to localize in the right flank with occasional pain in the right lower quadrant. She denies dysuria, gross hematuria, vaginal discharge, or painful intercourse. A urinalysis done in a walk-in clinic 1 week ago allegedly revealed red cells without pyuria or bacteriuria.

Figure 10-1. Continued.

No treatment was instituted. The patient finds that acetaminophen (Tylenol) minimizes the discomfort, which enabled her to continue to go to work.

The above problems are temporally related. Other than acetaminophen, she has attempted no treatment; other than the single visit to a clinic because of back pain, she has sought no medical attention and had no tests done. She came in today because the symptoms are interfering with her life and beginning to concern her that there might be something seriously wrong.

Problem 4: Hypothyroidism, treated
Three years ago, because of symptoms of cold intolerance and constipation, she was seen by a clinician who made the diagnosis of hypothyroidism. Since then the patient has taken 0.1 mgm of L-thyroxine (Synthroid) daily; last thyroid function studies were done 4 months ago and, according to the patient, were normal.

Past medical history (PMH)

Hospitalizations: Childbirth, normal vaginal delivery, 16 years ago; appendectomy, 30 years ago
Childhood illnesses: Measles, chicken pox, rubella, mumps; no history rheumatic fever
Immunizations: Routine and up-to-date; last DT, 4 years ago after minor skin trauma
Allergies: Mild fall seasonal rhinorrhea; no known drug allergies; has taken sulfa and penicillin without incident
Medications: L-Thyroxine, 0.1 mgm/day (see Problem 4); over-the-counter antihistamines in the fall; acetaminophen, 1–2 tablets a day for the past 3 months

Family history (FH)

Mother died at age 45 in automobile accident; Father, age 75, living and well. No siblings. One son, age 16, healthy. No known family history of heart disease, hypertension, or stroke. No known gout or renal stone. One grandparent known to have died of colon cancer at age 56.

Personal profile (PP)

The patient lives with her husband, an insurance executive, and her 16-year-old high school student son in their own home in a local suburb. The family is financially stable. The patient enjoys her 40–50-hour work week as an editor for a business magazine. She is completing a master's degree in history and is planning to teach and write when this is completed. She has a few close friends; no family in the area. She enjoys walking and does 2–4 miles every day. Her diet is generally well balanced; she rarely drinks milk and does not take calcium nor antacids. She has a 30 pack/year cigarette history and drinks, at most, 4–8 oz of wine a week if a social occasion presents itself. She has never used recreational drugs. She characterizes her life as pleasantly busy and stimulating. She is concerned because her current symptoms are making it difficult for her to enjoy her activities.

Review of systems (ROS)

Other than items noted above, the ROS is essentially negative. Two years ago, the patient had a suspicious lesion excised from the bottom of her right foot, which was diagnosed as a complex nevus. No follow-up was recommended.

Menstrual and sexual history
Periods continue at 28–30-day intervals; 3–4 days of moderate flow. There have been no changes. She is sexually active and monogamous with her husband. She has never been treated for a sexually transmitted disease. There has been some decrease in sexual activity over the past 3 months due to her fatigue. Patient's husband had a vasectomy 10 years ago, and she has not used supplemental birth control. Last pelvic examination and Pap smear were 6 months ago. Patient does not practice breast self-examination and has never had a mammogram.

There is no history of psychiatric disease or treatment.

Formulation of problem list from medical history

Active problems
Problem 1: Fatigue
Problem 2: Low-grade fever
Problem 3: Back and flank pain
Problem 4: Hypothyroidism, by history, under treatment
Problem 5: Hematuria x one, by history
Problem 6: Tobacco use, 30 pack/year history

Inactive problems
Problem 1: Seasonal rhinorrhea
Problem 2: S/P excision complex nevus, right foot, by history

Discussion of problem list

Active problems
Problems 1, 2, and 3 are the major symptoms gleaned from the HPI. Since, it is not possible to define at this point, they are listed by symptom.

Problem 5 also belongs to the HPI. It is added as a piece of presumed historic data and requires verification by the clinician at the walk-in clinic since it may have bearing on the remainder of the HPI.

Figure 10-1. Continued.

Problem 4, although not apparently contributing to the current symptoms, must be given a priority ranking, for data verification, for consideration in the course of any anticipated diagnostic or therapeutic intervention, and for the remote possibility that it may be related to the HPI. Because it is an ongoing problem, currently under treatment, it may logically be placed in the HPI as well as being considered active.

Problem 6, although likely not related to the HPI, certainly is a health concern for the patient, and at the very least demands some patient education intervention.

Inactive problems
These are listed because of their potential for recurrence or for consideration in any long-term management of the patient. For example, should her present illness require long-term therapy, awareness of the seasonal rhinorrhea will remind the clinician to consider any potential drug interactions when the patient resumes her seasonal antihistamines. The complex nevus, though very likely a resolved problem, needs to be observed for recurrence and must be noted for the sake of comprehensiveness.

Physical examination. This is a well-developed, well-nourished white woman who appears anxious but not acutely distressed.

Vital signs
BP: Both arms, sitting, 110/72
Pulse rate: 110 and regular
Temperature: 100 degrees orally
Respiratory rate: 20/min

Skin
Normal texture and turgor; color normal; no lesions noted except for well-healed surgical scar on sole of right foot

Lymph nodes
Cervical, submandibular, supraclavicular, axillary, and inguinal not palpable

Head
Normal hair distribution; no scalp lesions

Eyes
Sclera and conjunctivae normal; no lid lag; funduscopic examination normal bilaterally

Ears
Normal hearing; TMs normal bilaterally

Nose and throat
Entirely within normal limits (WNL)

Mouth
Good dentition and hygiene; no oral masses or lesions seen

Neck
Supple with full range of motion; thyroid nonpalpable without masses; trachea midline

Chest and lungs
Normal respiratory excursion and diaphragmatic motion; vesicular breath sounds throughout; fremitus normal; no rales nor rhonchi heard; no tenderness to percussion over ribs, sternum, nor spine; mild costovertebral angle (CVA) tenderness, right

Breasts
Symmetrical elevation of nipples without dimpling; mild bilateral cystic variants noted; no nipple secretion, masses, nor tenderness

Cardiac
PMI 5th intercostal space, 4 cm to left of midsternum; no heaves or thrills; A2 greater than P2 at base; S1 and S2 normal in all positions; no S3 nor S4, no murmer or click heard; rhythm sinus tachycardia at 110/min

Vascular
All pulses 2 + and equal throughout without bruit

Abdomen
Scaphoid; RLQ surgical scar; no bruits heard; bowel sounds normal; liver percusses to 6 cm; liver and spleen not palpable; right flank examination reveals fullness with tenderness and a soft mass deep and easily palpable, approximately 3 × 4 cm; renal tip not clearly appreciated

Musculoskeletal
Entirely normal

Neurologic
Mental status: Oriented × three
Cranial nerves (II–XII): WNL
Motor: DTRs 3 + and equal; no clonus; all muscle groups 4/5 and symmetrical; no Babinski elicited

Figure 10-1. Continued.

Sensory: Vibration, pain, proprioception intact
Cerebellar: Grossly normal upper and lower
Gait and station: Normal; no tremor

Back
Full range of motion; normal lordosis; no spinal tenderness

Pelvic and rectal
Introitus normal; speculum examination reveals no abnormalities; on bimanual, the uterus is consistent with age, freely mobile without mass or irregularity; both adnexae easily palpated and clear; ovaries normal in size and non-tender; rectovaginal examination confirms pelvic; no rectal masses; stool guaiac negative

Formulation of problem list from physical examination

Active problems   **Inactive problems**
Problem 7: Sinus tachycardia   **Problem 3:** S/P appendectomy
Problem 8: Right flank mass

Discussion of problem list

   On physical examination, two new problems have been observed, which were not apparent in the history: the presence of a sinus tachycardia and of a mass palpated in the right flank. These findings are added to the problem list derived from the medical history. Also, although the history indicates appendectomy, this was neglected as an addition to the inactive list earlier; it should now be added. (Why might this be an important bit of past medical history in this particular case?)
   There now exists a list of problems presented by L.P., cited at the level to which they are absolutely understood. This problem list is the basis for hypothesizing a differential diagnosis, planning a diagnostic workup, and using the results of the expanded data base to synthesize and reorganize the primary problem list as the clinical problem-solving process is put into action.

III. APPROACH TO THE DIFFERENTIAL DIAGNOSIS

   A. Formulating hypotheses. As clinicians obtain the medical history and do the physical examination, they consider, check, verify, and reject possible etiologies of the symptoms and signs encountered. Hypothesis formulation results in the list commonly known as the **differential diagnosis,** a composite of all of the possible etiologic bases for each of the problems that have been defined. The differential diagnosis remains speculative until one or more of the possibilities is proven to be the genesis of the problem. Clinicians must beware, however, of **premature closure.** Only hypotheses, not decisions, must be made until all of the information is collected.

   1. **From the medical history.** From the time the patient first presents with a chief complaint (CC), the clinician should begin to think in terms of pathophysiology. If the symptoms are vague or general, or the interviewer has not yet learned much about disease process, it is best to use the **seven parameters** (see Chapter 3 I C 2) to obtain information without attempting hypotheses. The more the interviewer has learned about pathologic processes, the more refined his or her hypothesis formulation will be.
      a. A young runner who presents with a CC of "pain in the foot," leads the interviewer to consider the anatomic area and the pathologic processes that are common to that area in the settings of youth and running.
      b. A CC of "pain in the foot" from a sedentary 75-year-old man would direct the questioner quite differently. (The medical student is apt to make very primitive attempts to juggle these possibilities.)

   2. **From the physical examination.** As the clinician moves to the physical examination, focus is guided by the information obtained in the history. If the patient's complaints are directed to the painful foot, the clinician will be more than usually meticulous about examining the area indicated. However, it is also necessary to consider **systemic disease** as the cause of a local symptom. If the examiner's level of knowledge precludes a clear-cut hypothesis derived from the history, he or she ought to approach the physical examination **generically,** by looking everywhere for clues. Hypothesis formulation should be used wisely, and premature closure should be avoided at all costs.

   B. Systems approach to differential diagnosis. After creating a problem list, the clinician must derive a differential diagnosis, the first step in converting problems to plans for intervention.

1. Most clinicians, including the most experienced, resort to "the books" to construct a list of diagnostic possibilities, which is both rational and sufficiently comprehensive to guarantee an efficient and effective approach to problem-solving. This can be the most interesting stage of the diagnostic process, but it must be both **adequately inclusive** and **reasonably exclusive**. Such results are usually best accomplished by a systems approach.

2. With the history, physical examination, and problem list, which constitute the primary data base, it is possible to proceed with the construction of a differential diagnosis, despite a limited understanding of the major body systems, which for the purposes of this discussion, include: skin, reticuloendothelial, cardiovascular, central and peripheral nervous, connective tissue, endocrine, gastrointestinal, musculoskeletal, renal–urinary, reproductive, respiratory, and psychiatric. Each clinician has a slightly different way of arranging a systems organization, but it is important that each has a defined method for constructing the differential diagnosis.

   a. **Systems.** The clinician now sorts through the above 12 systems, one by one, demanding of each: Could any, several, or all of the problems be related to this system? All possibilities should be listed.

   b. **Categories of dysfunction.** The clinician should consider whether the system under scrutiny could be involved with one or more of the following pathophysiologic processes: congenital, degenerative, metabolic, infectious, immunologic, functional, toxic, or traumatic.

   c. **Priorities.** Within each category of dysfunction, the priorities for further diagnostic and therapeutic inquiries should be determined.

      (1) **Prevalence.** This is an issue of commonality in the general population. How often may one expect to see the dysfunction in the world at large? Are we dealing with mosquitoes or with zebras?

      (2) **Probability.** How likely is it that this patient, of a particular age, sex, race, place of origin, and particular family and general health history, would have any of the categories of dysfunction listed?

      (3) **Likelihood of poor outcome.** If the diagnosis is not made now, how will the patient be affected? Missing a fractured rib as a cause of chest pain is a far less ominous error than missing an early pneumococcal pneumonia.

C. Generating a differential diagnosis from the problem list

1. The clinician should take each of the active problems in the problem list and construct a differential diagnosis based upon the information available. The following information should be gleaned for each problem:

   a. The system from which this symptom or sign could arise

   b. The category of dysfunction within each listed system that could account for the symptom or sign

   c. The priority of the dysfunction

2. To illustrate the application of the process, the first problem on the list generated for the case presented in Figure 10-1 will be worked through to a preliminary set of diagnostic possibilities in Figure 10-2.

Figure 10-2.

Sample Case: Generating a Differential Diagnosis from the Problem List

Problem 1: Fatigue

Systems
In the instance of this ubiquitous and vague symptom, essentially every system must be considered as a potential source; therefore, it is prudent to move quickly to the second question.

Category of dysfunction
Cardiovascular: Primary organ failure (e.g., myocardial compromise due to either infectious, metabolic, endocrine, degenerative, immunologic, toxic, traumatic, or (remotely) congenital causes). From this survey of pathophysiologic possibilities, the following list is generated:

1. Myocarditis
2. Endocarditis
3. Amyloidosis
4. Hemachromatosis
5. Hypothyroid cardiomyopathy

Figure 10-2. Continued.

6. Ischemic heart disease
7. Connective tissue disease, lupus, or polyarteritis
8. Alcoholic cardiomyopathy

This list has already been narrowed by some of the information available, but it remains broad to be pared as the clinician moves forward in the decision-making process. This same process of listing is invoked for each of the systems potentially implicated as a cause of fatigue.

Priority

In terms of **prevalence, probability,** and **potential for bad outcome** if not diagnosed or treated now, priorities for diagnosis and treatment must be established.

Myocarditis is sufficiently common to be considered. Also, in this particular patient there is a high-risk age, fever, and sinus tachycardia, all of which suggest myocarditis. Against this diagnosis is the duration of the symptom as well as its indolence.

Endocarditis is relatively common. Again there is fever and tachycardia plus a history of hematuria. The indolence is against the disease but does not rule it out. The absence of a murmur lessens the likelihood. The potential for fatal outcome in this treatable disease, however, makes it imperative that it remain on the list of considerations.

This same thought process should be applied to all of the cardiovascular possibilities until a reasonable assembly of primary considerations remains. The primary cardiovascular diseases to be put into the differential diagnostic list might rest at this level:

1. Subacute bacterial endocarditis
2. Viral myocarditis
3. Primary amyloidosis
4. Alcoholic cardiomyopathy
5. Cardiomyopathy of hypothyroidism
6. Idiopathic cardiomyopathy

Following the pattern set above for Problem 1, a full preliminary differential diagnosis scheme for this patient will be as follows:

Differential Diagnosis. Problem 1: Fatigue

1. Subacute bacterial endocarditis
2. Viral myocarditis
3. Alcoholic cardiomyopathy
4. Cardiomyopathy of hypothyroidism
5. Idiopathic cardiomyopathy
6. Primary amyloidosis (very unlikely)
7. Connective tissue disease
8. Parenchymal renal disease, including nephrolithiasis with chronic pyelonephritis, glomerulonephritis, and toxic nephritis
9. Hypernephroma
10. Depression and anxiety
11. Substance abuse

The identical process is used to establish a differential diagnosis for each of the remaining active problems. As each problem is considered, a subset of recurrent diagnoses will emerge. Each time a diagnosis recurs, the probability of its being the genesis of the patient's present illness is increased. This reordering of probabilities will dictate the sequencing of the diagnostic procedures planned, and the list of differential diagnostic possibilities will, thus, be narrowed systematically and the workup more tightly focused. This is clinical problem-solving in action, based upon the two initial components of the data base: the medical history and the physical examination.

IV. FORMULATING A PLAN

A. From differential diagnosis to plan. The plan develops from three basic determinations.

    1. Additional information

        a. In-depth history and physical examination. Fleshing out details in the history and fine-tuning the physical examination are cost-effective and productive uses of the clinician's time. These steps should antedate elaborate laboratory tests, since they may narrow diagnostic possibilities and save the patient unnecessary interventions and expense. The clinician should:

            (1) Return to the bedside to clarify details and delve further into symptoms
            (2) Review preexisting medical records or laboratory data
            (3) Talk to prior caretakers who might shed light on the problem
            (4) Confer with family members who may add important new information

        b. Consultation. If consultation might preclude expensive or dangerous procedures or prompt necessary early therapy, it is appropriate to request that help now.

    c. Laboratory tests. By looking at the differential diagnosis, the clinician can determine:
      (1) If preliminary laboratory tests would be helpful
      (2) Which tests could be done now
      (3) In what order will such tests best narrow the diagnostic field (see V for a detailed discussion of an approach to laboratory testing)
    d. Procedures. It is important to determine which procedures need be done now to refine the diagnostic possibilities, to provide for the safety of the patient, or to guide emergency treatment before the data base is complete. The decisions about procedures must be made primarily in terms of the potential hazard to a patient if they are not done or are delayed; for example, the febrile, convulsing child with a stiff neck needs a lumbar puncture much more urgently than he or she needs a complete blood count (CBC) or a complete social history.

2. Treatment. Questions about early treatment must be asked even as the diagnostic workup is considered. On occasion, both diagnosis and treatment must proceed simultaneously.
    a. Immediate interventions apply in two instances:
      (1) Life-threatening situations, such as cardiac arrhythmia, tension pneumothorax, status epilepticus, or massive bleeding, when diagnosis of the underlying disease process is less urgent than treatment of the symptom or sign
      (2) Patient comfort when symptoms are so disabling to the patient that humane considerations demand symptomatic treatment without a definitive diagnosis
    b. Therapeutic trials
      (1) Sometimes the institution of a therapeutic trial is prudent even while diagnostic workup is proceeding. For example, empiric antibiotic therapy can begin in a patient with a presumed infection while waiting 24–72 hours for results of cultures and sensitivities. This decision to institute therapy before arriving at a definitive diagnosis in the non–life-threatening situation is based upon the probability that therapy will alter the disease course before the pathology is labeled.
      (2) Therapeutic trial may be substituted for a definitive diagnostic procedure, when the diagnosis seems almost certain or the risks or costs of the test outweigh those of the therapeutic trial. For example, antigout treatment can be instituted when a patient presents with symptoms and signs highly suggestive of the diagnosis without waiting for serum uric acid levels, which are suggestive, but not definitive. If the working diagnosis is correct, the patient will become asymptomatic quickly; if incorrect, no harm will have been done as long as the other diagnostic possibilities are pursued concurrently.
    c. Watchful waiting is often the most difficult decision for the clinician, who is trained to intervene—to do something—and whose patient expects nothing less. Many of the problems with which patients present are self-limited, and prudent observation will allow time and "mother nature" to do their work. When the clinician has determined that "doing nothing" will not harm the patient, this approach should be strongly considered.

3. Patient education. Throughout the process of diagnosis and therapeutic interventions, a concern for the patient's queries and worries must be kept uppermost in the clinician's mind. It is the patient who comes with, and ultimately owns, the problem. He or she must be informed as decisions are made.
    a. Negotiating procedures
      (1) If the patient is conscious and aware, all interventions should be discussed before the fact. Reasons for any diagnostic intervention should be shared with the patient.
      (2) If there is hazard, discomfort, or expense to be incurred, the patient must not only be aware of, but agree to, what is planned.
    b. Communicating progress and prognosis. Patients are often reluctant to ask questions because of lack of knowledge, fear of being considered nuisances, respect for the clinician's time, or fear of potential bad news. The patient should know as much as he wants to know and be encouraged to ask questions.

B. Updating and revising the differential diagnosis. As new information is acquired or as the patient's clinical condition evolves, the clinician repeatedly revises and alters the provisional differential diagnosis.

    1. Reviewing new information. As new data from the laboratory, physical examination, or history are collected, thinking and planning must be adjusted accordingly.

2. **Assessing additional information needs**
   a. When new data are added to the chart and consequent revisions are made in the problem list, differential diagnosis, or management plan, the need to confirm or add to the growing data base must be considered. The decision to request new information derives from answers already supplied or diagnostic possibilities that have been enhanced or negated.
   b. A piece of information that does not fit the pattern must be either confirmed or rejected; for example:
      (1) If a patient presents with a typical clinical history of pneumococcal pneumonia, has gram-positive diplococci in the sputum smear, but does not grow *Streptococcus pneumoniae* on culture, the clinician must reconsider the diagnosis.
      (2) If the patient, now 36 hours into the appropriate regimen of penicillin, is afebrile and looking good, perhaps the negative sputum culture needs to be discounted.
      (3) If the clinical response to the treatment for pneumococcal disease has been disappointing, the Gram stain may have been misinterpreted. Alternative diagnostic possibilities must be entertained.

3. **Eliminating disproven diagnoses.** When the primary diagnostic studies show definitive evidence that one of the differential diagnostic possibilities has been ruled out, the record should reflect this. Negative information is helpful in narrowing the differential diagnosis.

4. **Revising the problem list.** In the excitement of chasing the diagnosis, the problem list should not be forgotten. It is the problem list from which the progress notes are written and from which new diagnostic possibilities may be derived.
   a. If it now appears that two or more problems are secondary to a single pathologic process, the record should be updated so that others caring for the patient can follow the progress of problem resolution.
   b. If the patient reports new problems, they are added to the list.
   c. If a problem changes or disappears, this is reflected in the problem list.

5. **Revising therapeutic plans.** Treatments may need to be stopped or altered if they:
   a. Are not helping the patient
   b. Are creating new problems
   c. Become irrational in the face of new diagnostic evidence
   d. Have succeeded in eliminating one or more of the problems or diagnostic possibilities

6. **Keeping the patient advised.** The patient should be informed of changes in plans or of new developments in the "case."

C. **The process of working from the differential diagnosis to a preliminary plan** is illustrated in Figure 10-3, using the sample case used in Figures 10-1 and 10-2.

Figure 10-3.

Sample Case: Working from the Differential Diagnosis to the Preliminary Plan

Problem 1: Fatigue

Subacute bacterial endocarditis

Further information from history and physical examination
1. Obtain history of any dental, GU, GI procedures, or IV drug use
2. Listen again for murmur
Laboratory studies and procedures
1. Blood cultures, CBC*
2. Echocardiogram*
Therapy: None now
Patient education
1. Discuss laboratory tests
2. Discuss echocardiogram

Viral myocarditis

---

*Note the recurrence of the same tests or procedures in more than one diagnostic consideration.

Figure 10-3. Continued.

Further information from history and physical examination
1. Check history for any antecedent viral illness
2. Listen again for S3, quality of heart sounds
Laboratory studies and procedures: Echocardiogram*
Therapy: None
Patient education: Discuss echocardiogram

Cardiomyopathy of hypothyroidism
Further information from history and physical examination: Get results of recent thyroid function tests
Laboratory studies, therapy, and patient education: None

Alcoholic cardiomyopathy

Further information from history and physical examination
1. Question again regarding patient's alcohol intake
2. Question family regarding patient's alcohol intake
Laboratory studies and procedures
1. Electrocardiogram (EKG)
2. Echocardiogram*
3. Red cell indices, CBC*
Therapy: None
Patient education: Discuss laboratory studies and reasons

Idiopathic cardiomyopathy. Covered in three possibilities discussed above under alcoholic cardiomyopathy

Connective tissue disease

Further information from history and physical examination
1. ROS pertinent to connective tissue disease
2. Recheck physical for signs of connective tissue disease
Laboratory studies and procedures
1. Antinuclear antibody (ANA)
2. Sedimentation rate
Therapy and patient education: As above

Renal disease

Further information from history and physical examination
1. Check with walk-in clinic regarding urinalysis
2. Review analgesic history
3. Reassess right flank mass
Laboratory studies and procedures
1. BUN, creatinine, serum calcium, phosphorus, uric acid, urine sediment, and urinalysis
2. Renal ultrasound or scan
Therapy: None
Patient education: Explain tests and procedures

Depression and anxiety. Low probability; hold for later consideration

Substance abuse. Review history; talk with family

Differential diagnosis and plan revision based on the new information

Further information from history and physical examination
All additional data collected above is negative except for a positive history of a routine dental hygiene visit 3 weeks before onset of symptoms.

Laboratory studies and procedures
1. CBC reveals a mild normochromic, normocytic anemia without an increase in WBCs.
2. All chemistries are normal.
3. EKG and echocardiogram are normal.
4. Blood cultures are negative at 48 hours.
5. Urinalysis is positive only for 10–15 RBCs/hpf.
6. Renal ultrasound reveals a solid mass, right kidney.

New differential diagnosis. Problem 1: Fatigue

1. Hypernephroma
2. Subacute bacterial endocarditis (highly unlikely)

---

*Note the recurrence of the same tests or procedures in more than one diagnostic consideration.

Figure 10-3. Continued.

The procedure for evaluating the differential diagnosis for each of the remaining problems is the same. The data collected on this first run allow the student to consolidate and subsume problems, to narrow the differential diagnostic possibilities, and to make the next step in planning for any additional diagnostic or therapeutic steps. The process illustrated for formulation of the initial plan is repeated as often as necessary to arrive at a definitive diagnosis and management plan.

V. APPROACH TO CHOOSING A LABORATORY DATA BASE. This section gives an overview of the basic principles essential to the use of laboratory studies and commonly used tests in primary assessment. It is important to note that **this overview supplements, but does not replace, disease-specific reviews**. The difference between screening asymptomatic individuals and the application of laboratory studies to problem lists and differential diagnoses are discussed. Some of the principles of test selection based on simple statistical analytical usefulness are reviewed and applied to the sample case (Figure 10-4).

Figure 10-4.

Sample Case: Choosing Primary Laboratory Procedures

To illustrate the approach to choosing a primary laboratory data base for L.P., the differential diagnosis compiled in Figure 10-2 for Problem 1 (fatigue) should be reviewed. For each of the diagnostic considerations, the possible laboratory tests must be examined based upon their **sensitivity, specificity,** and **risk:benefit ratio**.

Subacute bacterial endocarditis

CBC
1. **Sensitivity** is high for defining anemia, red cell morphology, and elevated WBC with left shift, all of which are expected in any valvular disease with systemic infection.
2. **Specificity.** No abnormality on CBC is disease-specific but taken as a part of the total data base, the CBC will be useful in enhancing or reducing the possibility of this diagnosis.
3. **Risk:benefit ratio.** Low cost and low risk to the patient make this test worth doing at this time.

Urinalysis
1. **Sensitivity** is high for the detection of red blood cells.
2. **Specificity** is low, since red blood cells in the urine may mean any number of things.
3. **Risk:benefit ratio.** Since the test is inexpensive, without risk, and may add useful information to the data base, it is indicated.

Electrolytes
Since this patient is alert and ambulatory and her condition is not metabolically critical, there seems to be no need to do electrolytes. These tests have no useful sensitivity or specificity in terms of this differential diagnostic possibility.

BUN and creatinine
Neither specific nor sensitive in terms of endocarditis; therefore, they are not useful in this diagnostic consideration.

Serum glucose
No indication

Serum enzymes
No indication

Cholesterol
No indication

Bilirubin
Since bilirubin might be elevated in the hemolytic process sometimes seen in subacute bacterial endocarditis, one might consider requesting this test. However, its specificity in the diagnosis considered is so limited that it does not seem indicated at this time.

EKG
This patient has an unexplained tachycardia, and primary cardiac disease is being considered. EKG will be very nonspecific in regards to this diagnostic possibility. As the workup progresses, the EKG may eventually become imperative.

Chest x-ray
This is a hard call. The sinus tachycardia raises the possibility of insipient cardiac failure, which the chest x-ray might help define. There is also the possibility of calcification, indicating underlying valvular abnormality, but the auscultatory examination does not suggest this. The chest x-ray cannot be expected to help much in refining this portion of the differential diagnosis.

Figure 10-4. Continued.

After thinking through the potential yield of each of the laboratory studies considered, the plan for differential diagnostic possibility, **subacute bacterial endocarditis,** might include: CBC, urinalysis, and (possibly) EKG. Blood cultures and echocardiogram become necessary if clinical judgment indicates that bacterial endocarditis is the primary diagnostic consideration. However, perusal of the list and review of the physical examination findings indicate that the **flank mass is of a higher magnitude of concern**.

Before writing orders for primary laboratory testing for this patient, the clinician uses the above decision-making process for each of the remaining diagnostic considerations. A **composite list** of the **primary tests** most likely to lead to a diagnosis most quickly, efficiently, and with the minimum of risk and cost is made. Pending the results of these first tests, the clinician may now write the orders and enter the laboratory diagnostic plan in the patient's progress notes.

Problem 1: Fatigue

Assessment—strongest differential diagnostic considerations
1. Subacute bacterial endocarditis
2. Hypernephroma

Still to be ruled out
1. Viral myocarditis
2. Alcoholic cardiomyopathy
3. Cardiomyopathy of hypothyroidism
4. Idiopathic cardiomyopathy
5. Primary amyloidosis
6. Connective tissue disease
7. Chronic renal disease
8. Depression and anxiety
9. Substance abuse

Plan
CBC, urinalysis, EKG, thyroid function studies, serum creatinine all ordered today. If indicated from EKG, will plan echocardiogram for this afternoon. Renal ultrasound scheduled for tomorrow A.M. Family conference regarding substance abuse and any indications of emotional or behavioral changes is scheduled for tonight.

Summary
Renal ultrasonography revealed a solid mass in the upper pole of the right kidney. Surgical exploration confirmed hypernephroma, which could account for the fatigue as well as the physical examination findings in the abdomen and the abnormal laboratory values. Sinus tachycardia and low-grade fever disappeared after recovery from the nephrectomy performed.

A. **Screening laboratory examinations**

1. **Asymptomatic patient.** Basic to the issue of routine laboratory screening should be an awareness that no consistent agreement exists among clinicians as to which laboratory tests should be done as "screens" in a population of asymptomatic and apparently healthy individuals. A number of groups have compiled data and made recommendations on the basis of ongoing studies (e.g., Frame, Breslin, American Cancer Society, and Canadian Task Force). Students should monitor these recommendations for changes and new rationales.

2. **General guidelines** given below are not intended to be definitive recommendations in screening asymptomatic patients. The following suggestions are arranged by **age-groups,** but **variations in life-style habits** (e.g., tobacco, alcohol, and substance use) and **family risk factors** should also be considered. When choosing laboratory tests for asymptomatic individuals, it is necessary to ask whether or not these tests will reveal anything that may alter the outcome for the patient.
    a. **Well child.** Refer to pediatric textbooks.
    b. **Adolescent.** There is no recommended routine other than that based in life-style issues and family history (FH) of genetic disease. (See V A 3 for gynecologic screening in this age-group.)
    c. **Young adult** (20–40 years of age). It is generally recommended that serum cholesterol be monitored at 4-year intervals from age 20–70.
    d. **Middle age** (40–50 years of age)
        (1) Cholesterol should be monitored as above.
        (2) Some clinicians suggest an EKG as a baseline during this period.
        (3) Most clinicians suggest that between the ages of 40 and 50 annual stool guaiac examinations should begin to screen for colon cancer, although this recommendation is in flux as new studies are completed.
    e. **Late adulthood** (60–75 years of age). Continue cholesterol and stool guaiac as above.

   f. Old age (over 75). No specific routine laboratory screens are suggested except possibly the continuation of stool guaiac studies.

   3. **Special surveillance.** There are particular situations related to life-style, FH, age, and sex that require attention that is somewhat more specific than the general screening noted above.
      a. Gynecologic surveillance
         (1) With increasing recognition of human papilloma virus (HPV) infection as a possible antecedent to premalignant changes in the uterine cervix, there has been a shift back toward the recommendation of **annual Pap smears in all sexually active women**.
         (2) It is necessary to keep abreast of the changing recommendations for *Chlamydia* screening in sexually active women, with or without symptoms.
      b. Breast cancer surveillance. The use of **mammography** in screening for breast cancer is also in a state of flux. At present, it is suggested that all women have a **baseline mammogram** between the ages of 35 and 50, and **annual mammograms** thereafter until age 65–70. Special considerations for the earlier institution of screening are applied to women with such **risk factors** as a prior breast cancer, a FH of breast cancer, and nulliparity.
      c. Other cancer surveillance. Helms and Weiner pointed out some of the **characteristics** of a successful **cancer screening program**.
         (1) Reliability. The chosen test should be specific and sensitive.
         (2) Effectiveness. Early detection should provide a positive effect on outcome; that is, there should be a treatment available for the disease being sought that makes early detection in the patient's best interest.
         (3) Economy. The benefit of the test should justify both the risk and the cost.

B. Symptom-related laboratory examinations

   1. **Choosing the appropriate tests.** Before ordering a laboratory test, the clinician should determine the following:
      a. Cost-effectiveness. Is this test the cheapest way—in time, money, and risk to the patient—to get the diagnostic answers to serve the patient best?
      b. Diagnostic effectiveness. Is this test sufficiently **specific** and **sensitive** to be indicated at this time?
         (1) Specificity. The percent of time that a positive test result correctly indicates that the patient does have the disease in question. A specificity of 90% means that there will be 10 false-positives per 100 patients tested.
         (2) Sensitivity. The percent of time that, when the test is negative, the disease is not present. A sensitivity of 95% means that there will be 5 false-negatives for every 100 patients who actually have the disease for which they are being tested.
      c. Risk:benefit ratio. Is this test sufficiently sensitive to be helpful in the indication of the presence of the disease being considered, and at the same time, sufficiently specific to preclude a futile chase, so that the risk of the test to the patient can be justified? For example:
         (1) Sending a blood sample to the laboratory for a hemoglobin determination when the diagnosis of anemia is being considered is highly sensitive, highly specific, of relatively low cost, and of no risk to the patient.
         (2) Careful consideration must be given to doing a coronary arteriogram on a patient whose condition precludes surgery even if a lesion is found and for whom the physical risk of the test is high.

   2. **Effective use of laboratory data.** If the laboratory result does not come out as predicted, the clinician must then decide whether or not the unexpected result warrants a **repeat test for confirmation, relegation to the "red herring" or "fluke" category,** or a **new investigative quest**. For example, if the CBC ordered on the patient expected to be anemic reveals a normal hemoglobin and hematocrit, but a very low white count, what does this do to the differential diagnosis and the next diagnostic step? If the anemia is still thought to be present, should the test be repeated, or should the health care team abandon the diagnosis of anemia and pursue the low white blood cell count?

C. Common laboratory procedures. This section is intended to be a review of common and frequently ordered tests as an illustration of general principles. For disease-specific indications and interpretations of these tests, the reader is referred to any standard textbook of medicine.

   1. **CBC.** The CBC usually includes the **hemoglobin, hematocrit, red cell indices, white blood cell count with differential,** and an estimate of the **platelet count**. This is a relatively inexpensive,

fully automated test (except for the differential count) with high specificity, sensitivity, and accuracy for the diagnosis of anemia, differentiation of large categories of anemia (e.g., micro-, normo-, and macrocytic anemias), and suggestion as to quantitative and qualitative abnormalities of white blood cells and platelets.

2. **Urinalysis.** The urinalysis may be ordered as a part of the routine **assessment** of **undifferentiated disease, to test diagnostic hypotheses,** or as a **follow-up in therapy**. Of most importance to the student of introductory clinical medicine is an understanding of the components of the test and their clinical usefulness.
    a. **Specific gravity** (usual range 1.010–1.035). This is an indirect measure of the kidney's ability to conserve or to dump body water and solute. False elevations of the specific gravity may occur with massive loads of solute, such as glucose or protein.
    b. **Protein, sugar, ketones, blood, and pH.** All are quickly tested by means of impregnated paper or "dipstick."
    c. **Appearance.** Color and turbidity are noted by visual inspection.
    d. **Sediment.** Cellular components and bacteria in the stained or unstained sediment indicate specific functional processes.

3. **Serum chemistries.** This group of tests, often grouped into panels, is probably one of the most useful, and yet most often abused, group of laboratory examinations available. There is a tendency to order a full panel without regard for the questions being asked about the patient's particular problem.
    a. **Electrolytes** [i.e., sodium (Na^+), potassium (K^+), and chloride (Cl^+)]. The role of the clinician is to determine from the list of problems and differential diagnostic possibilities whether any or all of the above chemistries will lead to a diagnostic resolution and a therapeutic plan. Serum electrolytes are highly specific and sensitive in a properly considered clinical situation but should be ordered with a particular question in mind.
    b. **Creatinine and blood urea nitrogen (BUN).** These are the two standard serum **assessments of renal function**.
        (1) **Creatinine** becomes elevated when the renal clearance drops below approximately one quarter of its normal capacity. The elevation of creatinine warrants investigation of the specific functional problems: circulatory impairment (prerenal), primary kidney failure (renal), or urinary tract obstruction (postrenal).
        (2) **BUN** is a less specific test for renal impairment as it may be elevated as a result of excessive absorption of urea nitrogen into the circulatory system, as well as from the inability of a diseased kidney to excrete urea.
    c. **Serum glucose.** This is a highly specific and sensitive test for **metabolic failure to handle carbohydrates**. The significance of an abnormal serum glucose must be interpreted in light of the metabolic status of the patient.
        (1) Elevation of fasting blood glucose levels usually indicates the presence of diabetes mellitus or glucose intolerance.
        (2) Low levels are more difficult to interpret but could suggest an insulin-secreting tumor or the excessive use of exogenous insulin.
    d. **Serum enzymes.** These tests are used to **verify or eliminate the probability of specific organ damage,** usually toxic, infectious, or ischemic. Students should be acquainted with the specificity of the various enzyme analyses and their usefulness in the diagnosis of liver, cardiac, bone, pancreatic, and muscle disease. The circumstances under which **false-positivity** occurs in these tests must be understood and taken into consideration when ordering them and using them to make diagnostic decisions.
    e. **Serum cholesterol** (see V A c)
    f. **Serum bilirubin.** This determination is useful in the consideration of either primary liver disease, extrahepatic biliary obstruction, or hemolytic disease.

4. **Electrocardiogram (EKG or ECG).** The decision to order an EKG presents one of the commonest dilemmas in choosing tests. Because it is harmless and "noninvasive," the tendency is to proceed at the most minimal provocation. The EKG, when fully processed, is a test that will cost the patient or his third-party payer between $75 and $100. This is a small price if the test is helpful in managing the patient's problems but not if it is ordered without specific purpose. The student should have a working knowledge of the electrophysiology basic to the interpretation of the test, the skill to apply the electrodes and record a 12-lead EKG, and a preliminary approach to "reading" the EKG. Minimally, he or she should know how to determine rate and rhythm, electrical axis, P-wave morphology, P-R interval, QRS interval, Q-T interval, QRS morphology, S-T segment position, and T-wave morphology.

    a. Because of its broad applicability in defining cardiac dysfunction, the EKG will likely be indicated in any patient in whom cardiac disease is considered.

    b. The test is also quite sensitive for detecting electrolyte abnormalities, although serum determinations of the electrolyte in question are much more specific.

    c. There are toxins and drug overdoses for which the EKG is crucial in following the patient for dangerous conduction problems.

    d. Certain metabolic and endocrine crises require the EKG as part of progress monitoring.

5. Chest x-ray. The chest film is one of the commonest laboratory procedures ordered. It is a noninvasive, safe, but relatively expensive (approximately $100) test. Like the EKG, it has a wide range of applicability in the evaluation of a patient suspected of having primary lung disease, lung disease secondary to cardiac failure, mediastinal disease, or less commonly, lung involvement in systemic or remote organ pathology.

REFERENCES

Medical Practice Committee—American College of Physicians. *Ann Intern Med* 95:729–32, 1981

Helms SR, Weiner RS: Cancer screening: the primary care physician's role. *Compr Ther* 11:6–9, 1985

STUDY QUESTIONS

Directions: Each of the numbered items or incomplete statements in this section is followed by answers or by completions of the statement. Select the **one** lettered answer or completion that is **best** in each case.

1. A 63-year-old white man comes in with a CC of "pain in the right calf when walking." The pain is always immediately relieved by rest. All of the items below should be recorded as active problems EXCEPT

(A) a 60 pack/year smoking history
(B) a serum cholesterol of 330 mg/100 ml (6 months ago)
(C) appendectomy at age 22
(D) FH of young cardiac deaths
(E) diet-controlled diabetes mellitus

2. The clinician is asked to evaluate a 24-year-old man for a bus driver's license application. Which one of the following historic items should be entered as Problem 1?

(A) Broken leg at age 16
(B) Jail sentence for marijuana possession at age 19
(C) Myopia (nearsightedness) sufficient to require glasses
(D) Strong FH of diabetes mellitus
(E) History of rejection from the armed forces because of an inguinal hernia

3. In the problem-oriented medical record, a problem listing of inactive should be made for any problem that

(A) requires further data collection now
(B) is of no importance to patient care
(C) is quiescent but of potential future significance
(D) is of historic interest only
(E) is of doubtful validity

4. A 77-year-old woman comes into the emergency room with a CC of "dizziness." Which one of the following problems should be relegated to the inactive list?

(A) high blood pressure for 20 years
(B) insufficient income to buy adequate food
(C) rapidly progressive unilateral hearing loss for the last 6 months
(D) cholecystectomy 4 years ago
(E) aortic valve replacement 2 years ago

5. All of the following statements about Pap smears of the uterine cervix are true EXCEPT

(A) the sample is considered inadequate if endocervical cells are not present
(B) annual Pap smear screening should begin for all women at age 16
(C) human papilloma virus infection may predispose to premalignant changes in the cervical cells on Pap smear
(D) a history of multiple sexual partners increases the risk of cervical malignancy
(E) after age 60, the frequency of Pap smear screening may safely be reduced to every 3–5 years

6. Each of the following parameters is critical in choosing any given laboratory test EXCEPT

(A) specificity of the test
(B) sensitivity of the test
(C) cost:benefit ratio of the test
(D) on site availability of the test
(E) patient willingness to undergo the test

7. The CBC is highly specific for each of the following abnormalities EXCEPT

(A) anemia
(B) polycythemia
(C) thrombocytosis
(D) leukopenia
(E) leukocytosis

8. The routine urinalysis (i.e., dipstick plus microscopic examination of the spun urine sediment) is highly sensitive for establishing the presence of each of the following conditions EXCEPT

(A) hematuria
(B) pyuria
(C) albuminuria
(D) cancer of the kidney
(E) acute glomerulonephritis

Directions: Each item below contains four suggested answers of which **one or more** is correct. Choose the answer

A   if **1, 2, and** 3 are correct
B   if **1 and** 3 are correct
C   if **2 and** 4 are correct
D   if **4** is correct
E   if **1, 2, 3, and 4** are correct

9. In the problem-oriented medical record, an active problem is defined as one which requires

(1) therapeutic action
(2) diagnostic action
(3) revision and update
(4) patient education action

Directions: The groups of questions below consist of lettered choices followed by several numbered items. For each numbered item select the **one** lettered choice with which it is **most** closely associated. Each lettered choice may be used once, more than once, or not at all.

Questions 10–14

For each age-group listed below, select the laboratory test that is most appropriate for screening asymptomatic patients.

(A) Serum cholesterol
(B) Annual EKG
(C) No routine laboratory screen recommended
(D) Annual CBC and urinalysis
(E) None of the above

10. Children from infancy to 2 years of age

11. Men from 10–20 years of age

12. Individuals from 20–40 years of age

13. Women from 40–60 years of age

14. Individuals over 75 years of age

Questions 15–19

For each of the case scenarios presented below, select the most likely diagnosis based upon prevalence in the population at large and probability in the individual case.

(A) *Neisseria gonorrhoeae* infection
(B) *Candida albicans* infection
(C) *Chlamydia* infection
(D) Human immunodeficiency virus infection
(E) None of the above

15. A sexually inactive 26-year-old woman with a 5-day history of a thick, curdy white, vaginal discharge and vulvar itching

16. A 26-year-old man with a thick, yellow, penile discharge who had a single sexual encounter with a prostitute 5 days ago

17. A 30-year-old intravenous heroin user who comes in with generalized lymphadenopathy

18. A 65-year-old widow who comes in with a history of vulvar itching without discharge

19. A 23-year-old sexually active woman who is asymptomatic but is found on pelvic examination to have a purulent cervicitis

ANSWERS AND EXPLANATIONS

1. The answer is C. [*II A 1–3*] Rational thought would dictate that the appendectomy 41 years ago has no relationship to the presenting complaint; however, since it represents the historic absence of an organ, it deserves to be included on the inactive list. The smoking history, elevated cholesterol, FH of cardiac events, and the presence of diabetes in this patient all constitute risk factors for vascular disease. Combined with the classic history for intermittent claudication, these vascular risk factors are prominent considerations in this patient's active problem list and may be directly related to the CC.

2. The answer is C. [*II B, C*] Since the task at hand is to determine this man's physical ability to drive a public conveyance, the primary concern is his vision. The presence of myopia and the need for glasses are paramount and should constitute the most important problem related to the task. The broken leg belongs on an inactive list; the history of marijuana use must be included but is of less significance today than is the myopia. The FH of diabetes is important to long-term care but is irrelevent to the bus driver's license as long as the candidate is not symptomatic. The inguinal hernia has importance to the patient but none to the bus company.

3. The answer is C. [*II C 2*] In formulating the inactive problem list, the clinician is concerned with a data base that can be used to guide current and future patient care. Therefore, even a past medical problem, now apparently resolved but with the potential of resurfacing or later creating confusion, must be recorded. By definition, there is no need to pursue further information at this time. Although the problem may be irrelevant to the HPI, it may be relevent to the long-term comprehensive care of the patient. Validity is not a priority issue for inactive problems.

4. The answer is D. [*II C 2*] The history of gallbladder removal 4 years ago is unimportant to the presenting problem, although it must be noted for the record in the event of future abdominal complaints. Any one of the four remaining problems listed could be implicated in the current problem. Uncontrolled high blood pressure may be associated with dizziness; cerebral vasoconstrictive or occlusive events, leading to vestibular dysfunction, may be secondary to hypertensive cerebrovascular abnormalities. Poor diet may lead to anemia or specific nutriment deficiencies, which could result in dizziness. The presence of unilateral hearing loss must be evaluated for the possibility of inner ear disease or eighth nerve tumor as the basis for the presenting complaint. Dizziness is a common symptom of aortic valve disease or prosthesis dysfunction.

5. The answer is B. [*V A 3 a*] There is no evidence to support the need for routine Pap smears in adolescents based on age. The time to begin this screen is with the onset of sexual activity, in the rare instance of vaginal symptoms, or with a history of DES exposure. Most cytologists worry that sampling is inadequate if endocervical cells are not present. There is good evidence now to indicate that women infected with the human papilloma virus have an increased risk for carcinoma in situ, as well as a more rapid progression from the dysplastic stage to carcinoma in situ. There is a significant correlation between number of sexual partners and early age of sexual activity with dysplasia and carcinoma in situ on Pap smear. The incidence of carcinoma of the cervix drops precipitously after menopause, leading most clinicians to reduce the frequency of Pap smears after age 60.

6. The answer is D. [*V B 1*] If a test is specific and sensitive for the diagnosis being considered, if it has a positive cost:benefit ratio, and the patient is willing to undergo the test, the basic criteria for the need for the test have been met. Once the test has met these criteria, the place where the test may be done becomes a nuisance factor but it does not justify abandoning it.

7. The answer is C. [*V C 1*] A rough estimate of platelets may be made from the stained blood smear; however, the diagnosis of thrombocytosis requires a full platelet count, which is not a part of the standard CBC and must be ordered as a separate test. Anemia is diagnosed definitively by a reduction in hematocrit, hemoglobin, or total red cell count—all of which are a part of the CBC. Polycythemia (too many red blood cells) is also specified in this test, as are leukopenia (too few white blood cells) and leukocytosis (too many white blood cells). The numerical standards of normal ranges for each of the above have been well established and are accurately assessed in the CBC with the noted exception of the platelet count.

8. The answer is D. [*V C 2*] Cancer of the kidney cannot be diagnosed by urinalysis. The urine in this disease may vary from completely normal (usual) to revealing the cancer cells (rare). Thus, the test is never sensitive and is rarely specific for the diagnosis. In contrast, hematuria (blood in the urine), pyuria (white blood cells in the urine), albuminuria (albumin in the urine) are straightforward observations; they are not diagnoses but indicators of problems, and they serve as clues for further investigation. The "telescoped" urine of acute glomerulonephritis—that is, a urine sediment containing red cells, white cells, albumin, red cell casts and renal cell casts—is highly suggestive, though not specific, for the diagnosis of acute glomerulonephritis.

9. The answer is E (all). [*Figure 10-2*] Maintenance of a dynamic active problem list requires attention to three actions—diagnostic, therapeutic, and patient education. It also demands constant revision and update as new information becomes available.

10–14. The answers are: 10-E, 11-C, 12-A, 13-A, 14-E. [*V A 1, 2*] None of the screening tests listed are appropriate for the pediatric age-group. For early pediatric screens, refer to a pediatric textbook. There are no routine screening studies currently recommended for the healthy, asymptomatic man from 10–20 years of age. At the present time, it is suggested that all individuals be assessed at regular intervals for serum cholesterol levels, beginning at age 20 (or earlier if there is a FH suggestive of early coronary artery disease or familial hyperlipidemias). Women over 40 years of age should have periodic mammograms, stool guaiacs, serum cholesterols, and Pap smears. Other than stool guaiacs, no routine screening tests are currently recommended for asymptomatic individuals over age 75.

15–19. The answers are: 15-B, 16-A, 17-D, 18-E, 19-C [*V B, C*] Sexual inactivity generally rules out gonorrhea and *Chlamydia* infections. The commonest pathogen of the vagina is *Candida,* and the description of the thick white discharge with itching is pathognomonic.

The onset of a yellow penile discharge within 5 days of a casual sexual encounter is gonorrhea until proven otherwise. A smear or culture of the discharge should be sufficient to establish the diagnosis. The treatment is penicillin unless contraindicated.

The intravenous drug user in the United States today is at high-risk for human immunodeficiency virus (HIV) infection. Generalized lymphadenopathy in such a person must be considered evidence for HIV infection until proven otherwise.

Vaginal pruritus in a postmenopausal woman is most commonly related to estrogen-deficient local mucosal changes. The absence of discharge mitigates against infection. A vaginal examination should confirm the presence of local mucosal atrophy, and local application of estrogen cream will alleviate the symptom.

Chlamydia infection is rapidly becoming the commonest sexually transmitted disease. It is usually asymptomatic in women. A cervical inflammatory process should be indication for further investigation or treatment for *Chlamydia.*

11
Communicating with Colleagues

Janice L. Willms, Anthony J. Ardolino
Henry Schneiderman, Linda R. Benedetto

I. INTRODUCTION. To facilitate the care of patients in today's complex health care system, communication among caretakers must be standardized, efficient, complete, and accurate.

   A. Written communication of all patient care activities comprises the **medical record**. This chapter reviews the format and content of the medical record, including the:

   1. **Primary data base** (initial history and physical examination)

   2. **Problem list**

   3. **Progress notes**

   4. **Medical orders**

   B. Legal ramifications. Consideration of the medical record as a **legal document** is discussed.

   C. Verbal communication among members of the health care team includes informal discussions and consultations and formal bedside rounds. The centerpiece of formal rounds is the **oral case presentation**. Guidelines and a format for this presentation are discussed.

II. WRITTEN MEDICAL RECORD. The transcription of the medical record may use either a traditional or problem-oriented format. The **traditional format** is designed for recording data rather than for problem-solving. It is primarily concerned with the rapid definition of a differential diagnosis. It does not contain a problem list and does not develop progress notes by problem. The **problem-oriented format** was proposed in the 1960s by Lawrence Weed, M.D. As with any new system, reactions to it have been mixed, and adoption of its theories and use has been varied. Because problem orientation emphasizes process as well as content, it is presented here as the standard for review.

   A. Overview of the problem-oriented medical record

   1. **Philosophy of problem orientation.** The problem-oriented medical record provides a framework within which changes in a patient's status and the progress of problem resolution are measured and communicated.

      a. Problem definition. By initiating the clinical assessment with a definition of the problems with which patients present, then working from these problems toward the need for and type of action required, the clinician begins the problem-solving process at its simplest level.

      b. Dynamics. The record generated by a problem-oriented system ideally remains dynamic and keeps problems patient-related rather than clinician-related. If first level problems are kept in view, such difficulties as **premature closure** and **excessive or irrelevent diagnostic workups** may be avoided. This active process stimulates continuous **reassessment of the patient's condition, refinement of diagnostic and therapeutic considerations,** and **hypothesis revision**. The problem list is revised based upon the dynamics of the "case," thus keeping every member of the health care team apprised of alterations in diagnosis and therapy.

   2. **Utility of problem orientation.** The structure of this system promotes better record-keeping and better communication with colleagues about the progress of a "case."

      a. Access to identified problems. If the problem list is altered as the patient's status changes, new providers are assured a review.

    b. Access to status change. Systematic and efficient review of changes in status become available to all health care providers.

    c. Access to problem revision. Active problems are kept in the forefront; changes in historic information, physical examination findings, and laboratory data are recorded where they can be quickly accessed.

  3. Problem-solving mentality. Proper use of the problem-oriented system demands that all of the providers involved in a patient's care understand both the format used by this system and the process of recording in this format.

B. Components of the problem-oriented medical record

  1. Medical history. For details on the acquisition of these data, see Chapter 3; for details on recording these data, see III A.

  2. Physical examination. For details on the acquisition of these data, see Chapter 6; for details on recording these data, see III B.

  3. Laboratory data. For details on the acquisition and recording of these data, see Chapter 10 V.

  4. Problem lists are usually recorded in two places: a face sheet on the front of the chart designed for this purpose and at the end of the recorded medical history and physical examination. For details on formulation and revision of the problem list, see Chapter 10 II and III.

  5. Primary assessment and management plan. A preliminary plan for assessment and management is recorded for each problem.

  6. Progress notes. For details on recording progress notes, see IV.

C. Activity of the problem-oriented medical record. The value of this system lies in the continuous updating and revising of its components.

  1. Format for revision. A standardized format for revision—understood and accepted by all members of the health care team—must be adopted. The active portions of the chart, which are assigned to the primary clinician and clinical consultants, are the problem list and the progress notes.

  2. Data sources for revision. From nursing notes, laboratory reports, vital signs recordings, and many other observations that indicate patient progress, the clinician must cull, synthesize, and record the important changes or significant stabilizations.

III. FORMAT FOR RECORDING THE HISTORY AND PHYSICAL EXAMINATION*

A. Recording the medical history

  1. Identifying data. This introduction to the written history includes the name, age, and sex of the patient and any demographic data that are pertinent to an accurate interpretation of the history to follow; for example, "Mr. John Jones is a 36-year-old white, male, steelworker who presents with. . . ."

  2. Chief complaint (CC). The CC is a direct quote or close paraphrase of the reason the patient states for the current presentation. Mr. Jones' CC might be recorded as: "I have been coughing and wheezing for 3 months."

  3. History of the present illness (HPI). The HPI is a narrative record of the development of the CC and any other ongoing problems that currently affect the patient. Mr. Jones' HPI might include the following:

    a. Derived from the presenting complaint. Problem 1: Cough and wheeze. A chronologic description of the course of the two related symptoms follows, each including the seven parameters (see Chapter 3). Any positive information from the pulmonary and cardiovascular review of systems, such as pertinent negatives and relevant general symptoms, environmental considerations, and allergy history are recorded here.

---

*For clarification of acceptable abbreviations in the problem-oriented record, see Appendix. For details of acquisition, see Chapters 3 and 6.

b. Derived from the history of concurrent disease. Problem 2: Any concurrent illness for which the patient is being treated or which must be considered in the assessment of the presenting complaint (problem 1) is recorded.

4. **Past medical history (PMH).** This may be recorded in tabular form and includes:
   a. **Surgical history:** Procedures, dates, and sequelae
   b. **Hospitalizations:** Reasons and dates
   c. **Major trauma:** Types of injury, dates, and sequelae
   d. **Childhood illnesses.** Routine (e.g., chickenpox) and unusual (e.g., rheumatic fever), which could have long-term implications
   e. **Immunization record and update,** especially the need for boosters
   f. **Allergies.** Environmental allergies with the source of symptoms as well as any history of untoward reactions to medications with designation of the medication and the symptoms interpreted as allergy are recorded; for example, "Mr. Jones had a reaction to penicillin, including swelling of lips and tongue with wheezing, requiring injection for control."
   g. **Major past illnesses.** Any illness that required long-term care or resulted in chronic therapy or disability with implications for the present or future should be recorded here. For example, "Radiation therapy for stage I Hodgkin's disease of the mediastinum 10 years ago; last follow-up chest film 1 year ago showed no recurrence."

5. **Patient profile (PP)** should include, but not necessarily be limited to, the following items:
   a. Living situation
   b. Occupational history
   c. Educational and financial status
   d. Support network
   e. Health habits, such as diet, exercise, and recreation
   f. Substance use, including alcohol, tobacco, and chemicals
   g. Life-style (e.g., "What do you do with your free time?")
   h. Patient concerns about the impact of current medical problems

6. **Family history (FH)**
   a. This includes a family tree of **medical problems,** including **ages** and **causes of death** of (at least) **one generation preceding proband, siblings of proband,** and **offspring,** if any. This information may be recorded as illustrated in Figure 11-1.
   b. The FH also contains an overview of such illnesses as heart disease, cancer, stroke, hypertension, and diabetes. Other familial diseases are also recorded here or, if indicated, in the HPI.

7. **Review of systems (ROS).** This section is conventionally recorded by system in the same manner in which it is acquired (see Chapter 3). For the student, it is important to record the specific symptoms pursued; as the student becomes more experienced, it will be sufficient to indicate a "negative" or "no symptoms elicited" under each system category.

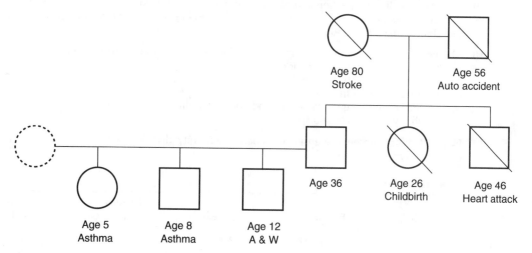

Figure 11-1. A genogram (family medical history).

B. Physical examination. The physical examination record is comprised of objective observations made by the examiner. This is a tabular recording and is abbreviated by standard designations (see Appendix). There is a variety of acceptable ways to organize the record of the physical examination, but each should include the following:

1. **Primary description and general appearance** provide the reader with a general picture of the patient, including **stance, demeanor, level of consciousness, levels of personal care and dress** (as indicators of physical or mental well-being), **unusual mannerisms,** or **evidence of discomfort or disability** on initial observation. A primary description of Mr. Jones might read: "Mr. Jones is a well-nourished, neatly dressed man who appears his stated age. He is in moderate respiratory distress and appears very anxious."

2. **Vital signs.** Four observations are recorded in tabular form and are as extensive as the problem requires. Mr. Jones' vital signs might be cited as follows:
   a. **Temperature:** 98° F by mouth
   b. **Pulse rate:** 120 and regular
   c. **Respiratory rate:** 32 and moderately labored
   d. **Blood pressure:** 140/88 both arms sitting; no pulsus paradoxus

3. **Skin.** This includes a description of **texture, turgor,** and **color** and is supplemented with any notable **lesions** anywhere on the surface of the body.

4. **Head and neck.** By convention, this segment includes a description of the **cranium, eyes, ears, nose, throat,** and **mouth,** and the **structures of the neck,** such as the trachea and thyroid gland.

5. **Lymphatics.** Unless it is noted with each region of the body, adenopathy is recorded and described here. If none is present, the examiner may simply state: "No adenopathy appreciated."

6. **Chest and lungs.** The structure of the chest wall and the findings on palpation, auscultation, and percussion of the anterior and posterior chest are described systematically.

7. **Cardiovascular.** Findings on auscultation and palpation of the heart are described. Mr. Jones' examination might read: "PMI located in the fifth intercostal space, 3 cm to the left of the left sternal border. No heaves or thrills felt. Rate 120; rhythm regular. S1 normal throughout. S2 increased in the 2nd left intercostal space. No S3 nor S4 heard. No murmurs, clicks, or rubs appreciated."

8. **Peripheral vascular.** A recommended format for quick reader assessment is shown in Table 11-1.
   a. **Pulses,** including carotid, femoral, and distal upper and lower extremity pulses are noted, especially for **symmetry.**
   b. The presence or absence of a **bruit** is recorded for the larger vessels (e.g., carotids and femorals).

9. **Breast and axillae.** Inspection and palpation of the breast and axillary nodes are recorded in this section, including the presence or absence of **dimpling, asymmetry, masses, pain, nipple secretion,** or **palpable nodes**.

10. **Abdomen.** The results of inspection, auscultation, and palpation are recorded here.
    a. Presence of abdominal scars or herniations
    b. Characteristics of bowel sounds; bruits (if heard)
    c. Percussion span of the liver
    d. Presence or absence of masses or tenderness, guarding, or rebound
    e. Palpability of the liver and spleen

11. **Extremities.** The presence or absence of edema, deformity, discoloration or other abnormality of any extremity is noted and described.

Table 11-1. Format for Recording Pulses

	Radial	Femoral	Popliteal	Dorsalis Pedis	Posterior Tibial
Right	4+*	4+	3+	4+	4+
Left	4+	4+	3+	4+	4+

*4+ = normal.

12. **Joints and back. Swelling, heat, redness,** or **tenderness** of any joint is described. The **range of motion (ROM)** of each of the major joints, including the spine, are recorded. If all joints move freely, it is appropriate to simply state: "ROM of all joints within normal limits."

13. **Neurologic examination.** This examination is divided into the following:
    a. **Cranial nerves.** If all were tested and normal, it is appropriate to record: "CN I (or II) through CN XII—normal." If there is an abnormality of one or more cranial nerves, the nerve and the abnormality are indicated: "CN VII—left lower facial droop; upper division intact."
    b. **Motor.** This includes **muscle strength** and **deep tendon reflexes,** which are most efficiently recorded as shown in Table 11-2 and Figure 11-2.
    c. **Sensory.** Depending upon the situation, this may include **proprioception** of peripheral joints, **vibratory sense** at peripheral joints, and discrimination of light touch and pain. If all sensory modalities are normal, the examination is recorded as "Sensory—within normal limits."
    d. **Cerebellum.** The screening functions for the cerebellum are usually the **Romberg position** ("held normally" or "falls to right side") and rapid and accurate repetitive movements of the upper and lower extremities, such as finger-to-nose and heel-to-shin.
    e. **Gait and station.** The patient's ability to walk normally or any deviation from normal in gait or stance are recorded.
    f. **Mental status.** At a minimum, the orientation in three spheres (person, time, and place) are noted and recorded as: "Oriented × 3" or "Oriented as to person and place but states date as 1882." For elicitation and recording of a more detailed neurologic examination than that deemed essential for screening, see Chapter 7 V.

14. **Male genital and rectal examinations.** Examination of the following are recorded:
    a. Penis, including foreskin and meatus
    b. Each testicle, epididymis, and cord structures
    c. Presence or absence of varicocele or hydrocele
    d. Rectal sphincter tone
    e. Prostate size, shape, and consistency
    f. Presence or absence of rectal masses
    g. Result of stool guaiac examination

15. **Female pelvic and rectal examinations.** All structures are described in detail. See Chapter 7 III for details of the observations to be made from this part of the examination.

Table 11-2. Format for Recording Reflexes

		Deep Tendon Reflexes				Superficial Reflexes	
	Triceps	Biceps	Brachio-radialis	Patellar	Ankle	Abdominal	Plantar
Right	2+*	3+	3+	2+	1+	2+/2+	↓
Left	2+	3+	3+	2+	1+ .	2+/2+	↓

*2+−3+ = normal.

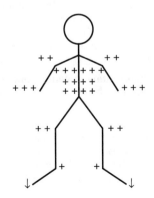

Figure 11-2. Stick figure shows an alternate method of recording reflexes.

IV. WRITING PATIENT PROGRESS NOTES

A. Definition of the SOAP format. The **progress note** is the element in the patient's record that allows the members of the health care team to communicate progress made toward resolution of each of the patient's problems. The progress note is recorded by problem, thus minimizing confusion, redundancy, and omission. It is the hourly or daily record of change.
S— Change in the patient's subjective complaints
O—Change in the objective data
A—Change in the assessment of the problem
P— Change in the management plan

B. Components of the SOAP format

1. **Subjective change.** This segment represents information obtained by querying the patient. How does the patient feel? Have there been any changes in symptoms or have new symptoms appeared? How is the patient dealing with the problem?

2. **Objective change.** Under this heading are the objective data, including vital signs and other physical findings relevant to the problem; new laboratory information; and observations by nurses or other caretakers.

3. **Assessment.** This section represents the impact of the foregoing information on the understanding of the problem under consideration. Is the condition worse? Better? Stable? Does it need to be redefined? Has it reached resolution?

4. **Plans** are divided into diagnostic, therapeutic, and patient education (see Chapter 10 II A).
   a. **No plan.** If there is no current plan or no change in the current plan, this is stated.
   b. **Action of plan deferred.** If the problem under consideration warrants no further diagnostic, therapeutic, or educational action now because it is overshadowed in importance by another problem, the fact that the action is deferred is indicated.
   c. **Change in plan.** If a new plan is to replace a former plan, the specific changes to be made are indicated. If recorded carefully, the update in thinking and acting on the problem is readily apparent to all individuals involved in the care of the patient or in the management of the particular problem.

C. Problems for SOAP. Not every problem needs to be explored in detail each time a progress note is written. Only problems that are dynamic or that are to be relegated to the resolved or deferred category are included. Any problem in which a change in any of the four elements has occurred needs to be updated. An example of SOAP used to revise and update a basic problem is shown in Figure 11-3.

V. WRITING MEDICAL ORDERS

A. General principles

1. **Legibility** is a very serious matter. Serious errors have resulted from illegible handwriting. For example, 5-fluorocytosine, an antifungal agent, is often abbreviated 5-FC; in one instance, illegible handwriting was read as 5-FU, an abbreviation for 5-fluorouracil, a cancer chemotherapy agent. The leukopenia that resulted from the administration of the wrong drug enhanced the growth of the fungus, and the patient died. Perhaps future technology will provide instantaneous and accurate transcriptions of the spoken word, but at present, most medical notes and orders are handwritten.

2. **Accuracy** is critical in communicating in general and in writing orders in particular. For example, "Do not draw blood from the left arm" is significantly different from "Do not draw blood from the right arm."

3. **Completeness**
   a. **Legal liability** assumes that what is recorded in the chart accurately reflects totality. There is a presumption that if it is not written down, it did not happen.
   b. **Precision.** The law, the public, and the profession demand that the clinician have the knowledge base and the data base to write orders that are explicit and clear.

Figure 11-3.

Progress Notes

A patient was admitted from the emergency room 24 hours ago with chest pain of uncertain origin. His primary problem list included: chest pain, cough, fever, and skin rash. Twenty-four hours of workup and observation have ensued. The team has just seen the patient and reviewed laboratory data available since last evening. The following **progress note** is generated as a result of this visit:

3/12/90

Problem 1: Chest pain
   S: Pain unchanged; still most severe with deep breathing and cough.
   O: Chest x-ray this A.M. reveals a new infiltrate in the area of the right middle lobe; otherwise unchanged. On auscultation, fine rales now audible in the right axilla with egophony over the same region.
   A: Suspect right middle lobe pneumonia.
   P: Diagnostic—Repeat sputum smear this A.M.
      Therapeutic—Defer until after smear repeated.
      Education—Patient informed of chest x-ray findings; spouse to be called this A.M.

Problem 2: Cough
   S: Cough worse; now raising thick green sputum; no blood seen.
   O: Lung findings as noted under problem 1.
   A: Suspect this symptom is directly related to the chest pain and represents right middle lobe pneumonia.
   P: Repeat sputum smear now; culture pending.

Problem 3: Fever
   S: Patient noted shaking chill and profuse diaphoresis during the night.
   O: Temperature spiked to 104° F at 2:00 A.M.; was 99° F at 6:00 A.M.; had acetaminophen at 3:00 A.M.
   A: Spiking fever likely secondary to pneumonia.
   P: As under problems 1 and 2.

Problem 4: Skin rash
   S: Patient reports that he climbed through the rough on the golf course 7 days ago, where he was told there was poison ivy. He knows himself to be highly allergic to ivy. The rash appeared 5 days ago.
   O: Increased number of blisters on both forearms and hands. Clearly linear. No new erythematous bases noted.
   A: Rash is not likely to be related to febrile illness and may be poison ivy.
   P: Diagnostic—Dermatology consult requested.
      Therapeutic—Pending dermatology consult.

Two days later, after confirmation of pneumococcal pneumonia and institution of appropriate antibiotic therapy, the following progress notes are made after the morning visit with the patient. Note that problems 2 and 3 have been subsumed under problem 1 and that problem 1 has been renamed to indicate the more refined understanding of the admitting problems.

3/14/90

Problem 1: Pneumococcal pneumonia, right middle lobe (problems 2 and 3 have been subsumed)
   S: "Feeling human again!" Only occasional twinge of chest pain. Still a lot of sputum, but it is becoming yellow in color.
   O: Afebrile for past 18 hours. Chest examine unchanged from yesterday.
   A: Pneumococcal pneumonia, apparently responding to intravenous penicillin therapy.
   P: Diagnostic—Repeat chest x-ray today; repeat white blood cell count in A.M.
      Therapeutic—If still improving this evening, plan shift to oral penicillin unless chest film reveals extension.
      Education—Patient and patient's wife informed of progress and probability of discharge in 24–48 hours.

Problem 4: Poison ivy dermatitis
   S: "Doesn't seem to be spreading any more and the new medication has helped the itching a lot."
   O: No new vesicles; some crusting on hands but no evidence of secondary infection.
   A: Poison ivy dermatitis, resolving.
   P: Continue local steroid cream three times a day. Will be seen by dermatologist again today.

B. Admission orders are written in the chart at the time a patient enters the hospital. In many teaching hospitals, orders are written only by housestaff (or by students with co-signature by housestaff). This reflects an educational philosophy that links authority to responsibility.

1. **"Done" orders** are written to create a record of when an act has been implemented; for example, "Draw two blood cultures. Done by HO" followed by the signature of the HO (see Appendix for common abbreviations).

2. **"Stat" and "now" orders** remove the relative discretion available to the nurse or other staff about when to carry out medical orders. They require immediate fulfillment, which takes a toll on busy professionals.
   a. The clinician should think twice before writing a "stat" order. For example, "Please draw blood for potassium level next draw" may result in equal speed and less disruption, particularly if the next routine blood-drawing is just 1 hour away.
   b. If a task must be done immediately, the clinician is best advised to carry it out personally rather than asking someone else.
   c. It is always wise to point out a stat order in person after writing it and to notify any person implicated (e.g., a radiology technician who is being asked to take an x-ray immediately).

3. A template for creating orders is shown in Table 11-3.

4. A sample set of admission orders is shown in Table 11-4. Components of admission orders follow:
   a. **Admit to hospital** is always the first order; it should specify the geographic site, the service, and the names of the attending and resident clinicians.
   b. **Admitting diagnoses** in the orders can be multiple.
      (1) They should reflect the clinician's working hypotheses at the time they are written. Thus, they can be explicitly tentative (e.g., "Rule out myocardial infarction").
      (2) They should not be so numerous or comprehensive as to repeat the problem list.
   c. **Condition** gives the first clear notion of the degree of urgency and expected outcome.
      (1) Choices include "critical," "moribund," "stable," and so on.
      (2) When the order "Do not resuscitate" (DNR) is written upon admission, based upon full and proper indications, it should also contain detailed information about interventions that are permissible.

Table 11-3. Template for Medical Service Orders

Date _____   Time _____

 1. Admit to:
 2. Diagnosis:
 3. Condition:
 4. Activity:
 5. Allergies:
 6. Diet:
 7. Vital signs:
 8. Other nursing measurements:
 9. Laboratory work (check off, specify as needed):
    a. Urine
    b. Blood
    c. Cultures
    d. EKG
    e. ABG
    f. Radiograph(s)
10. Interventions (nursing):
11. Interventions (other services):
12. Oxygen and other respiratory assistance:
13. Intravenous fluids and additives:
14. Medications, other:
15. Thank you.

   Signed: _____

   Printed name: _____

   Telephone and/or beeper number: _____

Table 11-4. Sample Set of Admission Orders

12-22-90   2300 hours

Resident clinician's admitting orders
1. Admit to: 7 North, to Dr. Schneiderman's service, Dr. Mankiewicz resident
2. Diagnoses: AIDS, *Pneumocystis carinii* pneumonia, and dehydration
3. Condition: Critical
4. Activity: Bed to chair until specified otherwise; please provide bedside commode.
5. **Allergy: penicillin;** please so label chart.
6. Diet: Regular; family and friends may bring food from home as well.
7. Vital signs: q4h WA and at least once qs; call HO for T > 103 or < 97, P > 125, RR > 30, SBP < 85. Please repeat P and BP if tolerated with patient seated qs.
8. Please measure I & O and record; weight q3d before breakfast
9. Urinalysis and culture with first voiding
10. Bloodwork (**done**); CBC with differential and platelet count; electrolytes, BUN, calcium, and creatinine
11. Blood cultures × 3 (**done**); please send any sputum produced for routine, fungal, and mycobacteria cultures.
12. Blood for K, BUN in A.M.
13. ABGs on room air (**done**)
14. CXR (**done**); Dx: AIDS, PCP
15. EKG (**done**); Dx: HIV; no clinical heart disease
16. Oxygen by nasal cannula, 4 L/min
17. Respiratory therapy to perform suctioning up to q1h WA PRN congestion
18. Co-trimoxazole, 160/800 mg IVPB q4h × 21 days
19. Multivitamins, 1 PO qd × 30 days
20. Zidovudine, 200 mg PO q4h × 14 days
21. D5NS, 250 cc/hr IV × 8 hours, then 75 cc/hr × 24 hr
22. Thank you.

Signed: _____

Printed name: _____Lynn Mankiewicz, M.D._____

Telephone and/or beeper number ____238-5876/4022____

---

    d. Activity ranges from complete bed rest to ambulation at will and without assistance.

    e. Allergies and any special **precautions** should be marked prominently. The order should stipulate measures intended to keep all personnel aware.

        (1) Reverse isolation (i.e., staff take extra measures to avoid infecting the patient with common flora) is sometimes used for patients who are neutropenic.

        (2) Standard isolation to protect staff and other patients from a contagious patient has become restricted to a few well-defined infectious diseases now that **Universal Precautions** in handling blood and body fluids have been mandated by law and widely implemented.

    f. Diet and any special nutritional consultations, requirements, or exclusions follow:

        (1) Restrictions of sodium, fat, protein, calories, fluid intake, or other parameters may be ordered in relation to medical needs.

        (2) Religious requirements may also be stipulated here (e.g., no pork products for devout Jews and Muslims).

        (3) Supplementation of any kind may be ordered here.

        (4) If there is no reason to add or subtract anything, the "default" setting is: "Diet: regular."

    g. Vital signs. Measurements of **pulse, blood pressure, respiratory rate,** and **body temperature** may be ordered to be taken as often as needed.

        (1) The **"while awake" restriction** is a mercy to patients. (Clinicians may also restrict other interventions, including procedures and some medicines, in the same way and for the same reasons.)

        (2) If only pulse and blood pressure tests are needed often, they should be ordered separately so that nurses do not take unnecessary temperature measurements as well.

        (3) The clinician can specify "Orthostatic measurements," "No rectal temperatures," or whatever else matches the needs for data and patient comfort.

   h. Nursing measurements of other types might include:
     (1) Measuring intake and output
     (2) Serial body weights
     (3) Urine specific gravity
     (4) Stool for occult blood
   i. Laboratory work can be voluminous, so it is useful to subdivide it.
     (1) Urinalysis is almost always ordered on admission. Urine can also be collected for drug levels, creatinine clearance, total protein over a 24-hour period, or specific endocrine studies.
     (2) Blood studies commonly include a complete blood count with differential white cell count and platelet count, electrolytes, blood urea nitrogen (BUN), glucose, and creatinine. Blood tests can also be ordered here.
     (3) Culture requests are specified by site and frequency if infection is in the differential diagnosis.
     (4) Electrocardiogram (EKG) is commonly ordered if there is consideration of heart disease, either past or current. Because an interpretation is part of this test, diagnostic information must be included at the time of ordering so that the interpreting clinician has a context within which to make sense of the findings.
     (5) Arterial blood gases (ABGs) have been separated from other blood work because the sample on which they are measured is collected in a different manner. They represent an overused test.
     (6) Imaging can include the routine PA and lateral chest radiograph, other plain films, ultrasound examinations of the heart (often called echocardiograms), computerized tomography (CT), magnetic resonance imaging (MRI), angiography, and newer modalities. As with the EKG, diagnostic information is required and should be specified on the order.
   j. Interventions by nursing staff include turning bed-bound patients; care of stomas, urethral catheters, and feeding tubes; wound care; and an array of other tasks.
     (1) Openness to nurses' suggestions about what the patient requires is a mark of wisdom in clinicians.
     (2) The clinician may ask to be called in certain situations (e.g., new or high fever).
     (3) Explicitness is particularly helpful when staffing is lowest (i.e., graveyard shift) or when manifestations of trouble are atypical.
   k. Interventions by other services
     (1) Requests for help from other services, such as respiratory therapy, physical therapy, and social service, require a consultation slip, which provides information about the patient and the goals of the consult.
     (2) Consultation from another discipline (e.g., orthopedics, radiotherapy, psychiatry, or pulmonary medicine) is formally requested here.
   l. Medication orders. The clinician can start with oxygen, followed by intravenous fluids and additives, which should be stipulated in considerable detail, including rapidity of administration. Nurses can correct oversights, but the clinician should give the nurses full details to ensure optimal patient care. Medication orders must include:
     (1) Name of the drug
     (2) Route of administration
     (3) Doses
     (4) Frequency
     (5) Duration
   m. Other medicines are then specified, including:
     (1) Chronic medications used prior to admission
     (2) Pain medicines
     (3) Antibiotics
     (4) Cardiovascular medicines
     (5) Antihypertensives
     (6) Urgent choices, such as thiamine in an alcoholic
     (7) Vitamin and hormonal supplements
   n. A statement of thanks to the nursing staff is indispensable.

5. Holding orders are written to cover a temporary situation. Most commonly, they pertain to a **patient who is not critically ill**.
   a. After a very brief assessment, the clinician orders:
     (1) Continuation of baseline medicines

(2) A diet (no meal will be served unless such an order is extant)
(3) Routine measurements of vital signs
(4) Initiation of laboratory studies

b. Holding orders are carried out during the few minutes to few hours during which the clinician must attend to more urgent cases before interviewing and examining the patient fully.

c. They must be reviewed and revised appropriately after a more complete assessment has occurred.

C. Medication orders have a number of additional special features.

1. Chronic medications should never be continued blindly. Renewal orders, or retranscription at the time of admission, offer opportunities to delete excess, unnecessary, or inappropriate choices.

2. Time-limited medication doses and courses are often most desirable.

   a. Pain medication, for example, must be rewritten frequently if the indication is dynamic (e.g., postoperative wound pain).

   b. Failure to stipulate time limits on medication orders is a major cause of inappropriate polypharmacy.

3. Analgesic orders, which are often written as "PRN" ("as needed"), should actually be written as "unless refused."

   a. Patients often have to ask for medicine ordered in this way, and nurses often have to refuse requests if the appropriate interval has not passed. Such interactions promote both inadequate pain control and drug-dependency behavior. The order should not be written PRN but as "unless refused." This puts the onus on the system, not the patient.

   b. If the pain is truly devastating, the clinician may specify "ATC" ("around the clock"), which alerts the staff to awaken patients for doses rather than to let them be awakened by excruciating pain.

4. Routine orders are sometimes written, or even printed, for bowel medication, minor pain medication, and sedative-hypnotic medication (i.e., sleeping pills).

   a. Sometimes clinicians merely check off items on preprinted forms and then sign. This is very convenient and saves time.

   b. Forms specifying advances in diet and activity postoperatively can also save time.

   c. The danger of these preprinted forms is in not considering individual needs related to each order every time. For instance, a routine sedative-hypnotic may produce fatal respiratory depression in a patient with advanced emphysema.

D. Renewal of home medications and treatments calls for the same skepticism and personal certainty as continuation of another clinician's orders.

1. Sources of error include mistakes of omission and commission by the patient, in addition to mistranscriptions and a host of others. The best strategy is to require that the medicine chest be emptied into a large plastic bag for personal inspection by the clinician. This allows discontinued and outdated products to be discarded, prescription items to be verified, and nonprescription or nonstandard treatments to be identified.

2. Opportunities for re-evaluation or investigation include the "medicine cabinet biopsy" described above and telephone calls to other providers and pharmacies. These steps are most important, unfortunately, when most difficult: the multiproblem patient with many health care providers (e.g., several specialists) and the patient with multiple medications.

3. Polypharmacy raises the question of **drug interaction**. In some institutions, the hospital pharmacy may automatically check for drug interactions. The simplest means of fulfilling this duty is to consider both the problem list and the medication list against a compilation of interactions.

VI. MEDICAL RECORD AS A LEGAL DOCUMENT.

The written medical record serves an important legal purpose in documenting the physician-patient relationship. Traditionally, the medical community conformed to general guidelines created by its own societies. Recent court rulings and legislation have resulted in more stringent regulations about the **content, confidentiality,** and **accessibility** of medical records.

A. Content issues

1. Medical records are mandated to be in a legible **written format**. These may be handwritten, typed, or computer-generated.

2. The records should be as **complete** and **accurate** a representation of the physician-patient relationship as possible. Completeness is essential for patient care, transfer of information to other health professionals, and in litigation (see VI D).

3. All entries must be **dated,** preferably **timed,** and signed (legibly).
   a. **The signature** should include at least a first initial and a full last name.
   b. **The title** of the health professional must be included (e.g., medical student, M.D., or R.N.).

4. **Medical orders** written or transcribed by a medical student, nurse, or other nonclinician must be **countersigned** by a clinician within 24 hours.

5. **Mistakes** in documentation **cannot be deleted** from the permanent record or **destroyed**.
   a. A single line can be drawn through the inaccurate information with the word "error" written above it. This correction should be signed.
   b. The original data should remain legible after the correction.
   c. Additional information cannot be added to this portion of the chart at a later period, unless the new information is dated, timed, and signed.

6. **Retention of medical records**
   a. Various state and local guidelines explicitly direct that records be kept for a **minimum of 5–10 years**.
   b. It is recommended that records be retained **indefinitely**.

B. Access to information

1. The medical record is considered a **confidential document**. This includes all medical, social, economic, and other data obtained during the physician-patient interaction.

2. The medical record is **"owned" by the clinician** or **hospital** generating the document.

3. **Patients have full access to their medical records** with few exceptions (see VI B 4).

4. **Release of information** must follow explicit legal guidelines.
   a. **Authorized representatives of the patient,** such as a lawyer or a family member, may request the patient's medical record.
   b. **Written permission from the patient** is required for a "release of information." The form must include the:
      (1) Patient's signature and date
      (2) Nature of the information to be released
      (3) Party to whom the information is to be released

5. Medical records can also be released under the following circumstances **without written permission:**
   a. To other health professionals actively involved with the patient's care
   b. In true medical emergencies
   c. For legitimate research purposes under the guidelines of appropriate review boards
   d. When requested by a court order or subpoena
   e. For quality assurance or authorized peer review

6. **Confidentiality** can be broken and appropriate third parties informed in certain clinical situations.
   a. In cases of suspected or proven **child abuse,** the clinician or hospital is legally bound to notify the responsible agencies, such as the municipal departments of youth services.
   b. Many **infectious diseases** (e.g., syphilis, gonorrhea, acquired immune deficiency syndrome [AIDS], and tuberculosis) must be reported to state health departments.

C. Informed consent. Essentially all surgical procedures and many other invasive diagnostic tests require informed consent from the patient.

1. **State and local guidelines** dictate which procedures require prior consent. The patient must be "informed" prior to the procedure.
   a. The patient must be told the purpose and the proposed outcome of the procedure.
   b. Side effects and potential unfavorable outcomes must be described.
   c. Options must be discussed, such as the consequences of not having the procedure or alternative testing available.

2. **The patient's consent** must be in **written format** with the **signatures of the patient,** the **individual performing the test,** and a **witness.** Standardized forms are usually employed.

D. Special legal considerations

1. **Medical malpractice** suits highlight the legal aspects of the medical record.
   a. The patient's lawyer has the right to review all records prior to bringing in a suit.
   b. Obviously, the accuracy of the record is paramount. Corrections or deletions raise the question of veracity.
   c. The health care provider's best defense is considered to be a thorough legible record that documents all discussions and interventions.

2. **Regulatory guidelines.** Federal, state, and local guidelines regulate the confidentiality and distribution in many clinical situations. These include:
   a. Drug and alcohol history
   b. Psychiatric history
   c. Accident or injury information
   d. Information regarding minors

3. **Computer-generated medical records** are becoming commoner and particularly problematic.
   a. Unauthorized access to computerized records is potentially more likely than access to written records. Great care must be given to authenticate the people seeking access to records.
   b. Tampering with and editing past records is also a potential problem.

E. Sensitive medical–legal issues

1. **Living wills**
   a. Various states have adopted living will legislation. These wills allow patients to decide the level of medical intervention provided to them should an untoward event occur.
   b. The living will can become part of the permanent medical record. The patient is free to change or remove this will at any time.
   c. While controversial and not universally accepted, living wills reflect an increased emphasis on the patient's wishes in determining medical care.

2. **DNR orders**
   a. Similar in intent to living wills, DNR orders limit potential or ongoing medical care to patients, depending upon their desires or underlying medical condition.
   b. To be implemented, the patient (if competent), appropriate family member, or conservator must give consent.
   c. State or institutional guidelines for DNR orders are developed by multidisciplinary committees usually comprised of clinicians, lawyers, philosophers, ethicists, clergy, and lay individuals.

3. **HIV testing and AIDS**
   a. The most controversial medical issues facing current health care providers are testing for the human immunodeficiency virus (HIV) and caring for patients with AIDS.
   b. Judiciary and legislative actions have controlled the reporting and confidentiality of this disorder.
   c. The medical and legal communities are balancing a need to protect public health with individual rights of privacy.
   d. As of this writing, there are no federal laws concerning the confidentiality of HIV testing and access to the medical records of HIV-positive individuals or AIDS patients. Readers are directed to their state and local regulatory bodies.

VII. ORAL CASE PRESENTATION

A. **Mastery of the oral case presentation.** Learning the skills necessary to present a case completely yet succinctly is a source of anxiety among medical students early in their clinical experience. Because there has typically been a lack of formal instruction in this essential skill, most medical students struggle to develop their own methods by listening to others and modeling their presentations after those given by senior colleagues. Once the framework that underlies the oral case presentation is mastered, the student should be able to present a clinical case effectively.

B. Value of the oral case presentation. The oral case presentation is a valuable method of communicating with colleagues about patients.

1. Medical professionals can infer organization in the array of facts with which they are presented if they are familiar with the structure of the case presentation.

2. A good case presentation describes recent events in the context of the patient's entire illness.

C. Principles of the oral case presentation

1. **Goals**
   a. **Completeness.** All relevant details of the case should be mentioned; this includes pertinent negatives as well as positive findings.
   b. **Brevity.** The presentation should be a rapidly moving summary of the case; facts should be stated succinctly.

2. **Duration.** The entire presentation must be structured with an awareness of time limitations. Since the average person is capable of attentive listening for approximately 7 minutes, oral presentations should not exceed 7 minutes in length.

3. **Level of detail.** The oral presentation should not be a recitation of the written hospital record, which is the repository for every detail of the patient's history and illness. The individual presenting the case should be aware of the details contained in the chart and be capable of commenting on these details if questioned but need not include everything in the rapidly moving summary.

4. **Classification of information within the oral presentation.** Information should be organized by its relevance to the primary problem rather than in the order in which it was obtained during the patient encounter; for example, a patient presenting with shortness of breath also has leg pain and swelling. Although the latter information was obtained during the ROS, it may be quite relevant to the present illness if deep venous thrombosis with pulmonary embolus is suspected as a cause of the patient's shortness of breath. For this reason, the student should present it as part of the HPI.

D. Format for the case presentation

1. **Opening remarks**
   a. It is essential to provide as much descriptive information as possible in the first sentence of the presentation so the listener will immediately have an impression of the patient. In one sentence, the student should describe the patient with respect to age, race, gender, relevant concurrent medical conditions, reason for presentation or hospitalization, and duration of the problem.
   b. Although the patient's CC is important and could be included in the written record, the opening remarks should help the listener to focus on the patient's main problems from the perspective of the medical profession; for example, a patient who states that she sought medical care because she "felt under the weather" might be described as "A 59-year-old white woman with a history of congestive heart failure and chronic obstructive pulmonary disease who is admitted for increasing shortness of breath."

2. **HPI.** The events leading to the patient's hospitalization or office visit should be included here.
   a. **Baseline health.** It is helpful to state what the patient's baseline is and when the patient began to deviate from that baseline; for example, "The patient was in good health until . . .," or "The patient was in her usual compromised health until . . . ."
   b. **Change in a chronic disease.** If this is an exacerbation of a chronic illness, the student should briefly describe the course of the chronic illness, the patient's level of functioning, and then describe more fully the events surrounding this episode.
   c. **Single problem HPI.** It is clear that if the patient has only one problem, the student will report events in the order in which they occurred.
   d. **Multiple active problems.** A difficulty arises when the patient has more than one active medical problem. In the case of multiple medical problems, the student must choose between the chronologic and the problem-oriented approaches.
      (1) **Chronologic approach**
         (a) **Features.** The sequence of events is reported in the order in which the events occurred.
         (b) **Advantages.** This approach leaves the listener with a strong sense of the time course of an illness.

      (c) **Disadvantages.** In patients with multiple medical problems, events relating to two or three different illnesses may be interspersed, leading to a disorganized and confusing narrative.

      (d) **Recommendations for use.** This approach is more useful in patients with few problems or in patients with numerous, closely related problems such that the timing of a single event may affect multiple problems.

   (2) **Problem-oriented approach**

      (a) **Features.** The problem-oriented presentation focuses on each of a patient's current problems separately. A chronologic sequence of events is then described for each problem.

      (b) **Advantages.** In the face of multiple problems, the problem-oriented presentation imposes some order for the listener and makes it easier for the listener to organize historic events.

      (c) **Disadvantages.** Often the time course is not as evident in the problem-oriented presentation as in a purely chronologic account. In addition, the problem-oriented approach can lead to a lengthy presentation if events are not summarized.

      (d) **Recommendations for use.** This approach is useful for patients with multiple problems and patients in whom it is unclear how numerous complaints are related.

3. **Other parts of the history.** PMH, FH, PP, and ROS are recited only to the extent that they contribute to the definition and management of the problems in the HPI.

4. **Physical examination.** The student should always begin a verbal report of the physical examination with vital signs and a general description of the patient's appearance. After this, the physical examination should be discussed only with respect to pertinent positives and negatives. Normal findings, which are not relevant to the patient's illness, may be dismissed by stating that examination of a particular organ system was "within normal limits," "unremarkable," or "benign."

5. **Laboratory values.** This category includes radiologic studies, EKG, ultrasound studies, and laboratory tests. By this time, most listeners will be entertaining a differential diagnosis, and the individual presenting the case should know which laboratory studies would be necessary to investigate each diagnosis. With this in mind, the student should report the pertinent normal and all abnormal laboratory data.

6. **Hospital course.** This is a brief summary of the major events that have transpired since the patient's admission. This includes **diagnostic studies** performed, **therapeutic modalities** initiated, the **patient's response** to therapy, and any **change in the patient's condition**.

7. **Summary.** A few sentences in length, the summary frames the patient's symptoms, physical signs, and laboratory abnormalities, and highlights the questions that the listener should address.

REFERENCES

Marks RM, Sachar EJ: Undertreatment of pain in medical inpatients with narcotic analgesics. *Ann Int Med* 78:173–181, 1973

Medical Letter: *The Medical Letter Handbook of Adverse Drug Interactions.* New Rochelle, NY, The Medical Letter, p 217, 1989

Seifer DB, Henry JB: The impact of technology on the clinical decision-making of house staff. *NY State J Med* 89:444–445, 1989

STUDY QUESTIONS

Directions: Each of the numbered items or incomplete statements in this section is followed by answers or by completions of the statement. Select the **one** lettered answer or completion that is **best** in each case.

1. A medical student is caring for an acutely ill patient in the hospital. After approval by her supervising clinician, she writes an order for a new medication. All the following statements about this process are true EXCEPT the

(A) supervising clinician must cosign the order within 24 hours
(B) order should be legible and written in ink
(C) medical student's first initial, last name, and title must be present
(D) entry into the chart should be dated and timed
(E) medical student's name, but not a signature, should be present

2. When medication requests are written on a patient's order sheet, the directions should routinely specify all of the following EXCEPT

(A) who is to administer the drug
(B) the dosage of the drug
(C) the route of administration
(D) the frequency of administration
(E) the name of the drug

3. When writing initial orders for analgesics, the most important consideration is the

(A) duration the medication is to be given
(B) addictive potential of the medication
(C) "placebo" potential of the medication
(D) pain control capability of the medication
(E) route of administration of the medication

4. Legally acceptable steps to correct a mistake in a medical record include all of the following EXCEPT

(A) obliteration of incorrect data
(B) the word "error" written above the incorrect data
(C) a single line drawn through the incorrect entry
(D) a signature at the place of correction
(E) a date at the place of correction

5. A 21-year-old male college student is seen and treated in a medical clinic. All of the following individuals or groups have a legal right to review the medical record of this encounter without the patient's permission EXCEPT

(A) a clinician seeing the patient in the same clinic 1 week later
(B) an emergency room clinician seeing the patient when he is brought in comatose after an automobile accident
(C) the patient's mother
(D) the medical clinic's quality assurance audit committee
(E) a clinician doing clinical research approved by the institution's human experimentation committee

6. Proper informed consent for a surgical procedure contemplated on a competent adult demands all of the following EXCEPT

(A) a written format
(B) the signature of the individual performing the procedure
(C) the signature of the patient
(D) the signature of the patient's next of kin
(E) the signature of a witness

7. The most important reason for limiting an oral case presentation to about 7 minutes is

(A) most clinical cases can be summarized in this length of time
(B) every student must learn to be succinct
(C) clinicians do not have the time for longer presentations
(D) the ability to concentrate on oral data is less efficient after 7 minutes
(E) Osler demanded that oral presentations be limited in this way

Directions: Each group of items in this section consists of lettered options followed by a set of numbered items. For each item, select the **one** lettered option that is most closely associated with it. Each lettered option may be selected once, more than once, or not at all.

Questions 8–12

For each piece of information presented, select the division of the medical history under which it should be entered after the admission history is acquired.

(A) PP
(B) FH
(C) HPI
(D) PMH
(E) None of the above

8. History of diabetes mellitus in spouse's family
9. Lack of health insurance coverage
10. Recent onset of leg swelling
11. All immunizations completed and up-to-date
12. History of exertional chest pain for 2 years

Questions 13–17

For each of the physical findings listed below, select the physical examination heading under which it should be recorded.

(A) Abdominal examination
(B) Neurologic examination
(C) General appearance
(D) Vital signs
(E) None of the above

13. Absent deep tendon reflexes (both knees)
14. Cyanosis of lips and fingers
15. Temperature of 99° F
16. Right costovertebral angle tenderness
17. Absent bowel sounds

ANSWERS AND EXPLANATIONS

1. The answer is E. [*V A, B; VI A 3, 4*] All individuals writing medical orders should date and time the orders and sign the order with a legible signature, including the first initial, last name, and title. The order should be written in ink for permanency. The supervising clinician should cosign the order within 24 hours.

2. The answer is A. [*V B 4 I*] Medication orders have implicit directions as to who will administer them, depending upon the routine of the institution. Only if there is to be an exception to this routine, is the administrator of the drug included in the orders.

3. The answer is D. [*V C 3*] The critical decision to be made when choosing and ordering an analgesic is its ability to control pain. All other considerations are secondary. If a patient has sufficient pain to require medication, a placebo is inappropriate. Concerns about the addictive potential and duration of use of drugs for pain need not be *initial* concerns but may require consideration later. The route of administration is a function of the drug chosen rather than a primary consideration.

4. The answer is A. [*VI A 5*] Under no circumstances should a mistake be removed from a patient's medical record. The legally acceptable correction includes a line drawn through the information that is in error, so that the original entry is still legible. This correction is labeled "error" by a notation above it, then the correction is signed and dated by the individual making it.

5. The answer is C. [*VI B 4–6*] Access to the medical records of the patient described in the question by clinicians involved in his legitimate care either in a scheduled visit or in an emergency situation do not need the patient's prior approval. Audit committees have automatic access to medical records, and clinicians doing clinical research are subjected to the institution's standards in reviewing such charts. Since the patient is an adult, his mother has no legal right to review the chart without her son's permission.

6. The answer is D. [*VI C 2*] A signature of a family member is not required on the informed consent form when the individual upon whom a procedure is to be performed is both adult (adult as defined by the laws of the state in which the consent is being obtained) and competent (conscious and mentally intact). The patient's consent must be in written format with the signatures of the patient, the individual performing the procedure, and a witness.

7. The answer is D. [*VII C 2*] Although it is true that most clinical cases can be summarized in 7 minutes, that students must learn to be succinct, and that clinicians do not have the time for long presentations, the most important reason for compressing the case presentation to 7 minutes is that the attention of listeners wanders and the purpose of the presentation—that is, assistance with problem management—is defeated. William Osler, the great turn-of-the-century clinician, may or may not have demanded this particular time limitation on oral case presentations.

8–12. The answers are: 8-E, 9-A, 10-C, 11-D, 12-C. [*III A 1–6*] The FH is intended to reflect the genetic background of the proband (patient). Although serious illness in a spouse might reflect social problems (PP entries), his or her family medical history has no immediate bearing on the patient's medical record.

Any social, financial, or other non–illness-related problem belongs in the PP. Although no health insurance may have an impact on decisions about the present illness, it is recorded as part of the PP.

Any current problem, even if it appears initially to be unrelated to the CC, must be entered as a problem in the HPI.

The immunization status is fixed and requires no immediate action; therefore, it is relegated to the PMH. Alternatively, it might be recorded in the ROS, although convention dictates otherwise.

Regardless of the nature of the presenting complaint, any concurrent problem that may impact upon the patient's present condition must be included in the HPI. Since the genesis or the status of the chest pain is not known, it belongs in the HPI until it can be determined whether the chest pain is stable or irrelevant.

13–17. The answers are: 13-B, 14-C, 15-D, 16-E, 17-A. [*III B 1, 2, 3, 10–13*] Deep tendon reflexes, a test of the integrity of the spinal circuit, are considered part of the neurologic examination. Even though primary muscle disease can affect the efferent loop of the circuit, examination results are recorded as a standard part of the neurologic examination.

Visible cyanosis of the lips and extremities is such an intimate part of the general picture of the patient that most clinicians would insist that it be part of the initial impression. Some clinicians might argue for recording color changes of the skin in the section on skin, but placed here, it is less likely to indicate the urgency of the patient's problem to a reader of the chart.

By tradition, temperature is recorded as one of the four components of vital signs.

By tradition, right costovertebral angle tenderness is recorded as part of the back examination, or much less frequently, the examination of the chest. The importance of adhering to tradition, even when it may defy reason, is to allow quick and easy access to the information required by other caretakers.

Bowel sounds are just what they are labeled—the noise made by intestinal peristalsis. Recording the status of the bowel sounds is always under the auscultatory component of the abdominal examination.

Comprehensive
Exam

Introduction

One of the least attractive aspects of pursuing an education is the necessity of being examined on what has been learned. Instructors do not like to prepare tests, and students do not like to take them.

However, students are required to take many examinations during their learning careers, and little if any time is spent acquainting them with the positive aspects of tests and with systematic and successful methods for approaching them. Students perceive tests as punitive and sometimes feel that they are merely opportunities for the instructor to discover what the student has forgotten or has never learned. Students need to view tests as opportunities to display their knowledge and to use them as tools for developing prescriptions for further study and learning.

A brief history and discussion of the National Board of Medical Examiners (NBME) examinations are presented in this introduction, along with ideas concerning psychological preparation for the examinations. Also presented are general considerations and test-taking tips as well as how practice exams can be used as educational tools. (The literature provided by the various examination boards contains detailed information concerning the construction and scoring of specific exams.)

National Board of Medical Examiners Examinations

Before the various NBME exams were developed, each state attempted to license physicians through its own procedures. Differences between the quality and testing procedures of the various state examinations resulted in the refusal of some states to recognize the licensure of physicians licensed in other states. This made it difficult for physicians to move freely from one state to another and produced an uneven quality of medical care in the United States.

To remedy this situation, the various state medical boards decided they would be better served if an outside agency prepared standard exams to be given in all states, allowing each state to meet its own needs and have a common standard by which to judge the educational preparation of individuals applying for licensure.

One misconception concerning these outside agencies is that they are licensing authorities. This is not the case; they are examination boards only. The individual states retain the power to grant and revoke licenses. The examination boards are charged with designing and scoring valid and reliable tests. They are primarily concerned with providing the states with feedback on how examinees have performed and with making suggestions about the interpretation and usefulness of scores. The states use this information as partial fulfillment of qualifications upon which they grant licenses.

The author of this introduction, Michael J. O'Donnell, holds the positions of Assistant Professor of Psychiatry and Director of Biomedical Communications at the University of New Mexico School of Medicine, Albuquerque, New Mexico.

Students should remember that these exams are administered nationwide and, although the general medical information is similar, educational methodologies and faculty areas of expertise differ from institution to institution. It is unrealistic to expect that students will know all the material presented in the exams; they may face questions on the exams in areas that were only superficially covered in their classes. The testing authorities recognize this situation, and their scoring procedures take it into account.

The Exams

The first exam was given in 1916. It was a combination of written, oral, and laboratory tests, and it was administered over a 5-day period. Admission to the exam required proof of completion of medical education and 1 year of internship.

In 1922, the examination was changed to a new format and was divided into three parts. Part I, a 3-day essay exam, was given in the basic sciences after 2 years of medical school. Part II, a 2-day exam, was administered shortly before or after graduation, and Part III was taken at the end of the first postgraduate year. To pass both Part I and Part II, a score equalling 75% of the total points available was required.

In 1954, after a 3-year extensive study, the NBME adopted the multiple-choice format. To pass, a statistically computed score of 75 was required, which allowed comparison of test results from year to year. In 1971, this method was changed to one that held the mean constant at a computed score of 500, with a predetermined deviation from the mean to ascertain a passing or failing score. The 1971 changes permitted more sophisticated analysis of test results and allowed schools to compare among individual students within their respective institutions as well as among students nationwide. Feedback to students regarding performance included the reporting of pass or failure along with scores in each of the areas tested.

During the 1980s, the ever-changing field of medicine made it necessary for the NBME to examine once again its evaluation strategies. It was found necessary to develop questions in multidisciplinary areas such as gerontology, health promotion, immunology, and cell and molecular biology. In addition, it was decided that questions should test higher cognitive levels and reasoning skills.

To meet the new goals, many changes have been made in both the form and content of the examination. These changes include reduction in the number of questions to approximately 800 on Parts I and II to allow students more time on each question, with total testing time reduced on Part I from 13 to 12 hours and on Part II from 12.5 to 12 hours. The basic science disciplines are no longer allotted the same number of questions, which permits flexible weighing of the exam areas. Reporting of scores to schools include total scores for individuals and group mean scores for separate discipline areas. Only pass/fail designations and total scores are reported to examinees. There is no longer a provision for the reporting of individual subscores to either the examinees or medical schools. Finally, the question format used in the new exams, now referred to as Comprehensive (Comp) I and II, is predominately multiple-choice, best-answer.

The New Format

New question formats, designed specifically for Comp I, are constructed in an effort to test the student's grasp of the sciences basic to medicine in an integrated fashion. The questions are designed to be interdisciplinary. Many of these questions are presented as a vignette, or case study, followed by a series of multiple-choice, best-answer questions.

The scoring of this exam also is altered. Whereas, in the past, the exams were scored on a normal curve, the new exam has a predetermined standard, which must be met in order to pass. The exam no longer concentrates on the trivial; therefore, it has been concluded that there is a common base of information that all medical students should know in order to pass. It is anticipated that a major shift in the pass/fail rate for the nation is unlikely. In the past, the average student could only expect to feel comfortable with half the test and eventually would complete approximately 67% of the questions correctly, to achieve a mean score of 500. Although with the standard setting method it is likely that the mean score will change and become higher, it is unlikely that the pass/fail rates will differ significantly from those in the past. During the first testing in 1991, there will not be differential weighing of the questions. However, in the future, the NBME will be researching methods of weighing questions based on both the time it takes to answer questions vis à vis their difficulty and the perceived importance of the information. In addition, the NBME is attempting to design a method of delivering feedback to the student that will have considerable importance in discovering weaknesses and pinpointing areas for further study in the event that a retake is necessary.

Since many of the proposed changes will be implemented for the first time in June 1991, specific information regarding actual standards, question emphasis, pass/fail rates, and so forth were unavailable at the time of publication. The publisher will update this section as information becomes available as we attempt to follow the evolution and changes that occur in the area of physician evaluation.

Materials Needed for Test Preparation

In preparation for a test, many students collect far too much study material only to find that they simply do not have the time to go through all of it. They are defeated before they begin because either they cannot get through all the material leaving areas unstudied, or they race through the material so quickly that they cannot benefit from the activity.

It is generally more efficient for the student to use materials already at hand; that is, class notes, one good outline to cover or strengthen areas not locally stressed and for quick review of the whole topic, and one good text as a reference for looking up complex material needing further explanation.

Also, many students attempt to memorize far too much information, rather than learning and understanding less material and then relying on that learned information to determine the answers to questions at the time of the examination. Relying too heavily on memorized material causes anxiety, and the more anxious students become during a test, the less learned knowledge they are likely to use.

Positive Attitude

A positive attitude and a realistic approach are essential to successful test taking. If concentration is placed on the negative aspects of tests or on the potential for failure, anxiety increases and performance decreases. A negative attitude generally develops if the student concentrates on "I must pass" rather than on "I can pass." "What if I fail?" becomes the major factor motivating the student to **run from failure rather than toward success**. This results from placing too much emphasis on scores rather than understanding that scores have only slight relevance to future professional performance.

The score received is only one aspect of test performance. Test performance also indicates the student's ability to use information during evaluation procedures and reveals how this ability might be used in the future. For example, when a patient enters the physician's office with a problem, the physician begins by asking questions, searching for clues, and seeking diagnostic information. Hypotheses are then developed, which will include several potential causes for the problem. Weighing the probabilities, the physician will begin to discard those hypotheses with the least likelihood of being correct. Good differential diagnosis involves the ability to deal with uncertainty, to reduce potential causes to the smallest number, and to use all learned information in arriving at a conclusion.

This same thought process can and should be used in testing situations. It might be termed **paper-and-pencil differential diagnosis**. In each question with five alternatives, of which one is correct, there are four alternatives that are incorrect. If deductive reasoning is used, as in solving a clinical problem, the choices can be viewed as having possibilities of being correct. The elimination of wrong choices increases the odds that a student will be able to recognize the correct choice. Even if the correct choice does not become evident, the probability of guessing correctly increases. Just as differential diagnosis in a clinical setting can result in a correct diagnosis, eliminating incorrect choices on a test can result in choosing the correct answer.

Answering questions based on what is incorrect is difficult for many students since they have had nearly 20 years experience taking tests with the implied assertion that knowledge can be displayed only by knowing what is correct. It must be remembered, however, that students can display knowledge by knowing something is wrong, just as they can display it by knowing something is right. **Students should begin to think in the present as they expect themselves to think in the future.**

Paper-and-Pencil Differential Diagnosis

The technique used to arrive at the answer to the following question is an example of the paper-and-pencil differential diagnosis approach.

> A recently diagnosed case of hypothyroidism in a 45-year-old man may result in which of the following conditions?

(A) Thyrotoxicosis
(B) Cretinism
(C) Myxedema
(D) Graves' disease
(E) Hashimoto's thyroiditis

It is presumed that all of the choices presented in the question are plausible and partially correct. If the student begins by breaking the question into parts and trying to discover what the question is attempting to measure, it will be possible to answer the question correctly by using more than memorized charts concerning thyroid problems.

● The question may be testing if the student knows the difference between "hypo" and "hyper" conditions.
● The answer choices may include thyroid problems that are not "hypothyroid" problems.
● It is possible that one or more of the choices are "hypo" but are not "thyroid" problems, that they are some other endocrine problems.
● "Recently diagnosed in a 45-year-old man" indicates that the correct answer is not a congenital childhood problem.
● "May result in" as opposed to "resulting from" suggests that the choices might include a problem that **causes** hypothyroidism rather than **results from** hypothyroidism, as stated.

By applying this kind of reasoning, the student can see that choice **A,** thyroid toxicosis, which is a disorder resulting from an overactive thyroid gland ("hyper") must be eliminated. Another piece of knowledge, that is, Graves' disease is thyroid toxicosis, eliminates choice **D**. Choice **B,** cretinism, is indeed hypothyroidism, but it is a childhood disorder. Therefore, **B** is eliminated. Choice **E** is an inflammation of the thyroid gland—here the clue is the suffix "itis." The reasoning is that thyroiditis, being an inflammation, may **cause** a thyroid problem, perhaps even a hypothyroid problem, but there is no reason for the reverse to be true. Myxedema, choice **C,** is the only choice left and the obvious correct answer.

Preparing for Board Examinations

1. **Study for yourself.** Although some of the material may seem irrelevant, the more you learn now, the less you will have to learn later. Also, do not let the fear of the test rob you of an important part of your education. If you study to learn, the task is less distasteful than studying solely to pass a test.

2. **Review all areas.** You should not be selective by studying perceived weak areas and ignoring perceived strong areas. This is probably the last time you will have the time and the motivation to review **all** of the basic sciences.

3. **Attempt to understand, not just memorize, the material.** Ask yourself: To whom does the material apply? When does it apply? Where does it apply? How does it apply? Understanding the connections among these points allows for longer retention and aids in those situations when guessing strategies may be needed.

4. **Try to anticipate questions that might appear on the test.** Ask yourself how you might construct a question on a specific topic.

5. **Give yourself a couple days of rest before the test.** Studying up to the last moment will increase your anxiety and cause potential confusion.

Taking Board Examinations

1. In the case of NBME exams, be sure to **pace yourself** to use time optimally. Each booklet is designed to take 2 hours. You should check to be sure that you are halfway through the booklet at the end of the first hour. You should use all your alloted time; if you finish too early, you probably did so by moving too quickly through the test.

2. **Read each question and all the alternatives carefully** before you begin to make decisions. Remember the questions contain clues, as do the answer choices. As a physician, you would not make a clinical decision without a complete examination of all the data; the same holds true for answering test questions.

3. **Read the directions for each question set carefully.** You would be amazed at how many students make mistakes in tests simply because they have not paid close attention to the directions.

4. It is not advisable to leave blanks with the intention of coming back to answer the questions later. Because of the way board examinations are constructed, you probably will not pick up any new information that will help you when you come back, and the chances of getting numerically off on your answer sheet are greater than your chances of benefiting by skipping around. If you feel that you must come back to a question, mark the best choice and place a note in the margin. Generally speaking, it is best not to change answers once you have made a decision, unless you have learned new information. Your intuitive reaction and first response are correct more often than changes made out of frustration or anxiety. **Never turn in an answer sheet with blanks.** Scores are based on the number that you get correct; you are not penalized for incorrect choices.

5. **Do not try to answer the questions on a stimulus–response basis.** It generally will not work. Use all of your learned knowledge.

6. **Do not let anxiety destroy your confidence.** If you have prepared conscientiously, you know enough to pass. Use all that you have learned.

7. **Do not try to determine how well you are doing as you proceed.** You will not be able to make an objective assessment, and your anxiety will increase.

8. **Do not expect a feeling of mastery** or anything close to what you are accustomed. Remember, this is a nationally administered exam, not a mastery test.

9. **Do not become frustrated or angry** about what appear to be bad or difficult questions. You simply do not know the answers; you cannot know everything.

Specific Test-Taking Strategies

Read the entire question carefully, regardless of format. Test questions have multiple parts. Concentrate on picking out the pertinent key words that might help you begin to problem solve. Words such as "always," "all," "never," "mostly," "primarily," and so forth play significant roles. In all types of questions, distractors with terms such as "always" or "never" most often are incorrect. Adjectives and adverbs can completely change the meaning of questions—pay close attention to them. Also, medical prefixes and suffixes (e.g., "hypo-," "hyper-," "-ectomy," "-itis") are sometimes at the root of the question. The knowledge and application of everyday English grammar often is the key to dissecting questions.

Multiple-Choice Questions

Read the question and the choices carefully to become familiar with the data as given. Remember, in multiple-choice questions there is one correct answer and there are four distractors, or incorrect answers. (Distractors are plausible and possibly correct or they would not be called distractors.) They are generally correct for part of the question but not for the entire question. Dissecting the question into parts aids in discerning these distractors.

If the correct answer is not immediately evident, begin eliminating the distractors. (Many students feel that they must always start at option A and make a decision before they move to B, thus forcing decisions they are not ready to make.) Your first decisions should be made on those choices you feel the most confident about.

Compare the choices to each part of the question. **To be wrong,** a choice needs to be incorrect for only part of the question. **To be correct,** it must be **totally** correct. If you believe a choice is partially incorrect, tentatively eliminate that choice. Make notes next to the choices regarding tentative decisions. One method is to place a minus sign next to the choices you are certain are incorrect and a plus sign next to those that potentially are correct. Finally, place a zero next to any choice you do not understand or need to come back to for further inspection. Do not feel that you must make final decisions until you have examined all choices carefully.

When you have eliminated as many choices as you can, decide which of those that are left has the highest probability of being correct. Remember to use paper-and-pencil differential diagnosis. Above all, be honest with yourself. If you do not know the answer, eliminate as many choices as possible and choose reasonably.

Vignette-Based Questions

Vignette-based questions are nothing more than normal multiple-choice questions that use the same case, or grouped information, for setting the problem. The NBME has been researching question types that would test the student's grasp of the integrated medical basic sciences in a more cognitively complex fashion than can be accomplished with traditional testing formats. These questions allow the testing of information that is more medically relevant than memorized terminology.

It is important to realize that several questions, although grouped together and referring to one situation or vignette, are independent questions; that is, they are able to stand alone. Your inability to answer one question in a group should have no bearing on your ability to answer subsequent questions.

These are multiple-choice questions, and just as is done with the single best answer questions, you should use the paper-and-pencil differential diagnosis, as was described earlier.

Single Best Answer–Matching Sets

Single best answer–matching sets consist of a list of words or statements followed by several numbered items or statements. Be sure to pay attention to whether the choices can be used more than once, only once, or not at all. Consider each choice individually and carefully. Begin with those with which you are the most familiar. It is important always to break the statements and words into parts, as with all other question formats. **If a choice is only partially correct, then it is incorrect.**

Guessing

Nothing takes the place of a firm knowledge base, but with little information to work with, even after playing paper-and-pencil differential diagnosis, you may find it necessary to guess at the correct answer. A few simple rules can help increase your guessing accuracy. Always guess consistently if you have no idea what is correct; that is, after eliminating all that you can, make the choice that agrees with your intuition or choose the option closest to the top of the list that has not been eliminated as a potential answer.

When guessing at questions that present with choices in numerical form, you will often find the choices listed in an ascending or descending order. It is generally not wise to guess the first or last alternative, since these are usually extreme values and are most likely incorrect.

Using the Comprehensive Exam to Learn

All too often, students do not take full advantage of practice exams. There is a tendency to complete the exam, score it, look up the correct answers to those questions missed, and then forget the entire thing.

In fact, great educational benefits can be derived if students would spend more time using practice tests as learning tools. As mentioned earlier, incorrect choices in test questions are plausible and partially correct or they would not fulfill their purpose as distractors. This means that it is just as beneficial to look up the incorrect choices as the correct choices to discover specifically why they are incorrect. In this way, it is possible to learn better test-taking skills as the subtlety of question construction is uncovered.

Additionally, it is advisable to go back and attempt to restructure each question to see if all the choices can be made correct by modifying the question. By doing this, four times as much will be learned. By all means, look up the right answer and explanation. Then, focus on each of the other choices and ask yourself under what conditions they might be correct? For example, the entire thrust of the sample question concerning hypothyroidism could be altered by changing the first few words to read:

> "Hyperthyroidism recently discovered in . . . ."
> "Hypothyroidism prenatally occurring in . . . ."
> "Hypothyroidism resulting from . . . ."

This question can be used to learn and understand thyroid problems in general, not only to memorize answers to specific questions.

In the Comprehensive Exam that follows, every effort has been made to simulate the types of questions and the degree of question difficulty in the various licensure and qualifying exams (i.e., NBME Comp I and FLEX). While taking this exam, the student should attempt to create the testing conditions that might be experienced during actual testing situations.

Summary

Ideally, examinations are designed to determine how much information students have learned and how that information is used in the successful completion of the examination. Students will be successful if these suggestions are followed:

- Develop a positive attitude and maintain that attitude.
- Be realistic in determining the amount of material you attempt to master and in the score you hope to attain.
- Read the directions for each type of question and the questions themselves closely and follow the directions carefully.
- Guess intelligently and consistently when guessing strategies must be used.
- Bring the paper-and-pencil differential diagnosis approach to each question in the examination.
- Use the test as an opportunity to display your knowledge and as a tool for developing prescriptions for further study and learning.

NBME examinations are not easy. They may be almost impossible for those who have unrealistic expectations or for those who allow misinformation concerning the exams to produce anxiety out of proportion to the task at hand. They are manageable if they are approached with a positive attitude and with consistent use of all the information the student has learned.

Michael J. O'Donnell

QUESTIONS

Directions: Each of the numbered items or incomplete statements in this section is followed by answers or by completions of the statement. Select the **one** lettered answer or completion that is **best** in each case.

1. An asymptomatic 65-year-old widow comes in for a complete physical examination. She has not been sexually active since her husband died 8 years ago and has not had a pelvic examination or Pap smear for 10 years. The clinician recommends a full gynecologic examination, but the patient refuses. The clinician should then do all of the following EXCEPT

(A) explain the importance of the examination in her situation
(B) describe the procedure and allow her to ask questions
(C) ask her to come back another day after thinking about it
(D) insist upon doing the full examination for medical–legal reasons
(E) negotiate to do a bimanual examination without speculum examination or Pap smear if the patient prefers

2. Acute appendicitis occurs with two age peaks, in children (including teenagers) and in the elderly. Which of the following statements accurately describes the presentation of acute appendicitis in the elderly?

(A) The CC is very specific
(B) The symptoms of the acute illness are influenced by other existing disorders
(C) Demented patients cannot give reliable symptoms to help with the diagnosis
(D) The presenting symptoms are similar to those in young patients
(E) The physical examination findings are similar to those in young patients

Questions 3–8

The clinician is sent to the hospital ward to do a workup on a newly admitted 32-year-old patient with the CC of abdominal pain and a working diagnosis of acute pancreatitis.

3. The primary data base should include all of the following information EXCEPT a

(A) complete medical history
(B) physical examination
(C) working problem list
(D) tentative plan
(E) final diagnosis

4. The clinician obtains an alcohol use history, which includes all of the following elements EXCEPT the

(A) amount of alcohol consumed daily or weekly
(B) type of alcohol consumed
(C) recent changes in alcohol use pattern
(D) FH of alcohol use
(E) duration of current alcohol use pattern

5. The clinician is suspicious that alcohol may play a role in the patient's current problem. The most significant danger of arriving at this conclusion too early is

(A) premature diagnostic closure
(B) incomplete problem list
(C) inappropriate laboratory testing
(D) limited differential diagnostic considerations
(E) delay in initiating treatment

6. The most important part of the physical examination on this patient is the abdominal assessment. All of the following maneuvers are likely to yield useful information EXCEPT

(A) palpation of the liver
(B) palpation of the gallbladder
(C) palpation for upper abdominal tenderness
(D) palpation of the abdominal aorta
(E) assessment of the bowel sounds

7. The clinician finds diffuse abdominal tenderness and guarding on examination as well as a liver span of 18 cm. The problem list should include all of the following conditions EXCEPT

(A) possible alcohol abuse
(B) abdominal pain
(C) acute pancreatitis
(D) abdominal tenderness and guarding
(E) hepatic enlargement

8. The clinician is asked to present this case to the ward attending. The presentation must include all of the following information EXCEPT the

(A) HPI
(B) alcohol consumption history
(C) patient's vital signs
(D) FH of alcohol consumption
(E) abdominal examination findings

(end of group question)

9. A clinician who is reviewing the hospital chart of a patient notes a gross error in the admission history and physical examination written 3 days before. In correcting the error, all of the following are acceptable procedures EXCEPT

(A) the original history and physical examination can be removed from the chart and replaced with the corrected version
(B) single lines can be written through the mistake and labeled as an error
(C) additional information can be added, as long as it is dated, signed, and marked as an addendum
(D) the original data should remain legible
(E) none of the above

10. The most appropriate time to initiate touching in the patient encounter is

(A) while taking the radial pulse
(B) while taking the blood pressure
(C) shaking hands on introduction
(D) while taking the oral temperature
(E) while palpating the scalp

11. A 1-week-old female infant is brought to the pediatrician's office for a weight check. The mother is concerned about the infant's breasts and vagina. The infant has a normal physical examination. All of the following findings are consistent with physiologic withdrawal of maternal hormones EXCEPT

(A) nipple discharge
(B) vaginal discharge
(C) breast engorgement
(D) labial ecchymoses
(E) vaginal bleeding

Questions 12–18

A medical student is asked to see a 30-year-old patient in the gynecology clinic who comes in for a routine examination.

12. The risk assessment and history for breast cancer should include all of the following factors EXCEPT

(A) history of fibrocystic breast disease
(B) FH of breast cancer
(C) parity history
(D) breast-feeding history
(E) history of nipple discharge

13. The most important element of the menstrual history in this patient is

(A) age of onset of menses
(B) frequency and duration of periods
(C) pain with menses
(D) any recent changes in menstrual pattern
(E) premenstrual symptoms

14. All of the following information is important in assessing the risk for cancer of the cervix EXCEPT

(A) age of onset of menses
(B) age of assumption of sexual activity
(C) number of sexual partners
(D) history of venereal warts (condyloma acuminatum)
(E) frequency of intercourse with a monogamous partner

15. The patient is expecting her period in the next few days. On examination, the medical student finds a tender, ballotable, mobile mass in the inferior left breast. The clinician should next

(A) order a mammogram
(B) reassure the patient
(C) have the patient return for re-examination in 2 weeks
(D) ask the preceptor to assess the finding
(E) ask for a surgical consultation

16. The medical student prepares to do the speculum examination and Pap smear. All of the following steps should be taken EXCEPT to

(A) label the slides for specimen reception
(B) wear gloves on both hands
(C) lubricate the speculum with water-soluble gel
(D) explain the procedure to the patient
(E) introduce the speculum above a finger at the vaginal introitus

17. Principles regarding the use of gloves for the pelvic examination include all of the following EXCEPT

(A) all genital examinations should be conducted with gloves
(B) the abdominal hand may be ungloved during the bimanual examination
(C) the rectal glove should be liberally lubricated with water
(D) gloves are protective for both patient and examiner
(E) gloves should be replaced between vaginal and rectal examinations

18. The rectovaginal examination is used to accomplish all of the following EXCEPT

(A) palpation of the rectovaginal septum
(B) palpation of the adnexal structures
(C) palpation of the posterior uterus
(D) palpation for rectal masses
(E) acquisition of stool specimen for blood analysis
(end of group question)

19. All of the following statements about the format for recording a medical history are true EXCEPT the

(A) CC is followed immediately by the HPI
(B) PP may be recorded in narrative, rather than tabular, form
(C) data are recorded in the order in which they were obtained in the patient encounter
(D) PMH includes allergies to medication
(E) FH may be recorded either graphically or in narrative form

20. A 29-year-old quadriplegic woman who is mentally intact is shifted in bed every 2 hours to prevent pressure (decubitus) ulcers. The clinician examines her at the end of 2 hours on her right side. She is feeling well, not coughing, and is afebrile. Examination of the lungs reveals dullness and crackles in the lateral half of the right lung field. The most reasonable interpretation of their cause is

(A) atelectasis secondary to mucus plugging
(B) pulmonary edema, which has localized due to gravitational forces
(C) compressive atelectasis
(D) hypostatic pneumonia from poor movement of secretions
(E) chronic pulmonary fibrosis

21. An 89-year-old woman with severe Alzheimer-type dementia presents with a CC of fever and a 1-day history of right lower quadrant abdominal pain. The patient is unable to recall her name or the date. Appropriate action at this time would be to

(A) presume the pain is a manifestation of her dementia
(B) begin a diagnostic workup to evaluate an abdominal process, such as acute appendicitis
(C) obtain a history from the patient's spouse and act upon this information
(D) presume that the pain could be anywhere and begin a general workup
(E) discount the symptoms and rely on objective data, such as a rectal temperature

22. Components of the PMH include all of the following EXCEPT

(A) immunization history
(B) obstetric history
(C) surgical history
(D) family history
(E) allergy history

23. Each of the following reflexes assess pyramidal tract function EXCEPT the

(A) Hoffman reflex
(B) Romberg reflex
(C) Babinski reflex
(D) Oppenheim reflex
(E) Chaddock reflex

Questions 24–26

An 82-year-old hemiparetic man is brought to a university hospital clinic for evaluation for admission to a nursing home. A second-year medical student is asked to do the preliminary assessment. The patient's frail, elderly wife and his son are with him.

24. The patient is strapped in a wheelchair, fully dressed. His eyes follow, but he does not respond to any questions. The failure to speak is likely due to

(A) anger at the situation
(B) hearing impairment
(C) central aphasia
(D) dementia
(E) all of the above

25. The medical student obtains a medical history from the patient's family. To proceed with the physical examination, what should be done next?

(A) Attempt the examination with the patient in the wheelchair
(B) Call for orderlies to move the patient to the examining table
(C) Ask the patient's son to assist the patient onto the table
(D) Query the patient's wife about the patient's ability to move himself onto the table
(E) Defer the physical examination to another time

26. Suddenly, the patient's wife begins to sob and asks to speak to the medical student alone. The student's best strategy is to

(A) ask the wife to leave the room and wait outside
(B) ask the son to take his mother from the room
(C) ignore the wife until the work with the patient is completed
(D) ask the son to remain with his father and take the wife outside to talk
(E) ask the wife to control herself until the examination of the patient is completed

(end of group question)

27. An 85-year-old man presents to an outpatient clinic for a complete history and physical examination. He considers himself to be "healthy" and offers no complaints. Which of the following is the **least** important component of the history to explore?

(A) PMH
(B) Social history
(C) FH
(D) Medication use
(E) Mental status examination

28. Innocent murmurs that may be heard in the school-age child include all of the following EXCEPT

(A) Still's murmur
(B) venous hum
(C) peripheral pulmonic stenosis
(D) carotid bruit
(E) pulmonary flow murmur

29. Questions about family violence should be included when all of the following information is in the medical history EXCEPT

(A) the HPI includes an accident or injury
(B) there is a history of drug and alcohol abuse
(C) the PMH includes a number of accidents or injuries
(D) the FH includes a pattern of family violence
(E) the ROS is negative

30. An 88-year-old woman displays increased confusion. On examination, she is found to have a rectal temperature of 35° C. What is the most appropriate response for the examiner to take?

(A) Assume the thermometer is not working correctly
(B) Ascribe the finding to age alone
(C) Consider hypothyroidism or other hypometabolic states
(D) Repeat the measurement orally
(E) Take an axillary temperature

31. Which of the following conditions is most likely to be accurately predicted from observation of the patient during the history and in the general appearance portion of the physical examination?

(A) Cardiovascular reserve
(B) Liver irritation
(C) Esophageal swallowing function
(D) Respiratory insufficiency
(E) Pancreatic insufficiency

32. A 22-year-old woman comes to the clinician with a history of increasing polydipsia and polyuria plus a 10 lb weight loss over the past 3 months, which is highly suspicious for diabetes mellitus. The most sensitive and specific test to order now is

(A) random serum glucose
(B) 5-hour postprandial serum glucose
(C) fasting (overnight) serum glucose
(D) urine glucose
(E) 30-minute postprandial serum glucose

33. Sexual histories are important for all of the following reasons EXCEPT

(A) STDs are on the increase
(B) sexuality is a concern for all age-groups
(C) patients may be uncomfortable initiating the topic
(D) medication compliance may be affected
(E) sexual practices are fairly standard for all age-groups

34. Admission orders on a new patient's chart must include all of the following information EXCEPT

(A) diet
(B) laboratory studies to be obtained
(C) informed consent for procedures
(D) vital signs to be monitored
(E) activity level to be allowed

Questions 35–39

A 35-year-old moderately mentally retarded woman is brought to the clinic by her group home leader because she has not had a menstrual period for 3 months. The clinician is asked to obtain a screening history and physical examination.

35. The patient turns away when the clinician tries to introduce himself. The best first strategy to deal with this situation is to

(A) leave the room with the attendant to obtain the history
(B) firmly insist that the patient speak
(C) sit down and converse with the attendant
(D) address questions to the patient, allowing the attendant to supply the answers
(E) attempt to engage the patient in conversation about her activities and interests

36. Eventually the student obtains a general medical history. Given the presenting problem, information about which of the following must also be obtained?

(A) Birth control measures
(B) Ongoing medications
(C) Opportunities for sexual activity
(D) Level of independent functioning
(E) All of the above

37. The clinician learns that the patient has recently started a medication that causes amenorrhea in some women. She is not protected against pregnancy. A physical examination should include all of the following EXCEPT

(A) a thyroid examination
(B) an abdominal examination
(C) a breast examination
(D) a detailed mental status examination
(E) a pelvic examination

38. The patient cries and will not allow her clothes to be removed for the examination. The best strategy is to

(A) inform the attendant that there is nothing more to be done
(B) suggest laboratory tests as an alternative to the examination
(C) consult the preceptor for suggestions
(D) get someone else to undress the patient and prepare her for the examination
(E) do the examination with the patient clothed

39. The patient's mother calls to ask what the clinician has decided is the cause of the amenorrhea. The clinician should

(A) supply the information requested
(B) tell the mother to get the information from the group home supervisor
(C) obtain the patient's permission to provide her mother with the information
(D) determine who is the legal guardian of the patient and supply information only to this party
(E) none of the above
(end of group question)

40. The clinician is unable to feel pulses in the superficial temporal arteries of a 78-year-old man who also has no palpable left foot pulses. The most important explanation is

(A) diffuse vascular obstruction from atherosclerosis
(B) simple age-related changes
(C) temporal (giant cell) arteritis
(D) inexperience of the examiner
(E) anatomic variation in pulse localization

41. Good questions to include in the sexual history include all of the following EXCEPT

(A) are you presently in a sexual relationship
(B) do you have any concerns about sexual activity
(C) have you ever been promiscuous
(D) have you ever had partners of the same sex
(E) has there been a change in your level of sexual activity

42. In doing an oral case presentation on ward rounds, all of the following identifying data should be included EXCEPT the patient's

(A) age
(B) sex
(C) race
(D) occupation
(E) marital status

43. In preparing a problem list for a new patient with a proven myocardial infarction, all of the following information should be relegated to the inactive problem list EXCEPT

(A) hysterectomy, 1976
(B) diabetes mellitus
(C) x-ray confirmed duodenal ulcer, 1984
(D) right hip fracture, 1988
(E) pneumococcal pneumonia, 1989

44. A pathologic finding in a healthy 14-year-old boy is

(A) Tanner stage III genitalia
(B) erupted second molars
(C) phimosis
(D) gynecomastia
(E) comedones

45. All of the following factors can cause a Folstein score to misrepresent the patient's actual cognitive function EXCEPT

(A) extensive formal education
(B) scant formal education
(C) serial repetition
(D) inherent test insensitivity
(E) inattention

46. In the course of a routine physical examination, the maneuver most likely to cause discomfort or pain for the patient is

(A) inspection of the tympanic membrane
(B) palpation of the breasts
(C) palpation of the thyroid gland
(D) palpation of the abdominal aortic margins
(E) palpation of the testicles

47. A 60-year-old male smoker presents with a complaint of pain in both calves while walking. The examiner makes a preliminary diagnosis of claudication pain from arterial insufficiency and embarks on a directed examination. All the following are useful components to evaluate the arterial system EXCEPT

(A) palpation of the femoral, popliteal, and dorsalis pedis arteries
(B) assessment of hair distribution on the legs
(C) noting capillary filling in the toe nails
(D) eliciting Homans' sign
(E) measuring blood pressure in both thighs

48. All of the following points are important in the oral presentation of a male patient with difficulty breathing EXCEPT the

(A) negatives in the cardiovascular ROS
(B) CC in the patient's own words
(C) dimensions or parameters of the presenting complaint
(D) normal elements of the pulmonary examination
(E) strong FH of breast cancer

49. A patient with chronic obstructive pulmonary disease presents to the clinician because she is having difficulty climbing the stairs to her third floor walk-up apartment. The clinician should discuss all of the following subjects with the patient EXCEPT

(A) frequency of symptoms
(B) severity of symptoms
(C) financial resources of the patient
(D) new medications in early stages of research
(E) other ADLs

50. If there are five new patients to see in the clinic, and there is only time to perform a mental status examination on four, which of the following patients is most appropriate to defer?

(A) A healthy 80-year-old man
(B) A 45-year-old woman with a long history of schizophrenia
(C) A 32-year-old man who is seropositive for HIV but who is otherwise well
(D) A 47-year-old male marathoner whose performance has declined
(E) A 17-year-old girl whose school performance has declined abruptly

51. An infant is seated on the floor of the examining room. As the clinician enters, the child is babbling "mama." When she sees the clinician, she pulls herself to a standing position but is unable to cruise to her mother. Her mother picks her up and distracts her with a game of peekaboo. The child's age is most likely

(A) 2 months
(B) 4 months
(C) 6 months
(D) 9 months
(E) 12 months

52. A slightly dizzy 82-year-old woman has a pulse of 85 supine and 100 sitting with blood pressure measurements of 120/60 supine and 110/50 sitting. She has a soft cardiac murmur and reports recent abdominal cramps and a fleck of blood in her last stool. Which of the following parts of the physical examination is most likely to prove injurious to her?

(A) Carotid palpation
(B) Breath-holding to characterize the murmur
(C) Rectal examination
(D) Assessment of gait
(E) Abdominal palpation

Questions 53–56

A 23-year-old pregnant diabetic woman comes into the emergency room with a CC of "sharp left-sided chest pain since this morning and difficulty getting my breath."

53. The problem list, based on history alone, should include all of the following EXCEPT

(A) diabetes mellitus
(B) chest pain
(C) acute pulmonary embolism
(D) pregnancy by history
(E) shortness of breath

54. On examination of the patient, the clinician finds a heart rate of 120/min, a respiratory rate of 32 with splinting, decreased breath sounds in the left hemithorax, uterine enlargement consistent with a gestation of 22 weeks, and a tender cord in the left calf. The problem list should now be modified to include all of the following items EXCEPT

(A) tender cord, left calf
(B) deep venous thrombosis, left calf
(C) tachycardia
(D) tachypnea
(E) intrauterine pregnancy, approximately 22 weeks gestation

55. The differential diagnosis for the presenting complaint of this patient's chest pain and shortness of breath should include all of the following EXCEPT

(A) acute pulmonary embolism
(B) spontaneous pneumothorax
(C) early pneumonia
(D) viral pleuritis
(E) acute myocardial infarction

56. Based upon the differential diagnosis, the clinician should order all of the following tests to be done immediately EXCEPT

(A) EKG
(B) arterial blood gases
(C) chest x-ray
(D) gynecologic consult
(E) ventilation/perfusion lung scan
(end of group question)

57. The clinician is asked to see a patient who is dying from the complications of AIDS. The hospital in which this clinician works observes Universal Precautions. The patient is not subject to reverse isolation. The clinician should wear disposable gloves for which of the following maneuvers?

(A) Abdominal palpation
(B) All physical examination maneuvers
(C) Phlebotomy
(D) Inspection of the oral cavity
(E) None of the above

58. A 62-year-old man who is admitted to the hospital for a workup of chronic diarrhea suddenly develops postural hypotension and tarry stools. The progress note following these new events should include all of the following information EXCEPT

(A) a statement about a change in the patient's perception of his symptoms
(B) the results of "stat" blood work
(C) the results of guaiac (occult blood) testing of the stool
(D) assessment of the patient's family situation for discharge home
(E) a plan for managing the blood pressure change

59. An appropriate screening test for a 40-year-old asymptomatic man who presents for a periodic health evaluation is

(A) hemoglobin and hematocrit
(B) serum cholesterol
(C) thyroid function tests
(D) serum electrolytes (i.e., sodium, potassium, chloride, bicarbonate)
(E) fasting serum glucose

60. A 45-year-old man with a long history of heavy alcohol consumption presents with an increasing abdominal girth, diffuse abdominal pain, and a fever. The examiner makes a preliminary assessment of ascites with bacterial peritonitis. Which of the following findings suggests an alternative diagnosis?

(A) Positive shifting dullness
(B) Hypoactive bowel sounds
(C) Positive fluid wave
(D) Positive Murphy's sign
(E) Positive rebound tenderness

61. A 65-year-old woman presents with a 3-day history of fever and a cough productive of green sputum. Percussion reveals dullness at the left lower lung field posteriorly. Chest x-ray shows a lobar consolidation in the left lower lung. All of the following findings would be expected at the left base EXCEPT

(A) decreased breath sounds
(B) coarse inspiratory and expiratory rhonchi
(C) vesicular breath sounds
(D) positive egophony
(E) increased vocal fremitus

62. An elderly patient complains of lethargy and weight loss. To screen for malnutrition, all of the following factors should be explored in the medical history EXCEPT

(A) changes in appetite, taste, or smell
(B) presence of chronic or acute medical conditions, which increase metabolic needs or increase nutrient losses
(C) self-imposed or prescribed diet regimens
(D) comparison of the patient's diet to the RDAs
(E) psychosocial or life-style changes that may have affected food acquisition, preparation, or eating

63. A patient in a coma is on a respirator (mechanical ventilation) because of loss of the neurologic drive to respiration. Which of the following features is of most help in determining the presence or absence of pulmonary pathology?

(A) Respiratory rate of 16 breaths a minute
(B) Coarse inspiratory–expiratory rhonchi heard diffusely over the lung fields
(C) Dullness to percussion at the left lung base
(D) Diffuse decrease in audibility of lung sounds over major airways
(E) Inability to assess tactile vocal fremitus adequately

64. A prostate of normal size excludes which of the following diagnoses?

(A) Prostatic hyperplasia
(B) Cancer of the prostate
(C) Hydronephrosis due to obstruction of the prostatic urethra
(D) Urinary incontinence due to prostatic disease
(E) None of the above

65. A student is very distressed by a patient encounter and wants to discuss it with a classmate. This is acceptable in all of the following circumstances EXCEPT when

(A) the patient's name is not used
(B) no one else is around
(C) the patient has given consent
(D) it is in the classroom, using only initials
(E) the classmate is directly involved in the care of the patient

66. A 45-year-old man is evaluated for depression. His PMH is significant only for a remote history of treatment for venereal disease. Complete eye examination reveals the following: Both pupils are small and equal; a light shined in each eye successively results in no change in pupillary size in either pupil. When the patient is asked to change focus quickly from a distant to a close object, the eyes converge and the pupils constrict. Which of the following statements about this man's condition is true?

(A) The pupils react to direct light
(B) The pupils react consensually to light
(C) Accommodation is intact
(D) There is evidence of a CN VI paralysis
(E) Nystagmus is present

67. A 90-year-old woman is brought to the emergency room by her son, who provided a CC of "For the first time in her life, my mother did not make a pot of coffee upon awakening. She is not herself." The patient herself offers no symptoms. She was previously in excellent health. The examiner should proceed with all of the following EXCEPT

(A) obtain a detailed medication list
(B) discount the son's information and rely on symptoms provided by the patient
(C) obtain a complete PMH
(D) perform a complete mental status examination
(E) perform a complete neurologic examination

68. The patient is a 55-year-old woman with diabetes and coronary artery disease. She continues to work at her secretarial position at an insurance company and lives with her husband in a two bedroom apartment. She is fatigued easily and takes frequent naps. She appears alert and well nourished. The above description includes all of the following factors EXCEPT

(A) diagnosis
(B) prognosis
(C) symptoms
(D) ADLs
(E) signs

69. Which of the following characteristics most strongly suggest that a murmur has an important pathologic cause and is not simply a benign flow murmur?

(A) Male sex
(B) Age over 90 years
(C) Diastolic timing
(D) Grade II rather than I intensity
(E) Location at left upper sternal border

70. A 20-year-old patient with Down's syndrome and mental retardation presents for a comprehensive physical examination. Accepted techniques to maximize the examination include all of the following EXCEPT

(A) allowing a family member to remain during the examination
(B) scheduling two or more sessions to complete the examination
(C) allowing the patient to move about while observing for gross and fine movements
(D) premedicating the patient with a sedative
(E) using visual aids to assess the patient's vision

71. *The Surgeon General's Report on Nutrition and Health* identified problems with overconsumption of all the following nutrients EXCEPT

(A) fats
(B) cholesterol
(C) complex carbohydrates and dietary fiber
(D) sodium
(E) protein

72. A 40-year-old man with a long history of heavy alcohol consumption presents with a change in mental status. The eye examination reveals the following: Pupils are equal and react to light and accommodation. Visual acuity is normal. The right eye cannot move laterally past the midline. All other fields of movement are intact for both eyes. Rapid fine movement in both eyes is elicited in upward gaze. All of the following statements about this man's condition are true EXCEPT

(A) CN II appears to be intact
(B) CN III appears to be intact
(C) vertical nystagmus is present
(D) CN IV appears to be intact
(E) CN VI appears to be intact

Directions: Each group of items in this section consists of lettered options followed by a set of numbered items. For each item, select the **one** lettered option that is most closely associated with it. Each lettered option may be selected once, more than once, or not at all.

Questions 73–76

For each of the case scenarios listed below, select the aspect of the therapeutic relationship that it best illustrates.

(A) Repetition
(B) Sharing common experiences appropriately
(C) Representational system mismatch
(D) Closed questions
(E) Improper introduction

73. A patient visits a clinician for the first time. The clinician enters the room and says, "I understand that you have chest pain. Tell me about it."

74. The patient says to the clinician, "I have been thrown by this illness; it has just knocked me for a loop." The clinician replies, "Yes, it looks like things are bleak for you now, but I think things will lighten up soon."

75. The clinician asks the patient, "Do you have dysuria?" The patient responds, "Excuse me?" The clinician repeats the question, "Have you been bothered by dysuria?"

76. A 35-year-old woman comes in complaining of stomach pain and nausea. The clinician enters the examining room and says, "I want to find out if you are pregnant. When was your last period?"

Questions 77–81

For each piece of data acquired or action anticipated, select the division of the progress note under which it should be recorded.

(A) S (subjective)
(B) O (objective)
(C) A (assessment)
(D) P (plan)
(E) None of the above

77. Pulse rate of 120/min

78. Increasing difficulty getting my breath

79. Stat EKG

80. Substernal chest pain for 2 hours

81. Unstable angina, accelerating

Questions 82–86

Match the data from each patient with the part of the history where it should be recorded (regardless of when the information is obtained).

(A) HPI
(B) PMH
(C) PP
(D) FH
(E) ROS

82. Patient is concerned about wife's health

83. Patient has occasional headaches

84. Patient has had IDDM for 5 years

85. Patient's father died at 54 years of age from a stroke

86. Patient has productive cough

Questions 87–91

For each finding in the physical examination, select the age-group in which it is most closely associated.

(A) Newborn
(B) Infancy (2 weeks to 12 months)
(C) Toddler (15 months to 4 years)
(D) School-age child (5–10 years)
(E) Adolescent (12–16 years)

87. Seborrhea

88. Caput

89. Flat feet

90. Thrush

91. Erupted permanent lower central incisors

Questions 92–96

For each clinical situation described below, select the single most useful laboratory test.

(A) EKG
(B) Chest x-ray
(C) CBC
(D) Echocardiogram
(E) None of the above

92. A 33-year-old lawyer with cough, fever, and pleuritic chest pain of 3 day's duration

93. A 62-year-old male construction worker with a 2-hour history of crushing substernal chest pain

94. A 23-year-old student with sudden onset (1 hour ago) of left sided chest pain and shortness of breath. Found to have absent breath sounds over the left hemithorax

95. A 40-year-old woman with a 3-hour history of "palpitations" who is found to have a heart rate of 160/min

96. A 72-year-old woman with a diffuse petechial rash

Questions 97–101

For each clinical situation described below, select the order that would be most appropriate.

(A) Measure vital signs every hour around the clock
(B) Record intake and output every shift, and weigh patient daily
(C) Administer O_2, 2 L/min by nasal cannula
(D) Test all stools for occult blood
(E) DNR if cardiac or respiratory arrest occurs

97. A healthy, lucid, and intelligent 27-year-old schoolteacher admitted for elective surgery makes out a living will, specifying that he does not wish to receive electric shock, cardioactive medicines, or mechanical ventilation.

98. A 34-year-old plumber with markedly symptomatic asthma is now improving.

99. A 62-year-old man with new acute renal failure is in the intensive care unit.

100. An 89-year-old man with end-stage dementia complains of unremitting epigastric pain.

101. An exhausted mountain climber comes in severely dehydrated and moderately hypotensive.

Questions 102–105

For each case presentation listed below, select a term that it best illustrates.

(A) Folk belief
(B) Personal biography
(C) Acute disease
(D) Mutual participation model

102. A 56-year-old woman presents with pneumonia. She admits to smoking two packs of cigarettes a day. The clinician is frustrated by the fact that smoking is a predisposing factor in pneumonia.

103. A 45-year-old smoker presents with emphysema. The clinician explains to the patient that the disease may be treated but not cured, and its natural history, especially if the patient continues to smoke, is a downhill course with increasing disability.

104. A patient with systemic lupus erythematosus comes to the clinician's office with an article from a nutrition-oriented lay health magazine that suggests a new treatment for her symptoms.

105. Many medical students have great expectations about the efficacy of modern medical care and the high moral character of the medical profession. However, when they are personally faced with the futility of modern medicine in dealing with chronic disease and disability and their own limited ability to impact on the health and well-being of many of their patients, they become cynical and frustrated, which may lead to the inappropriate use of medical care and very difficult relationships when they become patients.

Questions 106–110

For each case presentation listed below, select the diagnostic term that most appropriately describes it.

(A) Bradypnea
(B) Tachypnea
(C) Cheyne-Stokes
(D) Biot's
(E) Apnea

106. A comatose patient with a history of a drug overdose presents with a regularly irregular sine wave pattern of respiration.

107. A 17-year-old asthmatic patient in marked respiratory distress presents with a respiratory rate of 47.

108. An obese patient with a history of snoring has prolonged periods without respiratory efforts while sleeping.

109. A patient with severe head trauma following a motor vehicle accident presents with an irregularly irregular respiratory pattern.

110. A world class marathon runner is noted on a routine physical examination to have a respiratory rate of 10 at rest.

Questions 111–114

For each aspect of the physical examination, select the age-group in which this should be emphasized.

(A) Newborn
(B) Infancy (2 weeks to 12 months)
(C) Toddler (15 months to 4 years)
(D) School-age child (5–10 years)
(E) Adolescent (12–16 years)

111. Performance of the Ortolani and Barlow maneuvers

112. Elicitation of the parachute reflex

113. Examination of the thyroid gland

114. Conversation to elicit speech content and clarity

Questions 115–119

For each case presentation listed below, select the most responsible action to be taken.

(A) Notify the state health department or the Centers for Disease Control
(B) Notify the governmental agency responsible for youth services
(C) Notify the patient's spouse
(D) Maintain patient confidentiality
(E) Notify the patient's parents

115. An 18-year-old married man presents with an urethral discharge that is diagnosed as gonorrhea.

116. A 4-year-old boy presents with multiple contusions and a long history of trauma and broken bones.

117. A 16-year-old girl presents for birth control pills.

118. A 17-year-old intravenous drug user with *Pneumocystis carinii* pneumonia requests an HIV test, which returns positive.

119. A 16-year-old boy presents to discuss his alcohol and marijuana use, requesting counseling.

Questions 120–124

Match each case scenario listed below with the Kübler-Ross stage of coping with death that it best exemplifies.

(A) Denial and isolation
(B) Anger
(C) Bargaining
(D) Depression
(E) Acceptance

120. Mr. M, age 86, has been considerably more quiet during the last three visits than on previous visits. As recently as 2 weeks ago, he engaged in a lengthy discussion of his childhood and school years and the differences he observed in children today. He seems withdrawn; his eyes are often closed, though he does not seem to be sleeping. He is reluctant to engage in conversation, refuses visitors, even those special friends who have previously had unlimited access. Mr. M seems to prefer limited contact with family members. Not an openly religious person, Mr. M has recently asked for visits by the chaplain, but when visited, he engages in very limited conversation. He has asked for someone to remain in the room while he is falling asleep and occasionally awakes in a startled fashion, asking where he is. When questioned, he denies being frightened, says he is just waiting for a visitor and wondered if perhaps the visitor had arrived.

121. Mrs. P, a professional woman of some stature in the community, accuses others of misunderstanding and exaggerating the seriousness of her condition. She claims friends have abandoned her, though it was she who has refused their company. After a long and trusting relationship with her primary clinician, which was characterized by much self-education about health, illnesses, and treatment alternatives, she recently traveled to a nearby city for a consultation. She returned stating she feels much better and is sure there was a mistake in judgment regarding her prognosis. She confided that she had visited a faith healer while there but also spoke to specialists in her particular disease. She stated that the faith healer did not have much effect, since her symptoms had really disappeared by the time she had her scheduled visit.

122. Mrs. C is very cooperative and compliant. She denies pain and discomfort, and although she exhibits restlessness, she says she is "really feeling fine." She speaks repeatedly of her daughter's upcoming graduation from college and confides that she expects the young woman will soon announce her plans to marry the young man she has been dating, although the daughter denies any truth to this and states so frequently to her mother (the patient). Mrs. C was a regular volunteer at her local church and was responsible for laundering the altar linens weekly. Since she became ill, she has been unable to accomplish this task, which requires standing and ironing, but she has begun to embroider a new set since she had "promised" a long time ago to always do something for her church. In the past, whenever she neglected this promise, she had a spell of bad luck.

123. Mr. P, a laborer and avid sports fan and fisherman, was known by his friends and work colleagues for his affable good humor, easy going manner, and positive outlook. Recently he has been bitterly complaining about the "raw deal" he is getting. He feels that the nursing staff is purposely ignoring his needs and taking excessive breaks instead of tending to his needs and those of other patients. He has shouted for the nurse on duty, thrown his call button across the room, and left the floor demanding to see the hospital director or the chairman of the board. He stated that he believes that his company deliberately misled him in explaining his health insurance options, and he has engaged in long and agitated telephone conversations with the benefits counselors at his place of employment.

124. Miss J, a high school physical education teacher, coach, and member of the organizing committee of a community little league team has abruptly resigned from all her baseball activities. This action was taken in spite of her clinician's reassurances that these activities are not the least bit detrimental to her and, in fact, might be helpful. She has reported difficulty in falling asleep at night and consequent difficulty in waking in the morn-

ing. She has missed 5 days of school in the month and uncharacteristically "forgot" the monthly coach's clinic, which she had founded. Her classroom, usually extremely tidy, appears somewhat disorganized, with sports equipment scattered on bookshelves and books on the floor. Students have noticed that Miss. J is not her usual bubbly, outgoing self; she's "all inside herself" lately.

Questions 125–129

For each of the following patients listed below who have been hospitalized with an acute illness and are ready for discharge from the hospital, select the most appropriate disposition.

(A) Discharge home with visiting nurse follow-up in the home

(B) Discharge home with visiting nurse follow-up and Meals-on-Wheels delivered to the home

(C) Discharge home with follow-up only in outpatient office

(D) Consider temporary placement in a skilled nursing facility

(E) Consider permanent placement in a skilled nursing facility

125. A 65-year-old man with diabetes was hospitalized for a below-knee amputation of the left leg and a wound infection. He lives in a private home with his wife, son, and daughter-in-law.

126. An 80-year-old woman was admitted for an elective hip replacement for arthritis. She lives alone on the second floor of a two-family home.

127. A 75-year-old previously healthy man was admitted for an uncomplicated gallbladder operation. He lives alone in his own multilevel home.

128. An 80-year-old man with severe Alzheimer's disease was admitted with a fractured hip. He lives with his 78-year-old wife in a private home.

129. An 80-year-old woman with coronary artery disease and chronic obstructive pulmonary disease was admitted for pneumonia. She lives alone in her own apartment on the ground floor.

Questions 130–134

For each patient described below, select the neurologic function that can be best interpreted.

(A) Cerebellar function

(B) Function of CN III, CN IV, and CN VI

(C) Gross motor function

(D) Pyramidal tract function

(E) Function of CN IX and CN X

130. A 5-year-old boy runs into the examination room, climbs upon the examining table, jumps off, and lands on his feet.

131. A 7-year-old girl with cerebral palsy is noted to have bilateral Babinski reflexes.

132. An 8-year-old boy sways upon standing and is unable to walk.

133. A 38-year-old woman with cerebral palsy presents wearing a bib saturated with sputum.

134. A 17-year-old patient with mental retardation intently follows fish in an aquarium.

Questions 135–137

For each case presentation listed below, select the concept that it best illustrates.

(A) Mind–body split

(B) Hostile patient

(C) Overidentification

135. A student clinician meets a patient for the first time who was once a third grade teacher, is in full possession of her faculties, and is able to give the history as clearly as if she were teaching a history lesson. The match of student and clinician is good and the encounter proceeds easily. A classmate interviews the same patient a week later, and the encounter is a disaster. The second student had been a student of this teacher, and she could not cope with the implications of a serious problem in a beloved and once omnipotent person.

136. A 40-year-old man with severe heart disease whose ADLs are sharply curtailed becomes very angry as the student documents the items in the PP. It is very stressful for him to report the loss of valued work activities, relationships, and energy.

137. A 40-year-old woman has severe recurrent headaches. There are no findings on physical examination, and there is a poor response to medication.

Questions 138–142

For each of the case scenarios presented below, choose the most likely body system implicated.

(A) Musculoskeletal

(B) Renal–urinary

(C) Respiratory

(D) Reproductive

(E) None of the above

138. A 23-year-old runner comes to the outpatient department with a complaint of persistent pain in the left knee and calf since Sunday's marathon.

139. A 72-year-óld hypertensive man comes into the emergency room with acute shortness of breath, cyanosis, and rales throughout both lung fields.

140. A 32-year-old woman who has been taking high doses of calcium to prevent osteoporosis comes in with a 2-hour history of excruciating left flank pain.

141. A 25-year-old man comes to the clinic with a 3-day history of 10–12 loose stools a day, which began while he was camping in the Rocky Mountains.

142. A 27-year-old sexually active woman presents with a 2-month history of amenorrhea.

Questions 143–147

A second-year medical student is about to perform her first complete patient history on a 56-year-old woman. Arrange the following list of tasks in the most logical sequence for the medical student to follow.

(A) Obtain the HPI
(B) Obtain the immunization history
(C) Make introductions
(D) Obtain the CC
(E) Obtain a ROS

143. Step 1

144. Step 2

145. Step 3

146. Step 4

147. Step 5

Questions 148–150

For each clinical situation described below, select the order that would be most appropriate.

(A) Do not draw blood from left arm
(B) Do not take blood pressures supine
(C) Ambulate with assistance three times a day
(D) Measure electrolytes and blood sugar immediately
(E) Determine allergies

148. A retarded adult is brought in from an outing with automobile trauma. He is pleasant but nonverbal. The individuals accompanying him say, "This is his baseline mental status, I think; Mary usually works with him. Anyway, it is just the leg we are worried about."

149. A 19-year-old man is brought to the emergency room unconscious after passing out during a ball game. His parents report no prior incidents of this type.

150. A 38-year-old woman had a massive local excision for melanoma of the left arm a year ago. She is now 3 days postoperative for appendicitis.

ANSWERS AND EXPLANATIONS

1. The answer is D. [*Chapter 11 VI C*] A competent adult has the right to refuse any procedure. Under no circumstances should the patient be forced to comply or be pressured by the clinician's concerns. The clinician is protected from legal action if he or she clearly records that the decision not to do the examination was made by the patient. Usually, a careful explanation of the purpose and the need for the examination suffices to get the patient's consent. Sometimes patients are surprised when procedures they had not expected are suggested; usually they only need time to think about and prepare for the examination. In a sexually inactive woman of age 65, the greatest concern is palpation of the ovaries, not the Pap smear since the incidence of carcinoma of the cervix drops after menopause, especially in a woman with as few risk factors as this patient appears to have. However, ovarian disease increases significantly in incidence after menopause. Therefore, isolated bimanual palpation of the adnexal structures and uterus would be a reasonable compromise.

2. The answer is B. [*Chapter 9 I B 1, 2 a*] Appendicitis is just one example of several diseases that present differently in elderly patients than in young patients. Acute illness in elderly patients tends to produce diffuse or multiple complaints, and the symptoms are often different from the classic presentation. Physical findings, such as peritoneal findings, may be absent in elderly patients. Demented patients often give reliable symptoms that aid in the diagnosis. Other preexisting diseases can influence the symptoms of acute illness.

3. The answer is E. [*Chapter 10 II; IV A 1*] The data base always includes a complete medical history, physical examination, problem list, and usually a preliminary plan. The primary data base should never include a definitive diagnosis because the supporting data have not been obtained. It is potentially hazardous to jump to a final diagnosis as a part of primary data collection.

4. The answer is D. [*Chapter 4 III*] The FH of alcohol consumption is important in long-range planning for the patient and his or her children, but it is of little importance to the management of the immediate problem. The details of the patient's own drinking habits are key to consideration of his or her current symptoms.

5. The answer is A. [*Chapter 10 II–IV*] Arriving at a "knee-jerk" diagnosis is dangerous in the most experienced hands and potentially deadly when done by the novice. It is nice record-keeping to have a full problem list, a fully developed differential diagnosis, and a cogent laboratory plan, but none of this can occur if premature diagnostic closure has precluded further considerations.

6. The answer is D. [*Chapter 6 III O*] The probability of a 32-year-old having abdominal aortic disease as the basis for his abdominal complaints is remote. On the other hand, general assessment for signs of acute inflammation or viscus perforation are rational and essential. For further information on assessment for the complaint of abdominal pain, see any standard surgical textbook.

7. The answer is C. [*Chapter 10 II A*] At this stage of the data collection, symptoms and signs are known at a level that does not allow a diagnosis. The problems should be listed at the level at which they are absolutely definable.

8. The answer is D. [*Chapter 11 VII C, D*] The oral case presentation should include all of, but no more than, the data necessary for resolution of the patient's immediate problems. The FH of alcohol consumption is a second level of information, which is not critical to the immediate management of the acutely ill person being discussed.

9. The answer is A. [*Chapter 11 VI A 5*] In correcting an error, it is acceptable to write a single line through the material, as long as it remains legible. Additional information can be added as long as it is dated and clearly marked as new information. It is legally unacceptable to remove and replace existing documents in a hospital chart.

10. The answer is C. [*Chapter 1 IV B 1*] Upon first meeting a patient, the student should offer his or her hand as a courtesy and to establish the first physical contact. Acquiring the radial pulse or the blood pressure, as well as palpating the scalp are relatively nonthreatening first physical contacts, but they come much later in the encounter. Taking the oral temperature does not involve touching the patient.

11. The answer is D. [*Chapter 8 III A 5 b, 7 b (3)*] Beginning several days after birth, the infant may manifest signs of withdrawal of maternal hormones. These signs may include breast swelling, nipple secretion of a milky substance (in both boys and girls), labial swelling, vaginal discharge, or bleeding. These may last for several weeks. Vaginal or scrotal ecchymoses are seen in breech presentations and result from intrauterine pressure on the presenting part.

12. The answer is A. [*Chapter 3 I G 2 i; Chapter 7 II A 1 a*] FH of breast cancer, parity history, breast-feeding history, and history of nipple discharge are all important factors to be explored when reviewing the risk for breast cancer. Fibrocystic disease has no known association with an increased risk of breast cancer.

13. The answer is D. [*Chapter 3 I G 2 n (2)*] Change in the established pattern of the menses is a clue to the possibility of serious disease and indicates a need for further workup. The other symptoms listed in the question, such as frequency and duration of periods, pains, or premenstrual symptoms, are important in terms of management.

14. The answer is E. [*Chapter 3 I G 2 n*] Sexual monogamy and the frequency of intercourse therein are not known to be cancer risk factors. The other choices listed in the question (i.e., age of onset of menses, age of assumption of sexual activity, number of sexual partners, and history of venereal warts) have all been implicated as cervical cancer risk factors.

15. The answer is D. [*Chapter 10 IV A 1 b*] Although the experienced clinician may choose, based on his or her sense of the mass discovered in the 30-year-old patient, to pursue diagnosis rapidly or reassess, this is not the perogative of the student in this setting. It is important to get help.

16. The answer is C. [*Chapter 7 II B 3 b (1)–(3)*] Lubrication of the speculum with a water-soluble gel will confound the reading of the specimen in the cytology laboratory. Only water can be used as a lubricant.

17. The answer is C. [*Chapter 7 II B 3 b (3) (b), c (1) (b), d (1) (c)*] The use of gel for the rectal examination is imperative, unlike the speculum examination which is introduced prior to the Pap smear and thus cannot be lubricated with gel. All genital examinations should be conducted with gloves as gloves are protective for both the patient and the examiner. The abdominal hand may be ungloved during the bimanual examination, and gloves should be replaced between vaginal and rectal examinations.

18. The answer is B. [*Chapter 7 II B 3 d (2)*] Review of pelvic anatomy will reveal that the adnexae cannot be adequately assessed from the rectum; however, the rectovaginal examination can assess the rectovaginal septum, posterior uterus, and rectal masses, and can be used to acquire a stool sample.

19. The answer is C. [*Chapter 11 III A 1–7*] There is considerable flexibility in the format for recording the PP and the FH; tabular, graphic, or narrative forms are all acceptable. The reader needs to know where to seek information about allergies to medication; thus, this information is a standard part of the PMH. Since the CC directs the reader's attention to the HPI, they should be recorded sequentially. The written record is formalized to guide all readers; therefore, regardless of the order in which the information is obtained, it must always be recorded in the order dictated by the framework.

20. The answer is C. [*Chapter 7 III D 1*] The lung on the side on which a hypomobile individual lies tends to be compressed and partially atelectatic. This transient phenomenon is reversed with rather prompt re-expansion when the pressure is released, and it is a source of crackles that do not represent any threat to the patient. While patients with profoundly impaired mobility do have difficulty clearing secretions, such phenomena would almost inevitably produce symptoms, such as cough or dyspnea, or signs, such as fever. Pulmonary edema is incompatible with a comfortable patient. Pulmonary fibrosis is almost never unilateral.

21. The answer is B. [*Chapter 9 I B 2 c (3), 7 a*] The most appropriate action in dealing with the 89-year-old woman with dementia who presents with abdominal pain would be to presume that the pain is real and to act accordingly. While demented patients have significant problems with memory, they are often able to provide accurate descriptions of acute symptoms. While a spouse's information may be important to corroborate this information, it should not be used to discount it.

22. The answer is D. [*Chapter 3 I E 2 c, f, g, k; F*] The PMH is obtained to ascertain any medical information that relates to the patient's present or future health. It does not concern other members of the family, which should appear in the FH, a separate and distinct part of the history.

23. The answer is B. [*Chapter 6 III T 6 d, 7 a–d*] The classic test for the pyramidal tract is the Babinski reflex, but in patients where this is difficult to elicit, the Oppenheim reflex or the Chaddock reflex manifests the same function. The Hoffman reflex assesses the pyramidal tract function in the upper extremities. The Romberg reflex is a test of cerebellar function.

24. The answer is E. [*Chapter 7 III F; V D*] Any one or more of the factors listed in the question could contribute to this patient's failure to answer questions. Angry withdrawal, deafness, dementia, and inability to speak due to a brain abnormality are all possible in an elderly, neurologically impaired patient who is in a strange environment. The examiner's task is to determine which of the factors is operative by obtaining information from the family and by physically examining the patient.

25. The answer is D. [*Chapter 7 III B*] The medical student does not have enough information to know how best to transfer this patient. However, he or she cannot conduct the examination while the patient is dressed and strapped in the sitting position. If the patient can move himself onto the table, allowing him to do so will help preserve his dignity. Only if it is known that he cannot, should others be called on to help the patient.

26. The answer is D. [*Chapter 7 III B*] The medical student should keep in mind that the patient's wife can offer comfort and information needed to help assess whether the patient should be placed in a nursing home. By helping the wife to cope with the emotional impact of the situation, the medical student will be better able to gather important information about the patient and his home environment. The patient is likely to be disturbed by his wife's distress, which could further complicate the student's task. Thus, it is best that the student address the wife's distress and then proceed with the examination.

27. The answer is C. [*Chapter 9 I B 5*] In assessing elderly patients, the PMH and medication use provide essential information concerning chronic conditions and current medical risks. In this supposedly "healthy" man, the social history will yield the most important data regarding his disposition. A complete mental status examination should be performed in all complete evaluations of elderly patients to establish a baseline or to detect subtle deficits. A FH would be important for this gentleman's offspring but would have little value in evaluating and caring for an 85-year-old individual who has outlived any important inherited or familial disorder.

28. The answer is C. [*Chapter 8 III A 5 d (2), C 5 b (1)–(3), D 3 c*] A variety of innocent murmurs are heard throughout childhood. Peripheral pulmonic stenosis, an innocent murmur heard in the newborn, disappears by 3 months of age. Thus, the diagnosis is confirmed retrospectively when the murmur is no longer audible. This murmur is a midsystolic murmur, which is heard with equal intensity in both sides of the chest, because it originates from the peripheral pulmonary arteries. The other innocent murmurs of childhood listed in the question (i.e., Still's murmur, venous hum, carotid bruit, and pulmonary flow) may all be appreciated in the school-age child.

29. The answer is E. [*Chapter 4 VII A*] Accidents or injuries in the present or past should increase suspicions of family violence. Drug and alcohol abuse are associated with family violence, and family violence tends to run in families.

30. The answer is C. [*Chapter 9 II B 1 a*] Body temperature should not drop to 35° C in the absence of decreased metabolism, uncontrolled vasodilation (i.e., shock), or environmental deprivation (i.e., accidental hypothermia). Oral and axillary temperatures are lower than rectal temperatures, so they would not clarify this patient's hypothermia. While all measuring instruments should be inspected periodically for malfunction, the patient described in the question needs the clinician's immediate attention.

31. The answer is D. [*Chapter 6 III A 1–5*] The patient who is dyspneic at rest or with the minimal moving that occurs with a physical examination is recognized readily. Cardiovascular reserve is only detected with more intense activity. An irritated liver is seldom evident until punch tenderness is elicited or blood tests are done, although in severe cases pronounced jaundice may be observed on greeting the patient. Similarly, only in the worst cases of esophageal dysfunction will the patient be seen having difficulty with saliva during the interview and examination, and pancreatic problems are most unlikely to be detected this way.

32. The answer is C. [*Chapter 10 V C 3 c*] The most definitive diagnosis of diabetes mellitus has been shown to be an elevated fasting serum glucose. The random glucose—that is, glucose drawn without regard to the last glucose intake by the patient—is essentially impossible to interpret (it is not specific). The 5-hour postprandial glucose may be normal in an early diabetic, so it does not meet the criterion of sensitivity. The renal handling of glucose is sufficiently variable within normal serum glucose ranges so it is insufficiently specific for the diagnosis of diabetes. The range of normal 30-minute postprandial glucose in the serum is sufficiently variable among normals that it is also not sufficiently specific to establish the diagnosis of diabetes mellitus.

33. The answer is E. [*Chapter 4 II B 2*] Sexual histories should be part of all medical histories as sexuality is an important issue throughout the life span. While sexuality is a concern of all age-groups, there is a great variety of human sexual behavior. Sexual functioning can be affected by many health conditions and medications but may not be reported without inquiry by the clinician. With the increase of STDs, a sexual history and counseling about prevention should be provided for all individuals at risk.

34. The answer is C. [*Chapter 11 V B 4; VI C*] Admission orders are written in the chart at the time a patient enters the hospital; they are essentially directives to the nursing (nonclinician) staff. Informed consent is a separate document in the patient's record and should be obtained when the clinician plans a surgical procedure. It is not requested on the order sheet.

35. The answer is E. [*Chapter 7 IV*] It may eventually be necessary to try any or all of the approaches suggested in the question but the student must first attempt to establish rapport with the patient. Despite the label of retardation, it is sometimes possible to obtain valuable information if time is taken to gain the patient's trust. The remainder of the encounter will be markedly improved by taking a few minutes early on to gain the patient's confidence.

36. The answer is E. [*Chapter 7 IV C 1–3*] Amenorrhea in a 35-year-old woman must be considered a symptom of pregnancy until determined otherwise. Mentally retarded individuals may engage in sexual intimacy without full awareness of the implications. It is important to assess this patient's freedom in her environment and her self-care activities. Birth control protection and other medications are obviously important for their implications in this situation.

37. The answer is D. [*Chapter 7 IV C 1–3; V A 1–3*] In searching for causes for amenorrhea, the thyroid gland, the abdomen, and the pelvis must be assessed. The breast examination may give clues as to pregnancy, as well as being prudent because of the woman's age. A detailed mental status examination in this circumstance is of little value. The patient is known to be retarded, and a mental status evaluation will merely frustrate her and perhaps make the more important parts of the focused examination difficult.

38. The answer is C. [*Chapter 7 IV A 1*] This is a situation in which the novice needs experienced advice. Jumping to the laboratory without a physical examination is costly and often blindly nonproductive. A physical examination cannot be adequately done on a fully clothed patient, but forcing the examination is detrimental to both the clinician and the patient. The preceptor should be consulted in this case.

39. The answer is D. [*Chapter 11 VI B 4 a*] Before any information is transmitted, the guardianship or legal representative of incompetent patients must be known to the clinician. The clinician should also be acquainted with the laws of the community regarding medical care and information-sharing with guardians of mentally retarded individuals. Often the placement of a retarded individual in a group home setting shifts the legal responsibility to the officials of the home or to the state. It is important to know the rights of the clinician and the patient in this situation.

40. The answer is C. [*Chapter 9 II B 7 c*] Even in persons with widespread atherosclerosis and extremes of age, superficial temporal artery pulses are usually preserved. If they cannot be felt, one must consider temporal arteritis since this eminently treatable condition can cause irreversible blindness if the diagnosis is not made in time. If the clinician feels inept, a more senior clinician can be consulted. The location of the superficial temporal artery pulses varies only slightly from host to host.

41. The answer is C. [*Chapter 4 II B 1–3*] Questions in the sexual history should be nonjudgmental and generally open-ended to obtain accurate and valid information. It is also important for clinicians to use neutral terms when discussing sexual behavior. Labeling behavior promiscuous is both imprecise (i.e., more than one partner may be "promiscuous" to some people whereas more than ten partners may be "normal" to others) and judgmental.

42. The answer is E. [*Chapter 11 VII D 1 a, b*] Although marital status should be recorded in the full written history and physical examination, it is of insufficient medical importance to warrant inclusion in the more terse and directed oral case presentation. Age, sex, race, and occupation have potential medical implications and are critical elements of the verbal picture being drawn by the presenter.

43. The answer is B. [*Chapter 10 II C 1, 2*] The presence of diabetes must be kept in mind at all times in the management of the patient, regardless of the nature of the presenting problem. The hysterectomy and hip fracture are legitimate inactive problems and of no concern now, but they must remain as part of the patient's comprehensive medical history. The duodenal ulcer may recur, so it must be noted. The pneumonia is not a problem now, but since pneumococcal disease *may* indicate a specific lack of resistance to this organism, it must be carried forward on the inactive problem list.

44. The answer is C. [*Chapter 8 III B 7 c, C 7 b, E 5 b; Table 8-5*] During infancy, phimosis (tightness of the foreskin so that it cannot be drawn back from over the glans penis) is physiologic. By age 3, most boys (90%) have a fully retractable foreskin. Therefore, phimosis is a pathologic finding in the adolescent and requires surgical correction. Tanner stage III genitalia indicates that the male is in midpuberty. Gynecomastia (in boys) and comedones (blackheads) are common findings in the adolescent. Second molars erupt during early adolescence (ages 12–13).

45. The answer is C. [*Chapter 7 V D 4*] Unduly high scores for the level of cognitive function often occur with individuals who have extensive formal education, which diminishes the sensitivity of the Folstein test in detecting dysfunction; the same effect does not occur with repeated test administration. The test was designed to achieve a high level of specificity, and the price was relatively low inherent sensitivity. Poorly educated individuals tend to lose points independently of cognitive skills, as do uninterested subjects; these underperformances can produce false-positive results, reducing test specificity.

46. The answer is D. [*Chapter 1 IV B 1 b, 2*] The deep abdominal pressure necessary to delineate the aortic margins is mildly painful to most patients. Patients should be warned that the examination will be uncomfortable. Skillful and careful insertion of the otoscope speculum should be painless unless the ear is infected. Breast examination properly done does not cause pain unless the breast is diseased or the patient is immediately premenstrual. Thyroid palpation should never cause pain. Gentle palpation of the testicles causes a sensation described as "visceral" but not painful.

47. The answer is D. [*Chapter 6 III L 1, 2*] Direct measurement of the arterial system includes palpation of all arteries, including the femoral, popliteal, dorsalis pedis, and posterior tibial arteries of the legs. Further information can be obtained by measuring blood pressure in both thighs. Indirect measurement of arterial integrity includes assessment of the hair distribution on the legs. Arterial insufficiency is associated with decreased hair and thinning of the skin of the lower extremity. By compressing and releasing finger nails and toe nails, peripheral vascular integrity can be assessed indirectly. Homans' sign is a finding of dubious significance but is a test of deep venous thrombosis.

48. The answer is E. [*Chapter 11 VII D 3*] Since the purpose of the oral case presentation is to provide the data essential to assessment of the problem at hand, a history of breast cancer in a male patient's family is irrelevant to a complaint of breathing problems. As breathing difficulty may arise from either cardiovascular or pulmonary problems, full disclosure of historical and physical examination information pertinent to these systems, both positive and negative, is indicated. In every case presentation, it is necessary to state the patients' CC as they describe it (to avoid misinterpretation of the symptom) and to define all of its characteristics as outlined in Chapter 3.

49. The answer is D. [*Chapter 4 VIII A 2, B*] The patient needs consultation about how to manage the effect of her illness on her daily routine. This includes an assessment of the direct symptom effect, other daily behaviors affected, and the resources of the patient to change her living situation if the symptoms cannot be more effectively managed. A discussion of medications that may or may not be of value to the patient is not appropriate to this visit unless initiated by the patient.

50. The answer is D. [*Chapter 7 V A 1–3*] The marathoner is most likely experiencing an age-related decline in performance, and although he might need assessment of mood and affect to determine how he is coping with this, it is not an urgent problem; thus, his mental status examination could be safely deferred. The elderly are most apt to be mislabeled as to cognitive state and ought to have baseline mental status examinations. Patients with histories of mental illness or of physical illness that can include prominent cognitive deficits, such as HIV, share this need. Sharp decline in school performance can be a principal sign of depression in a child or teen, and identification of this can sometimes prevent a tragic suicide.

51. The answer is D. [*Chapter 8 III B 9 a (5)*] The 9-month-old sits alone well, pulls to stand, but may not yet cruise (walk around holding on to furniture for support). The 9-month-old child babbles mama, dada nonspecifically and is able to easily transfer small objects from one hand to another. The ability to play games, such as peekaboo, reflects the emergence of the concept of object permanence.

52. The answer is D. [*Chapter 9 II B 1 c*] In the presence of established orthostatic hypotension (or its equivalent, orthostatic tachycardia) in the sitting position, the patient should not stand up, as this may reduce perfusion to the brain and other vital organs; the clinician must defer not only standing measurements of pulse and blood pressure, but also other maneuvers requiring the standing position until they can be taken safely. All the other elements listed in the question (i.e., carotid palpation, breath-holding, rectal examination, and abdominal palpation) rarely produce complications, but the 82-year-old patient described in the question is at no special risk.

53. The answer is C. [*Chapter 10 II B 1*] Although the clinician may strongly suspect pulmonary embolism on the basis of the acute symptoms, there are not enough data to make this diagnosis, and incriminating it at this early date would constitute dangerous premature closure. Chest pain and shortness of breath, as the presenting complaints, should constitute the first two problems as this is the level at which they are definitive. The history of diabetes and of pregnancy, since each is a concomitant medical problem, should be retained as a part of the active problem list.

54. The answer is B. [*Chapter 10 II D; III A–C*] A tender cord is suggestive, but not diagnostic, of deep venous thrombosis. Superficial thrombophlebitis without deep venous thrombosis is common in pregnancy and has very different prognostic and therapeutic implications than the latter diagnosis. At this point in the assessment of the patient, the clinician must resist the temptation to arrive at diagnoses and stay with the observable findings: tender cord, increased heart and respiratory rate, and the objective finding of an enlarged uterus with fetus.

55. The answer is E. [*Chapter 10 III A–C*] The patient's sex, age, and the nature of the chest pain are all inconsistent with myocardial infarction. Pulmonary embolism is a hazard of pregnancy and presents with pleuritic chest pain and shortness of breath. Any young patient presenting with chest pain and shortness of breath with chest splinting could have either early pneumonia or viral (coxsackievirus B) pleurodynia. In this setting, it is important to rule in or out the potentially life-threatening diseases: embolism, pneumothorax, and pneumonia. The least likely diagnosis is the benign viral pleuritis.

56. The answer is D. [*Chapter 10 IV A 1 d*] Even though the patient is pregnant, the presenting problem does not directly involve the pregnancy. At some point, the obstetrician may need to get involved, but the acute problem is one for an internist. An EKG, in this situation, may support the diagnosis of pulmonary embolism if specific alterations are present. The arterial blood gases will indicate both diagnostic possibilities and also the need for oxygen therapy. (A low Po_2 in conjunction with a normal Pco_2 in this clinical setting would be supportive evidence for pulmonary embolism.) The gases are most important in following the patient's progress in this situation. Chest x-ray is necessary here to determine the presence or absence of pneumothorax or pneumonia and to serve as parenchymal basis for the critical ventilation/perfusion scan—the best currently available noninvasive test for pulmonary embolism.

57. The answer is C. [*Chapter 1 IV B 1 d*] Universal Precautions demand that gloves always be worn to draw blood from any patient to reduce the risk of direct contact with the patients' body fluids. Touching normal skin surfaces, such as an abdominal palpation, is of no risk to the examiner. Inspection of the oral cavity does not involve direct physical contact. Only under conditions of strict reverse isolation is gloving required for all maneuvers to reduce the risk of spread of skin organisms to a compromised patient.

58. The answer is D. [*Chapter 11 IV A, B*] The progress note is the hourly or daily record of change in a patient's condition or in management plans that affect the patient both immediately and over time. The appearance of a dramatic alteration in status takes precedence over such things as discharge planning and preempts long-range planning discussions in the progress note. Plans for management, results of emergent studies, and the patient's subjective symptoms are critical to understanding and communicating status changes.

59. The answer is B. [*Chapter 6 IV D 1*] The only blood test recommended for both men and women at any age is a serum cholesterol obtained every 5 years. Hemoglobin and hematocrit are not warranted for men but may be important in menstruating women. Thyroid function tests are unnecessary on asymptomatic men but may be tested in asymptomatic older women. Serum electrolytes are never recommended as a routine. Fasting serum glucose is also not recommended routinely and should be ordered only if symptoms warrant it.

60. The answer is D. [*Chapter 6 III O 5 c*] A positive Murphy's sign would suggest gallbladder disease. The finding of a positive fluid wave and a positive shifting dullness implies the presence of acidic fluid within the abdomen. Peritonitis often presents with hypoactive bowel sounds and would be evidenced on the physical examination with positive rebound tenderness.

61. The answer is C. [*Chapter 6 III K 4 a–e*] The patient in the question presents with a history, physical examination, and chest x-ray consistent with acute bacterial pneumonia. The least likely finding would be normal or vesicular breath sounds at the involved lung segment. Pneumonia characteristically presents with coarse rhonchi, a positive E to A change (egophony), increased vocal fremitus, and may present with decreased breath sounds at that site.

62. The answer is D. [*Chapter 4 V B 1–3, C 1–3*] The RDAs are frequently used as standards to compare the adequacy of an individual's intake of nutrients. However, these recommendations are developed to estimate the needs of healthy populations. The elderly are a very diverse population in terms of health status. The RDAs do not take into account the multiple medical problems of the elderly, which may affect nutrient needs.

63. The answer is C. [*Chapter 7 III D 2*] On a ventilator, the respiratory rate is set by the machine, not by the host's brain's responses to blood oxygen and CO_2 levels. This patient has needed a respirator precisely because such responses are ineffective due to the brain dysfunction. Thus, tachypnea, which is otherwise a very important and often sensitive sign of respiratory trouble, cannot be found. Rhonchi of the type described often reflect the noisy flow of gas delivered from the machine to the host's airways and, therefore, may lack significance. Localized dullness is distinctly abnormal and implies lung or pleural disease. Poor audibility of lung sounds may reflect the patient's inability to breathe with the open mouth on command, due to both the respirator and the coma; the same hindrances beset attempted fremitus.

64. The answer is E. [*Chapter 9 II B 3 c (2)*] The examiner can palpate only the posterior aspect of the prostate. This is where most, but not all, cancers of the prostate originate. All the effects of the prostate on the urinary tract are anterior, where the organ surrounds the prostatic urethra and, thus, may occur despite a normal posterior portion. Localized hyperplasia of the median bar at this site is a well-known cause of prostatic symptoms in this setting.

65. The answer is B. [*Chapter 1 III B 1, 2, 4*] While it is appropriate for a student to seek support after a distressing encounter, the patient should never be identified unless the classmate is also involved in the patient's care or unless the patient gives consent.

66. The answer is C. [*Chapter 6 III F 2, 3*] The patient described in the question presents with the Argyll Robertson pupil, a condition seen in tertiary syphilis. The patient's eyes show that the pupils do not react to direct light, nor consensually to light. The ability of the eye to converge and the pupils to constrict when changing focus to a close object implies that accommodation is intact. No evidence is given regarding CN VI, which would be determined by extraocular motions. Nystagmus is rapid movements of the eye in various fields of gaze. Information regarding nystagmus is not given in this clinical case.

67. The answer is B. [*Chapter 9 I B 1, 2*] The case described in the question demonstrates the often subtle nature of the CC in elderly individuals, especially in cases of mental status changes. The differential diagnosis in this case is broad. The clinician should exclude a medication effect, obtain a thorough history including the PMH, and perform a complete physical examination with emphasis on the neurologic examination and mental status. The son's observations are crucial in this case and should not be ignored. This example is based on an actual case. The patient had a spontaneous subdural hematoma, which was evacuated, and she returned home in excellent condition.

68. The answer is B. [*Chapter 1 V A 1–6*] Symptoms are any problems experienced by the patient, which may be used to identify the underlying pathology. Signs are physical indications of the disease, which may be visible to anyone or specifically to the clinician. Diagnosis is the underlying cause of any signs or symptoms. ADLs are a measure of a patient's level of functioning. Prognosis is the predicted course of a disease or condition.

69. The answer is C. [*Chapter 9 II B 7 a*] Most or all diastolic murmurs are significant. Over half of all elderly patients have murmurs, many of which are totally benign. The locale and intensity of these murmurs vary, but only an intensity of III or greater should be taken as independent evidence of importance.

70. The answer is D. [*Chapter 7 IV A 1–3, B 1–3*] To perform a comprehensive physical examination on a patient with mental retardation, adequate time must be allowed, which may be extended over more than one visit. Asking someone with whom the patient is familiar to remain often calms the patient during the procedure. Much information is obtained by observing the patient moving freely. Vision is a difficult part of the examination to test and is best accomplished by observing the patient's response to visual stimuli. While occasionally done, premedicating a patient with a sedative is very controversial and not widely acceptable medical practice.

71. The answer is C. [*Chapter 4 V A 4*] Most Americans need to change the distribution of calories contributed by the macronutrients: protein, fat, and carbohydrate. Fat intake should be reduced to 30% of total calories, and carbohydrate intake should be increased to 50%–60% of total calories. Diets that are high in protein and fat from animal sources are also usually high in saturated fat and cholesterol (cholesterol is only found in foods of animal origin).

72. The answer is E. [*Chapter 6 III F 2, 3, T 2 b–d*] The eye examination of the patient presented in the question is consistent with the diagnosis of Wernicke's encephalopathy from thiamine deficiency. Pupillary responses and visual acuity implies that CN II is intact. The only abnormality on extraocular movement is that the lateral rectus muscle in the right eye, controlled by CN VI, is abnormal. This implies that CN IV and CN III are intact. Rapid fine movement is present in upper gaze, implying vertical nystagmus.

73–76. The answers are: 73-E, 74-C, 75-A, 76-D. [*Chapter 2 I B 1 a, b; II D 2, 6 a, 7*] The clinician should introduce him- or herself immediately to the patient and ask how the patient wants to be addressed. He or she should then provide a clear statement of the purpose of the interview, state how long it will take, explain the examinations to be performed, and discuss the expected outcomes.

The clinician may find it helpful to mirror the patient's language style to improve rapport. However, communication works more easily when the representational systems match.

Repetition is rarely helpful. However, restating a question, using different words, may help to clarify the question for the patient. However, if the patient in the question does not understand what dysuria means, simply repeating the question will not clarify the meaning.

Closed questions should be used to clarify or guide a patient after a sufficient data base has been collected. They are not used appropriately to elicit initial information.

77–81. The answers are: 77-B, 78-A, 79-D, 80-A, 81-C. [*Chapter 11 IV B 1–4*] The observation of a quantitative measurement, such as the pulse rate, is always recorded as objective data. Any symptom reported by the patient is recorded as subjective data. The clinician's decision to order a test is a part of the plan. The definition of a syndrome or a diagnosis is a clinical decision made by the clinician and recorded under assessment, since it represents an impression or interpretation of information.

82–86. The answers are: 82-C, 83-E, 84-A, 85-D, 86-A. [*Chapter 3 I C 1 a, 4, D 3 a, e, F 1 a, 2, G 1 a, 2 c*] The relationship an individual has with a spouse is an integral part of the PP, and a patient's concern for a spouse's health is one domain of the relationship. It can significantly alter how the patient will deal with his or her own illness.

Occasional headaches are a common ailment. Without a major change in the description, severity, or frequency, headaches should be noted in the ROS.

IDDM is an active problem. Even if this is not the primary reason for admission, the clinician must have full knowledge (i.e., all the seven parameters) of the disease so that treatment and adjustment for stress can be made.

The FH is important so that familial and genetic diseases can be screened. Knowing that the patient's father died of a stroke at an early age may very well alter the screening and treatment of hypertension.

A productive cough is an active problem; it, therefore, becomes part of the HPI, and all seven parameters of the cough need to be described.

87–91. The answers are: 87-B, 88-A, 89-C, 90-B, 91-D. [*Chapter 8 III A 4 b (2), B 3 c, 4 e, 7 b (2), C 8 a, D 2 b (1)*] The young infant commonly manifests several skin eruptions, such as infantile acne and seborrhea. Seborrhea is a yellow-tinged, greasy, scaly eruption, which typically begins during the first few months of life. When located on the scalp, it is called "cradle cap." The face, eyebrows, and skin folds may also be involved.

Pressure on the newborn head during labor and delivery may result in a variety of swellings and asymmetries. A caput represents edema of the scalp tissues. This is an ill-defined area of swelling, which crosses the midline and is usually found on the top or back of the head.

Most toddlers appear to have flat feet. This appearance is due to the presence of fat pads, which obscure the longitudinal arch of the foot. This appearance is not predictive of true flat feet, which are sometimes seen in older children.

Candida albicans infection is common during infancy. The two commonest manifestations of *Candida* infection are thrush and *Candida* diaper rash. Thrush appears as white plaques on the tongue or buccal mucosa. Unlike formula or breast milk, these plaques do not scrape off easily with pressure from a tongue blade.

Shedding of primary teeth begins around 6 years of age, usually with the loss of the lower central incisors. Eruption of permanent dentition begins within 1–2 years after shedding begins. Delayed eruption of permanent teeth is usually either hereditary or due to delayed shedding of primary teeth.

92–96. The answers are: 92-B, 93-A, 94-B, 95-A, 96-E. [*Chapter 10 V C*] The combination of symptoms, such as cough, fever, and pleuritic chest pain, in a young person are highly suggestive of pneumonia, a diagnosis best confirmed by chest x-ray.

Crushing substernal chest pain is the classic symptom of myocardial infarction. The EKG may be definitive and, if not, is certainly essential to monitoring the course of the illness or beginning the process of "ruling out" the most dangerous diagnostic possibility.

The combination of historical data and physical findings (i.e., sudden onset of shortness of breath) are most consistent with spontaneous pneumothorax. It is essential for the proper care of the patient to establish that pneumothorax is present and to determine the degree of the lung compromise.

A heart rate of 160/min demands a definition of the conduction problem present. The proper choice of therapeutic intervention requires a knowledge of the source of the tachycardia (atrial or ventricular), which can usually be defined from a rhythm strip or a 12-lead EKG.

Petechial rashes are secondary to platelet problems until proven otherwise. This woman's problem may be either inadequate platelet numbers or dysfunction of platelets. The most important test in this situation is a platelet count.

97–101. The answers are: 97-E, 98-C, 99-B, 100-D, 101-B. [*Chapter 11 V B*] Orders not to resuscitate should be based on the expressed wishes of the patient or a legally and morally suitable surrogate, not on any outside party's assessment of prognosis or quality of life. Oxygen is generally beneficial to individuals who are short of breath and free of complications. Individuals with major fluid deficits or unstable renal function can be managed better by recording intake and output and frequent weighing. Stool testing for occult blood is a standard monitoring technique for patients with acute abdominal pain. The exhausted mountain climber ought not to be subjected to the sleep interruption that attends hourly vital signs around the clock. One might seek frequent vital sign measurements with observation of respiratory rate in between (something that does not risk awakening the sleeper).

102–105. The answers are: 102-C, 103-D, 104-A, 105-B. [*Chapter 5 I C 1 a, 2, 3, D 2 b*] Pneumonia is an acute disease whose successful treatment follows an objective rational approach. However, clinicians may become easily frustrated by some aspect of the treatment or symptoms. A smoker with emphysema has two chronic problems and a mutual participation model is best used in providing care. The frustration of both the clinician and the patient may parallel each other and lead to difficult interactions. The patient with lupus who believes that proper nutrition can cure her disease has a folk belief. The patient's views of health and illness can be a serious barrier to communication in the clinical setting. The personal biography of the medical student leads to the potential for a difficult dyad.

106–110. The answers are: 106-C, 107-B, 108-E, 109-D, 110-A. [*Chapter 6 III B 5 a, b*] A comatose patient with a history of a drug overdose who presents with a *regularly* irregular sine wave pattern of respiration has Cheyne-Stokes respirations, which are seen in a variety of comatose patients and are not by themselves prognostically important. A 17-year-old asthmatic patient with a respiratory rate of 47 is experiencing tachypnea (respiratory rate over 16), which implies great distress. Apnea is prolonged periods without respiratory effort, which is seen in a variety of clinical situations, particularly obesity. A patient with severe head trauma who presents with an *irregularly* irregular respiratory pattern has Biot's respirations, which imply significant brain derangement and a very poor prognosis.

111–114. The answers are: 111-A, 112-B, 113-E, 114-C [*Chapter 8 III A 8 b, B 9 b, c, C 4 d, E 3 e*] Examination for congenital hip dislocation begins in the newborn nursery and continues throughout infancy. The Ortolani and Barlow maneuvers are the most important components of the newborn hip examination. After the first few months of life, movement of a dislocated or dislocatable hip, in or out of the acetabulum becomes increasingly difficult. At that point, the ability to fully (almost to 90°) and equally abduct the hips (while they are in 90° of flexion) becomes very important in this evaluation.

Primitive reflexes supply information about the neuromaturation. Like other developmental milestones, primitive reflexes have predictable times of appearance and disappearance. The parachute reflex is elicited in an infant beginning at approximately 6–9 months. Absence of this reflex after 12 months is abnormal, as is a response that involves only one side of the body.

Inspection and palpation of the neck is a routine part of all pediatric physical examinations. Thyroid disease is commoner, however, in adolescents than in the younger age-groups. Thyroid examination includes inspection of the gland while standing in front of and to the side of the patient. This is followed by palpation, which is performed with the examiner standing behind the seated patient.

Language development is a major developmental issue for the toddler. History from the parent may elicit information related to content and clarity of speech; listening to the child in the examining room may be used as an opportunity to confirm the history. At age 2 years, approximately one-half of the toddler's speech should be intelligible; by age 4 years, the child should be understood most of the time.

115–119. The answers are: 115-A, 116-B, 117-D, 118-A, 119-D. [*Chapter 11 VI B 4, 6, D 2, E 3*] Gonorrhea tests and AIDS diagnoses must be reported to state or federal health departments. If child abuse is suspected, the clinician must contact the appropriate governmental agency responsible for youth services. In general, teenagers' use of birth control pills or alcohol drug use should be kept confidential. A patient's spouse or parents do not need to be notified.

120–124. The answers are: 120-E, 121-A, 122-C, 123-B, 124-D. [*Chapter 4 IX D 1–5*] Mr. M's change to a more quiet demeanor needs to be differentiated from a depression or feelings of isolation. His self-limited verbal and physical interactions coupled with his desire to have someone present, but not necessarily interacting with him, is also a clue to the fact that he may be nearing death. It is not uncommon for a patient to express some religious concerns at this time.

The changes Mrs. P has recently made in her closest relationships (i.e., friends, clinician) and her belief that these friends are overreacting to her illness are clues to the fact that she is denying her illness at this time. It is important to differentiate denial from anger, which is a later stage. Her statement that a mistake in judgment has been made and her report that the symptoms disappeared before she went for consultation are further clues of her denial.

Mrs. C seems to be attempting to "strike a bargain" with God by taking on, finally, a task she had been postponing for many years. Her compliance and cooperation are attempts to be "a good patient" and not invoke the anger of anyone with whom she must interact. She is trying to invoke good luck by not continuing past behaviors that she feels have brought her "bad luck." It is important to evaluate Mrs. C's denial of pain to be sure it is not a generalized denial as in stage 1. In light of her other behaviors, it is more likely that she in fact is no longer using denial but has moved on, beyond anger, trying to bargain for the best outcome possible, not only for herself, but for her daughter as well.

Mr. P's change in outlook and feeling sorry for himself must be differentiated from depression. Unlike the depression stage however, Mr. P is active and not withdrawn; he is actively complaining to anyone and making sure his needs are not ignored. He is pursuing with energy his belief that he was mislead by his employer. He is demanding in his desire to communicate to persons in authority so he can let them know what a raw deal has come his way. It is important to note that he chooses not to make the clinician an object of his feelings; an individual in this stage would be reluctant to cut off the relationship or risk engendering the displeasure of the very person whose attention he or she may come to depend upon. This is in contrast to the denial stage when the clinician is often the most direct object of the patient's displeasure.

Miss J's resignations should be seen differently from Mrs. P's refusal to see old friends, because Miss J has also reported difficulty in falling asleep and difficulty upon awakening. Her forgetfulness and uncharacteristic disorganization are also clues. The most revealing statement is the one from her students, who observe her over the longest periods of time. Their view of her as "all inside" herself is most indicative of depression; the person in denial or in anger, or bargaining would more likely be viewed as "all outside themselves."

125–129. The answers are: 125-A, 126-D, 127-C, 128-E, 129-B. [*Chapter 9 I A, B; II A, B*] The cases described in the question illustrate the crucial role of the social history in caring for elderly patients. The 65-year-old man who had a below-knee amputation will need skilled nursing to monitor the wound infection and the diabetes. However, he appears to have adequate social support for all other ADLs. The 80-year-old woman admitted for a hip replacement has a presumably temporary problem with ambulation. Her ability to care for herself in a second floor home would be next to impossible, and temporary placement would be appropriate. The 75-year-old man hospitalized for a gallbladder operation should function well at home without in-home care despite the fact that he lives alone. The 80-year-old man with Alzheimer's disease has a progressive disease, coupled with a new hip fracture, which will compromise his ability to remain home with an elderly spouse. The 80-year-old woman with heart disease and COPD will need skilled nursing and may suffer nutritionally while she is recuperating and living alone.

130–134. The answers are: 130-C, 131-D, 132-A, 133-E, 134-B. [*Chapter 6 III F; T 2 h, 6 d, 7 a; Chapter 7 IV D 3*] Gross motor function is best assessed through observation and history. Babinski reflexes are a test of pyramidal tract function. A positive Romberg test and poor gait are indicative of cerebellar dysfunction. Difficulty swallowing, as often occurs in cerebral palsy, implies CN X dysfunction, which presents with excessive drooling. In patients with mental retardation, it is difficult to do a complete test of the eyes. Information is obtained best by watching the patient follow something with their eyes.

135–137. The answers are: 135-C, 136-B, 137-A. [*Chapter 5 II B 1 b; II C 1 a, D 1 a*] The student who interviewed her third grade teacher overidentified with her patient. Because of her emotional involvement, she confused her personal needs with the needs of her patient. The patient with heart disease is hostile and angry as part of his mourning process for lost activities. It is very stressful to report loss of valued work activities, relationships, and energy. The woman with severe headaches is being treated in a system that has a mind–body split. Patients who do not have a clear organic basis for their physical symptoms are highly suspect to both their caretakers and themselves.

138–142. The answers are: 138-A, 139-E, 140-B, 141-E, 142-D. [*Chapter 10 III B 2 a*] Young adults are commonly seen for traumatic injuries to the muscles and joints, especially those individuals who are strenuously physically active. The temporal relationship to the marathon should alert the clinician to the high probability of a musculoskeletal problem.

Despite the fact that this 72-year-old man presents with what appear to be respiratory problems, the history of hypertension, the acuteness of the problem, and the deoxygenation all suggest cardiac failure manifested as acute pulmonary edema in which the failing system is the cardiovascular with the respiratory system being only secondarily involved.

Flank pain may be generated from the gastrointestinal tract, the pelvic organs (reproductive), or the urinary system. The history of high calcium intake and the magnitude of the pain is most suggestive of ureteral stone, a common complication of excessive calcium intake in otherwise healthy individuals.

Acute diarrhea must be related to the gastrointestinal system, either as a primary infectious or inflammatory disorder or secondary to endocrine or systemic disease. The acuteness of the problem and its temporal relationship to a mountain camping trip are suggestive of an ingested organism, which has caused local bowel symptoms.

Amenorrhea in a healthy sexually active woman is pregnancy until proven otherwise. The primary system to be considered here is the reproductive, and the first tests are those for pregnancy. If pregnancy is disproven, then further consideration of less common causes for amenorrhea may be pursued.

143–147. The answers are: 143-C, 144-D, 145-A, 146-B, 147-E. [*Chapter 3 I A, C, E 2 f, G*] All interactions are preceded by a formal introduction and role clarification. The CC is the patient's agenda and, thus, needs to be addressed first as the interview begins. The CC defines the first problem to be followed up in the HPI. By convention, the immunization history is part of the PMH, which should be taken after the HPI but always before the ROS, which is the final check list of the medical history.

148–150. The answers are: 148-E, 149-D, 150-C. [*Chapter 11 V*] Group home workers who are not the primary caregivers are only occasionally aware of specific allergies of their patients. However, this information must be determined since antibiotic or other chemical therapy may be required in the course of treatment of the injuries and their complications.

Hypoglycemia and dehydration are likely in the teenager who passes out during a ball game. Both are likely causes of new syncope, and because they have specific treatments, they should be pursued.

After axillary surgery, it is important to avoid using the ipsilateral arm for blood pressure readings, intravenous lines, or blood drawing, but there is no such proscription if it is only the arm itself upon which there was surgery. This patient, however, must be encouraged to ambulate with assistance at least three times a day after abdominal surgery.

Appendix: Abbreviations That Are Useful in Recording Histories and Physical Examinations

Terms in italic are foreign words, most often Latin; their translations follow immediately in parentheses. Other parenthetic entries are self-explanatory. Entries separated by commas represent unrelated terms, any of which may be signified by the abbreviation; interpretation of the abbreviation thus depends on context. Capitalizations employed are those considered most widely accepted, most clear, and easiest to use and remember. Periods are not used after medical abbreviations. Although some terms are marked as applying equally to singular and plural forms, there are many others that are used more or less indiscriminately to abbreviate both singular and plural forms.

The ampersand (&) is treated here as though it were the word "and" for purposes of alphabetizing these abbreviations. By contrast, numbers are treated as nonexistent in alphabetizing here.

–A–

a	*ante* (before)
A2	aortic component of the second heart sound
AA	Alcoholics Anonymous
AAA	abdominal aortic aneurysm (sometimes abbreviated A^3, or AAAA for atherosclerotic abdominal aortic aneurysm)
AAL	anterior axillary line
A & W	alive and well
ab	abortion [spontaneous (i.e., a miscarriage) or otherwise], antibody
ABc	antibiotic
abd	abdomen, abduction
ABG	arterial blood gas
AC	air conduction
Ac phos	acid phosphatase
ac	*ante cibum* (before meals)
ACEI	angiotensin-converting enzyme inhibitor
ACTH	adrenocorticotropic hormone
add	adduction
ADH	antidiuretic hormone
ADL	activities of daily living
ad lib	*ad libitum* (as desired, by the patient not the staff)
AF	atrial fibrillation
AFB	acid-fast bacillus (synonymous with mycobacteria)
ag	antigen
AI	aortic insufficiency
AIDS	acquired immune deficiency syndrome

AJ	ankle jerk (Achilles reflex)
AKA	above-knee amputation
Alk phos	alkaline phosphatase
ALL	acute lymphocytic leukemia
ALS	amyotrophic lateral sclerosis
am	*ante meridiem* (the morning)
AMA	against medical advice, American Medical Association
AMI	acute myocardial infarction, anterior myocardial infarction
AML	acute myelogenous leukemia
ANC	absolute neutrophil count
Ao	aorta
AP	anteroposterior, angina pectoris
ARC	AIDS-related complex
ARDS	adult respiratory distress syndrome
ARF	acute renal failure (sometimes misused for acute respiratory failure)
AROM	active range of motion
AS	aortic stenosis
ASA	acetylsalicylic acid (i.e., aspirin)
ASAP	as soon as possible
ASMI, ASWMI	anteroseptal wall myocardial infarction
AV	aortic valve, arteriovenous, atrioventricular
AVF	arteriovenous fistula
AVM	arteriovenous malformation

AVN	atrioventricular node
AVR	aortic valve replacement
AWMI	anterior wall myocardial infarction

–B–

B	bruit, black [with M(an) or W(oman)], basophil (in differential counts), band forms (in differential counts)
B-I	Billroth I operation (i.e., gastroduodenostomy)
B-II	Billroth II operation (i.e., gastrojejunostomy)
Baso	basophil
BBB	bundle-branch block [with R(ight) or L(eft), blood–brain barrier]
BC	blood culture, bone conduction
BCG	bacille Calmette-Guérin (tuberculosis vaccine)
BCP	birth control pill(s)
BE	barium enema; base excess (an obsolescent term)
bid	*bis in die* (twice daily)
bili	bilirubin
bili, T & D	bilirubin, total and direct
BJ	biceps reflex(es)
BKA, BK	below-knee amputation
BM	bowel movement, bone marrow
BMT	bone marrow transplant(ation)
BP	blood pressure
BPD	bronchopulmonary dysplasia
BPH	benign prostatic hyperplasia
BRBPR	bright red blood per rectum
BRJ	brachioradialis reflex(es)
BRP	bathroom privileges
BS	bowel sounds, breath sounds, blood glucose
BSO	bilateral salpingo-oophorectomy
BSU	Bartholin's and Skene's glands and the female urethra
BUN	blood urea nitrogen
bx	biopsy (singular or plural)

–C–

C	degrees Celsius, centigrade
c	*cum* (with)
CA	cancer
Ca	calcium
CABG	coronary artery bypass graft
C & S	culture and sensitivity testing
CAD	coronary artery disease
CBC	complete blood count(s)
CC	chief complaint(s), creatinine clearance
cc	cubic centimeter(s), cell count
CCB	calcium channel blocker
C/C/E	cyanosis/clubbing/edema
CCU	coronary care unit, critical care unit(s)
CDC	United States Federal Government Centers for Disease Control
CF	cystic fibrosis
CHD	congenital heart disease
chemo	antineoplastic chemotherapy
CHF	congestive heart failure
CHO	carbohydrate
CLL	chronic lymphocytic leukemia
CMV	cytomegalovirus
c/o	complains of, complaints of
COPD	chronic obstructive pulmonary disease
Cor	heart
CPC	clinicopathologic correlation (or a conference about same)
CPR	cardiopulmonary resuscitation
Cr	creatinine
CRF	chronic renal failure
crypto	cryptococcosis, cryptosporidiosis
CSF	cerebrospinal fluid
CT	computerized tomography
CV	cardiovascular
CVA	costovertebral angle, cerebrovascular accident (the latter is a misnomer for a stroke)
CVP	central venous pressure

CXR	chest radiograph	**Echo**	echocardiogram
cysto	cystoscopy	**ECT**	electroconvulsive therapy
	–D–	**EDC**	estimated date of confine-ment (expected date of delivery of a baby)
D	deceased		
d	deciliter (also abbrevi-ated dl)		
DBP	diastolic blood pressure	**EEG**	electroencephalogram
d/c	discontinue(d), discharge	**EGD**	esophagogastroduode-noscopy
D & C	dilatation of the uterine cervix and curettage of the endometrium		
		EMG	electromyogram, electro-myography
ddx	differential diagnosis	**ENT**	ear, nose, and throat
diff	differential cell count	**EOM**	extraocular movement(s) [EOMI means all EOM are intact; EOM F & C means all EOM are full and conjugate]
dig	digoxin		
DIP	distal interphalangeal (joint)		
DJD	degenerative joint dis-ease (osteoarthrosis)		
		Eo(s)	eosinophil(s)
DKA	diabetic ketoacidosis	**ER**	emergency room, estro-gen receptors
DM	diabetes mellitus, dias-tolic murmur		
		ETOH	ethanol
DNR	do not resuscitate if cardiac or respiratory arrest occurs	**ETT**	exercise tolerance test, endotracheal tube
			–F–
D/NS	dextrose and saline solution, usually for intravenous adminis-tration	**F**	degrees Fahrenheit, female
		FB	foreign body
DOA	dead on arrival	**FBS**	fasting blood glucose level
DOB	date of birth		
DOE	dyspnea on exertion	**Fe**	iron
DOSS	dioctyl sodium sulfosuc-cinate (a stool softener)	**FET**	forced expiratory time
		FH	family history
DP	dorsalis pedis artery and its pulse	**flex sig**	flexible sigmoidoscopy
		F→N	finger-to-nose test
DPH	phenytoin	**FROM**	full range of motion
DPT	diphtheria, pertussis, and tetanus immunization	**FUO**	fever of undetermined origin
DTRs	deep tendon reflexes (a misnomer for muscle stretch reflexes)	**Fx**	fracture, function
			–G–
DTs	delirium tremens	**G**	gravida
DU	duodenal ulcer	**g**	gallop
DVT	deep venous thrombosis	**G & D**	growth and development
D & W	dextrose and water solu-tion (usually for intra-venous administration)	**GA**	general appearance
		GB	gallbladder
		GC	gonorrhea (or its causa-tive microbe)
dx	diagnosis (singular or plural)		
dz	disease(s)	**GI**	gastrointestinal
	–E–	**gm**	gram
E	eosinophil(s) [in differen-tial counts]	**GNID**	gram-negative intra-cellular diplococci (usually GC)
ECG	electrocardiogram (often abbreviated EKG)	**GNR**	gram-negative rod(s)

GPC	gram-positive cocci
GSW	gunshot wound
G-tube	gastrostomy (feeding) tube (also abbreviated GT)
gtt	drop(s)
GTT	glucose tolerance test
GU	genitourinary, gastric ulcer
GXT	graded exercise tolerance test (for coronary disease)
gyn	gynecology, gynecologic, gynecologist

–H–

H	hydrogen
h	hour(s)
HA	headache
H & E	hemorrhage(s) and exudate(s); hematoxylin and eosin histologic stain
H & P	history and physical examination and record of same
hb	hemoglobin
HBab	hepatitis B antibody
HBP	high blood pressure
HBsAg	hepatitis B surface antigen
HCG	human chorionic gonadotropin
hct	hematocrit
HCTZ	hydrochlorothiazide
HEENT	head, eyes, ears, nose, (mouth and) throat
heme	blood, hematology
Hg	mercury
HH	hiatus hernia
HIV	human immunodeficiency virus
HMD	hyaline membrane disease
HNP	herniated nucleus pulposus (disc disease)
HO	house officer (intern, resident, or in some contexts, postresidency fellow)
HPI	history of present illness
HR	heart rate
H→S	heel-to-shin test
hs	hour of sleep (at bedtime)
HS	heart sound(s)

HSM	hepatosplenomegaly, holosystolic murmur
HT	hypertension
hx	history
hypo	hypotension, hypodermic

–I–

I	iodine, intake, radiographic pulmonary infiltrate (used only after an abbreviation for a lung lobe)
I & D	incision and drainage
I & O	fluid intake and excretory and other output
ICP	intracranial pressure
ICS	intercostal space
ICU	intensive care unit
ID	infectious disease(s)
IDDM	insulin-dependent diabetes mellitus
Ig	immunoglobulin
IM	intramuscular
IMI	inferior wall myocardial infarction
INH	trademark (isonicotine hydrazaine) for one brand of isoniazid
IP	interphalangeal, intraperitoneal
IUD	intrauterine contraceptive device
IUP	intrauterine pregnancy
IV	intravenous(ly)
IVDA	intravenous drug abuse(r)
IVF	intravenous fluids, in vitro fertilization
IVP	excretory urogram, intravenous push
IVPB	intravenous push, intravenous piggyback
IWMI	inferior wall myocardial infarction

–J–

JAR	junior assistant resident
J-tube	jejunostomy tube
JVD	jugular venous distension
JVP	jugular venous pressure

–K–

K	potassium
kg	kilogram(s)
KJ	knee jerk(s)
KOH	potassium hydroxide
KS	Kaposi's sarcoma

–L–

L	left, lymphocyte (in differential counts), lobe, liter
LA	left atrium, left arm, left anterior
L & A	light and accommodation reactions
LE	lower extremity (singular or plural), lupus erythematosus
LIH	left inguinal herniorrhaphy
LIQ	lower inner quadrant (usually refers to the breast)
LLL	left lower lobe
LLQ	left lower quadrant
LLSB	left lower sternal border
LMD	local medical doctor (sometimes abbreviated PMD for private medical doctor)
LMP	last menstrual period
LN	lymph node(s)
LOC	level of consciousness, loss of consciousness
LOQ	lower outer quadrant (usually refers to breast)
LP	lumbar puncture
LSB	left sternal border
LUL	left upper lobe
LUQ	left upper quadrant
LV	left ventricle
LVH	left ventricular myocardial hypertrophy

–M–

M	mother, mononucleated cell (monocyte or other) [in differential counts]
m	murmur
MAI	*Mycobacterium avium-intracellularis*
MAL	midaxillary line
MCL	midclavicular line
MD	physician, muscular dystrophy
MG	myasthenia gravis
Mg	magnesium
mg	milligram
MI	myocardial infarction
MICU	medical intensive care unit
min	minute(s)

ml	milliliter
MMR	measles, mumps, and rubella vaccine/vaccination
MN	midnight
mo	month(s)
Mono	mononucleosis, mononuclear cell
MP	metacarpophalangeal
MR	mitral regurgitation, mental retardation or mentally retarded
MRI	magnetic resonance imaging
MRM	modified radical mastectomy
MS	mitral stenosis, multiple sclerosis, morphine sulfate
MSE	mental status examination
MSL	midsternal line, a part of the anterior midline of the body
MSR	muscle stretch reflex(es)
MV	mitral valve, mechanical ventilation
MVA	motor vehicle crash (often miscalled an accident)
MVR	mitral valve replacement

–N–

N	nerve, normal
NA	no answer, not applicable
Na	sodium
NAD	no acute distress, no active disease
NAS	no added salt
NG	nasogastric
NH	nursing home
NIDDM	non–insulin-dependent diabetes mellitus
NKA	no known allergies
NKDA	no known drug allergies
NPO	*nil per os* (nothing by mouth)
NS	normal (0.9%) saline solution
NSAID	nonsteroidal anti-inflammatory drug (refers particularly to prostaglandin inhibitors)
NT	nontender
NTG	nitroglycerin
N & V	nausea and vomiting

NYHA	New York Heart Association*	**PCN**	penicillin
		PCP	*Pneumocystis carinii* pneumonia
–O–		**PCV**	packed cell volume (= hematocrit)
O₂	oxygen		
OA	osteoarthritis	**PDx**	physical diagnosis
Ob	obstetrics	**PE**	physical examination, pulmonary embolism
OB	occult blood (usually referring to stool testing)	**PEG**	percutaneously placed gastrostomy tube
OD	overdose, *oculus dexter* (right eye)	**PERRL**	pupils equal, round, and reactive to light
OGTT	oral glucose tolerance test (seldom indicated in diagnosis of diabetes mellitus)	**PFTs**	pulmonary function tests
		PGL	persistent generalized lymphadenopathy
OH	occupational history	**PH**	past history
OI	opportunistic infection	**PI**	present illness, history of present illness (also HPI)
OM	otitis media		
OOB	out of bed	**PIP**	proximal interphalangeal [joint(s)]
OPD	outpatient department		
OR	operating room	**plt(s)**	platelet(s)
ORL	otorhinolaryngology	**pm**	*post meridiem* (afternoon or evening)
Ortho	orthopedic(s), orthostatic		
OS	opening snap, *oculus sinister* (left eye)	**PMD**	private medical doctor
		PMH	past medical history
OT	occupational therapy	**PMI**	point of maximum impulse, posterior wall myocardial infarction
OWNL	otherwise within normal limits		
–P–		**PMN**	polymorphonuclear leukocyte(s)
P	pulse rate, pupil, phosphorus, parent, para, polymorphonuclear leukocyte(s) [in differential counts]	**PND**	paroxysmal nocturnal dyspnea
		PO	*per os* (by mouth)
p	post (after)	**poly**	polymorphonuclear leukocyte(s)
P2	pulmonic component of second heart sound	**POMR**	problem-oriented medical record
PA	posteroanterior, pernicious anemia	**post**	autopsy (a noun, not a verb)
P & A	percussion and auscultation	**PP**	patient profile
		PPD	tuberculosis skin test; pack per day of cigarettes smoked
PAC	premature atrial contraction		
Pap	Papanicolaou-stained cytologic smear (usually of uterine cervical cells but can be of any tissue or fluid)	**prn**	*pro re nata* (as needed)
		PROM	passive range of motion, premature rupture of fetal membranes
		pt	patient
path	pathology, pathologic	**PT**	posterior tibial (artery and pulse), physical therapy
pc	*post cibum* [after meal(s)]		

---

*A classification for cardiac disease severity, with class I representing asymptomatic; class II, symptom(s) only with marked exertion; class III, symptom(s) with slight exertion; class IV, symptom(s) at rest.

PTA	prior to admission	**s & s**	sign(s) and symptom(s)
PUD	peptic ulcer disease	**SAR**	senior assistant resident
PVC	premature ventricular contraction	**SBO**	small bowel obstruction
PWMI	posterior wall myocardial infarction	**SBP**	systolic blood pressure, spontaneous bacterial peritonitis

–Q–

Q	perfusion	**SC**	subcutaneous(ly)
q	*quisque* (every) [frequently combined with a number and "h" (e.g., q2h means "every 2 hours")]	**SCM**	sternocleidomastoid
		SDAT	senile dementia of the Alzheimer type
		SEM	systolic ejection murmur
		SG	specific gravity
		SH	social history
qd	every day	**SLE**	systemic lupus erythematosus
qh	every hour		
qid	four times a day	**SOB**	shortness of breath*
qod	every other day	**s/p**	*status post* (after)
qs	every nursing shift (each of which lasts 8 hours)	**SQ**	subcutaneous(ly)
		STD	sexually transmitted disease(s)

–R–

R	respirations, right	**SVT**	supraventricular tachycardia
RA	right arm, right anterior, rheumatoid arthritis	**sx**	symptom(s)

–T–

RBC	red blood cell(s)	**T**	temperature, fever
RDS	respiratory distress syndrome (of the newborn)	T_4	thyroxine, hyperthyroid(ism)
resp	respiration, respiratory	**TA**	superficial temporal artery
resp rx	respiratory therapy		
RLL	right lower lobe	**Tab**	therapeutic abortion
RLQ	right lower quadrant	**TAH**	total abdominal hysterectomy
RML	right middle lobe		
ROM	range of motion	**T & A**	tonsillectomy and adenoidectomy
ROS	review of systems		
RR	respiratory rate	**TB**	tuberculosis (also abbreviated tb and tbc)
RSB	right sternal border		
RT	radiotherapy	**T & C**	type and crossmatch (blood)
RUL	right upper lobe		
RUQ	right upper quadrant	**TFT**	thyroid function test(s)
RV	right ventricle	**TIA**	transient (cerebral) ischemic attack
rx	therapy, treatment		
		TJ	triceps reflex(es)

–S–

s	*sine* (without)	**TLC**	tender loving care
S1	first heart sound	**TM**	tympanic membrane(s)
S2	second heart sound	**TMJ**	temporomandibular joint
S2A	aortic component of the second heart sound	**TNG**	(tri-)nitroglycerin
		toxo	toxoplasmosis, *Toxoplasma gondii*
S2P	pulmonic component of the second heart sound	**TP**	total protein
S3	third heart sound	**TUR, TURP**	transurethral resection of the prostate
S4	fourth heart sound		

---

*There is also rumored to be another interpretation of this abbreviation, but the authors cannot find what it is.

TVF	tactile vocal fremitus	**V/Q**	ventilation/perfusion ratio
Txn	transplantation	**VS**	vital sign(s)
	–U–		**–W–**
U	upper		
U/A	urinalysis	**W**	Caucasian [with M(an) or W(oman)]
UA	uric acid		
UE	upper extremity (singular or plural)	**WA**	while awake
		WBC	white blood cell(s) or white blood cell count
UGI	upper gastrointestinal (tract, bleeding, or radiographs)	**WD**	well developed
		wk	week(s)
UI	urinary incontinence	**WN**	well nourished
UIQ	upper inner quadrant (usually refers to breast)	**WNI**	within normal limits
UOQ	upper outer quadrant (usually refers to breast)	**wt**	weight
			–X–
UQ	upper quadrant	**X**	times
URI	upper respiratory tract infection	**x**	except
		xrt	radiotherapy
US	ultrasound, ultrasonic		**–Y–**
UTI	urinary tract infection	**Y**	year(s)
	–V–	**YO**	year old
VD	venereal disease(s)		

Index